Healing

Moves

Healing

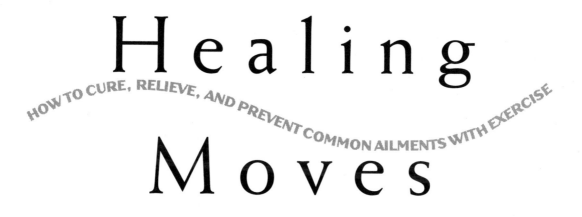

HOW TO CURE, RELIEVE, AND PREVENT COMMON AILMENTS WITH EXERCISE

Moves

Carol Krucoff and Mitchell Krucoff, M.D.

Illustrations by Adam Brill

HARMONY BOOKS

NEW YORK

Published by Harmony Books, New York, New York. Member of
the Crown Publishing Group.

Random House, Inc. New York, Toronto, London, Sydney, Auckland
www.randomhouse.com

Harmony Books is a registered trademark and Harmony Books colophon is a trademark of
Random House, Inc.

Printed in the United States of America

Design by Chris Welch

Library of Congress Cataloging-in-Publication Data
Krucoff, Carol.
Healing moves : how to cure, relieve, and prevent common ailments with exercise /
Carol Krucoff and Mitchell Krucoff.
Includes index.
1. Exercise therapy—Popular works.   I. Krucoff, Mitchell.
II. Title.
RM725.K78 2000
615.8'2—dc21 99-41779

ISBN 0-609-60222-5

10 9 8 7 6 5 4 3 2

To Nelson Ostrinsky and Sylvia Krucoff:

Your memories illuminate our lives.

Acknowledgments

We would like to express our sincere gratitude to the many people who helped support and inspire us in the creation of this book.

Our wise and wonderful agent, Muriel Nellis, believed in us from the start and provided essential guidance along the way. Peter Guzzardi, our editor, offered a clear vision of what this book should be and expertly helped nurture it—and us. Illustrator Adam Brill created a splendidly diverse "company" of characters to artfully demonstrate the healing moves.

Thanks, too, to the numerous exercise scientists, physicians, and fitness professionals who have served as sources for Carol's *Bodyworks* column and, thus, for this book. In particular we want to express our deep appreciation to experts from the Cooper Institute for Aerobics Research, the American College of Sports Medicine, the Melpomene Institute, the American Council on Exercise, IDEA: The Health & Fitness Source, and the Aerobics and Fitness Association of America. We also want to thank Carol's editors and colleagues at the *Washington Post*, in particular Abigail Trafford, Lexie Verdon, and Greg Mott.

We are grateful to Hanshi Jesse Bowen for showing us the way of karate, and we want to thank the entire Karate International of Durham family for their fellowship and support. Thanks, too, to the inspired yoga teaching of Susan Delaney and Tracy Bogart of Triangle Yoga in Chapel Hill.

We also owe a large debt of gratitude to our wonderful family and to our dear friends, for all their love and encouragement. Most especially, we wish to thank our incredible children, Max and Rae, for being understanding about deadline pressures and for the daily delight they bring into our lives.

Contents

Healing
Moves

Harnessing the Healing Power of Movement

Since ancient times, healers have recognized the curative power of physical activity. Yet only recently has scientific evidence confirmed the widespread belief that movement heals.

Today, virtually every form of medicine recognizes these basic truths:

1. Simple exercise can have profound healing effects.
2. Specific "healing moves" can help fight illness and enhance health.

These concepts are embraced by traditional healers and modern scientists, Eastern practitioners and Western physicians, alternative- and conventional-medicine advocates alike. At a time when patients and health-care providers are searching for safe, effective, and inexpensive therapies, healing moves provide an ideal self-care strategy to help prevent, relieve, and sometimes even cure disease.

Solid scientific research documents exercise's therapeutic power. Over the last few decades, study after study has shown that moving regularly enhances health, while inactivity impairs it. Physical activity can help some diabetics come off insulin and some hypertensives quit their high-blood-pressure medication. It can lower cholesterol, ease arthritis pain, lift depression, relieve anxiety, and help asthmatics breathe more easily. It can slow the aging process and boost both the length and the quality of life.

Movement enhances the heart's ability to pump blood, the lungs' capacity to fill with oxygen, the metabolism's ability to burn fat, and the immune system's defensive power. In fact, virtually every bodily system becomes stronger and more efficient with regular exercise. A growing amount of research indicates that getting regular physical activity may be the single most important thing you can do to prevent disease and promote good health.

This may surprise some people in our prescription-oriented society, where we're constantly searching for wonder drugs and taking the "high-tech" road to health. In contrast, our healing moves are low tech, low risk, low (or no) cost, and readily available. All it takes to harness the curative power of movement is time. Despite widespread misconceptions, healing movement doesn't take a lot of time, and it's not even necessary to sweat. Accumulate 30 minutes of moderate physical activity most days of the week—that is the simple prescription for good health touted by the *U.S. Surgeon General's Report on Physical Activity and Health.*

The delightful surprise (as those who exercise regularly will confirm) is that the time you spend moving is generally repaid in full by the energy, relaxation, and pleasure that physical activity brings. Unfortunately, too many people have come to think of exercise as a distasteful chore, often because of bad experiences, misconceptions about exercise, a poor body image, or frustrating athletic endeavors. The challenge, then, is to cast off past negative notions about movement—like the hazardous myth of "no pain, no gain" or the false idea that "you have to be thin to be fit." Instead, it's time to go out and play—to recapture the joy of motion we had as children, when "recess" (i.e., movement) was our favorite subject.

In fact, the most healing moves of all are those involved in just about any physical activity you enjoy. You can pick from a wide array of options: dancing, walking, swimming, skating, martial arts, cycling, tennis, yoga, to name a few. As the yogis say, "Follow your bliss." Because exercise does more than just boost your physical health—it can enhance your mental and spiritual health as well. The best way to achieve the full spectrum of "body and soul healing" accessible through movement is to approach this powerful therapy with the excitement and pleasure we knew in childhood, running outside on a beautiful day to play with friends. Instead of a dreaded "workout," exercise then becomes a much anticipated "play break" that can be a highlight of your day.

It's important, too, to recognize that moving regularly is not just about looking better. That's a merely a side benefit. Moving is about feeling better. We are physical animals, and daily exercise is essential to our health. In previous generations people's days were filled with physical activity, but today we must find ways to fit movement into our lives. Our parents and grandparents needed to walk regularly and perform many other physical tasks to get through their days. But now we sit on our bottoms most of the time, and our main exercise is pushing buttons. In many buildings, we can't even use our muscles to open the doors or climb the stairs if we want to: doors fly open as if by magic and elevators are the only route upstairs. In a world where we can do everything—from shopping to mowing the lawn—sitting down, we must make time to move.

If we don't, the consequences are grimly clear. Inactivity is a central contributor to

America's top killers: heart disease, some cancers, stroke, hypertension, diabetes, and osteoporosis. And it plays a major role in a host of other common health problems, from back pain to depression. Regular exercise can reduce the risk of all these ailments, and for some of these conditions, exercise not only inhibits or delays disease progression but can actually reverse the illness—often more safely and more effectively than drugs or surgery. "If exercise could be packed into a pill," sums up a report from the National Institute on Aging, "it would be the single most widely prescribed, and beneficial, medicine in the nation."

HEALING MOVES THROUGH TIME

Throughout the ages, many great minds have recognized that movement heals. Around 400 B.C., the Greek philosopher Plato wrote that "lack of activity destroys the good condition of every human being while movement and methodical physical exercise save and preserve it." His contemporary Hippocrates, who is considered the father of medicine, wrote that "food and exercise, while possessing opposite qualities . . . work together to produce health." These concepts came back into vogue during the Renaissance. In 1553, Spanish physician Christobal Mendez wrote the *Book of Bodily Exercise*, which affirmed that "the easiest way to preserve health, and with greater profit than all other measures put together, is to exercise well." Italian physician Bernardino Ramazzini noted in 1713 that

workers such as cobblers and tailors "suffer from general ill-health . . . caused by their sedentary life." New York physician Shadrach Ricketson, who authored the first American text on hygiene and preventive medicine, wrote in 1806 that "a certain proportion of exercise is not much less essential to a healthy or vigorous constitution, than drink, food, and sleep." And Edward Stanley, Earl of Derby, penned a maxim in the mid-1800s that is often repeated today: "Those who think they have not time for bodily exercise will sooner or later have to find time for illness."

At the turn of the twentieth century, however, this commonsense appreciation for the health benefits of movement began to decline. Tuberculosis was the scourge of the day, and rest was the popular remedy. Avoiding exertion came into vogue as a way to treat other illnesses, too. The discovery of penicillin in 1928 ushered in the age of antibiotics, and the powers of these wonder drugs seemed to eclipse the importance of simple preventive health measures like exercise. By the 1930s, bed rest was the accepted treatment for a wide range of conditions, including pregnancy, heart attack, nervous disorders, back pain, and arthritis. Exercise was often viewed as risky. Combine that philosophy with increased reliance on (and fascination with) technology—the automobile for transportation, the television for amusement, and the computer for everything—and it's no surprise that at the turn of twenty-first century we've become an overweight, out-of-shape society, battling a host of illnesses related to inactivity, such as heart disease, hypertension, diabetes, colon cancer, osteoporosis, and geriatric frailty.

Public health officials started sounding the alarm about our lack of fitness in 1953, when a disturbing report showed that more than 56 percent of American schoolchildren failed to meet even a minimum fitness standard required for health, compared to an 8.3 percent failure rate for European children. President Dwight Eisenhower invited athletes and exercise experts to a meeting in 1955 to examine the issue in more depth. His own cardiologist, Paul Dudley White, was an avid fitness enthusiast who shocked the nation by advising the president to exercise after he'd suffered a heart attack. Photos of Eisenhower golfing after his heart attack helped allay the public's fear that exercise was somehow risky and introduced America to the notion that physical activity can help prevent and treat disease. When John Kennedy became president in 1961, one of his first actions was to call a conference on physical fitness and young people. Less than a decade later, Dallas physician Kenneth H. Cooper coined the term *aerobics* in his 1968 best-seller by that title, and our modern "fitness revolution" was launched.

Since that time, there has been an explosion of scientific research documenting the dramatic health benefits of exercise. Despite some critics' dismissal of fitness as merely a fad, attention to exercise's therapeutic powers has continued to grow, fueled by swelling scientific support. The evidence of exercise's effectiveness is so strong that, in the last ten years alone, virtually every major public health organization has endorsed a program of regular moderate physical activity. In 1996, the culmination of these efforts was the *U.S. Surgeon General's Report on Physical Activity and Health*, which summa-

rized the extensive scientific literature documenting the health benefits of exercise and urged everyone in our sedentary society to get off their dangerously-widening rear ends. Yet despite widespread awareness that exercise is good for health, less than one-quarter of all adults exercise regularly and even today's kids spend most of their days in sedentary pursuits.

HEALING MOVES AROUND THE WORLD

Healing Moves offers a modern version of an ancient, global insight into wellness, health, and treatment of illness. Eastern medical systems have long recognized the health benefits of exercise and the hazards of inactivity. Traditional Chinese medicine views physical activity as essential to the proper flow of *chi*, or life energy, throughout the body, which proponents credit with boosting health and preventing disease. When *chi* is blocked by problems such as poor posture, nervous tension, or sedentary existence, illness results. That's why millions of Chinese greet the dawn by performing ancient self-healing exercises designed to develop and direct the body's *chi*, such as tai chi and qi gong. Used in China to treat a variety of ailments, including cancer and multiple sclerosis, these exercises are currently the subject of scientific scrutiny in the United States and have been linked to numerous positive health outcomes, such as reductions in blood pressure, improved balance, and pain relief.

Exercises designed to activate the body's own healing mechanisms are also central to the Indian medical system of Ayurveda, which prescribes the physical poses of hatha yoga as a means of achieving optimum health and treating specific ailments. From an Ayurvedic perspective, the purpose of exercise is to relieve stress, cleanse the body of toxins, boost circulation and digestion, and "tune up" the entire system. It is also considered an essential means of uniting body and mind, with particular emphasis on the breath and breathing to forge that link. The word *yoga* itself means union. A central goal of the practice is to link body and mind and to unite mortal human beings with the eternal divine. The physical poses of hatha yoga were created about five thousand years ago, in part to aid in spiritual development. By practicing hatha yoga, devotees were able to develop the strength, flexibility, and discipline necessary to sit still in a quiet, healthy manner fundamental to reaching deep levels of meditation.

In fact, the goal of many Eastern physical techniques—including most martial arts—isn't to break boards or build buff abs. Rather, they are spiritual disciplines designed to unleash the full human "wellness" potential. The process of adopting the daily practice of regular exercise yields a valuable "side effect," enhanced physical health, which cultivates and is further supported by a blossoming of mental and spiritual health as well.

One reason Westerners have begun to appreciate the dramatic health benefits of exercise is that more and more of them have been practicing these Eastern physical disciplines over the past thirty years. Yoga was popularized in the United States in the 1960s and 1970s, when the Beatles jetted to India to commune with the maharishi. Martial arts hit the American mainstream in the 1970s with the movies of jeet kune do master Bruce Lee. Today, enrollment in yoga and martial arts classes is soaring as "stressed-out" Americans flock to exercise forms that offer more depth and meaning than simple aerobics.

The American medical community has been slower to appreciate and endorse the vital role daily physical activity contributes to health, not so much through antagonism as through neglect. Only about 30 percent of physicians effectively counsel patients about regular physical activity, estimates the Centers for Disease Control and Prevention in Atlanta, which has embarked on programs to increase that proportion to at least 50 percent. Despite the well-documented health benefits of exercise, the surgeon general's report noted that "many [health care] providers do not believe that physical activity is an important topic to discuss with their patients and many lack effective counseling skills."

Patients themselves are leading the way in educating their doctors. Exercisers who've come to rely on their daily "fix" of physical activity won't tolerate doctors who tell them to stop running or cycling when they encounter a medical problem. Instead, committed exercisers will find a specialist in the booming field of sports medicine who will help them stay as active as possible while treating the condition so they can return to their preferred form of exercise. Once catering only to elite athletes, today's sports medicine doctor is far more likely to treat recreational athletes.

In truth, we are all athletes in the game

called life. The challenge of athletics—to play well and to have fun—is a worthy goal for each of us and has profound effects on our health.

HEALING MOVES FOR ALL

A central message of *Healing Moves* is that everybody—regardless of age or ability—needs and deserves to be physically active. Movement isn't just for the benefit of the young, the beautiful, and the strong. It's for people in wheelchairs, tots in diapers, pregnant women, cancer survivors, and people of every age, with virtually every health condition and skill level. Exercise is more than just a health responsibility, like brushing our teeth. It's a pleasurable, precious gift that people can give themselves. Taking 30 minutes each day to be present in your body, to breathe deeply, and to propel yourself through space is one of life's great joys, enriching body, mind, and spirit. In our sedentary, push-button age, it's vital that we all embrace healing moves. *The general principle of simply choosing to move more, when faced with a choice between moving more and moving less, represents a health-oriented discipline that must be learned and practiced by all who live in the twenty-first century.*

Current trends in health care are helping fuel the "healing moves" vision. Modern patients insist on taking an active role in their own treatment, and exercise works well for such independently health-minded persons. For providers, activity prescriptions are very cost-effective. A fit patient population means a better bottom line for insurance companies and health-care providers. This is one reason why a growing number of health-care systems are constructing state-of-the-art wellness and fitness centers to help their members stay healthy and reduce the need for expensive drugs and services. An estimated five hundred hospitals in the United States now have complete fitness centers catering to people in the community, and the number continues to grow.

Exercise is also holistic, addressing more than just a specific symptom or a particular disease. Activity benefits the whole person, physically, mentally, and spiritually—a great boon in a world of accelerated information processing, time consumption, stress, and depression. As the baby boomer population ages, the value of maintaining function through regular exercise will become more visibly important than ever before. The average American's life expectancy was less than fifty years in 1900 and just 4 percent of the population ever reached 65. Today, life expectancy is seventy-six years, and 12 percent of Americans are sixty-five or older. By 2025, one in five Americans—62 million people—will be sixty-five or older. The key medicine that will keep aging individuals out of nursing homes and help them maintain independent, high-quality lives is exercise. Some health professionals call this "upstream medicine" because exercise empowers people to swim against the typical current of infirmity and reliance on the health-care system with age.

Today's health-care consumer and a growing number of health-care practitioners are unafraid to look "outside the envelope" for ways to prevent and treat disease, as evidenced by the landmark November 1998 "alternative-medicine theme issue" of the *Journal of the American Medical Association.* Four out of ten Americans used alternative-medicine therapies in 1997, *JAMA* noted. Total visits to alternative-medicine practitioners increased by almost 50 percent from 1990 and exceeded the visits to all U.S. primary-care physicians.

While exercise is sometimes classified as a form of alternative medicine, we do not consider it an alternative practice to be used instead of mainstream medicine. Rather exercise *is* medicine, best used as a complementary therapy that works effectively in conjunction with many traditional treatments. For example, the best medicine for a breast cancer patient may start with a high-tech procedure, such as a mastectomy and chemotherapy. However, appropriate exercise is an essential complementary therapy because healing moves can help the breast cancer patient recover from the disease and its treatments by restoring her range of motion, combating weight gain or loss from anticancer drugs, relieving depression, fighting fatigue, enhancing immunity, improving strength and appetite, and boosting self-esteem.

Exercise is a very natural intervention because it is something our bodies are designed to do. The engineering of the human being is complex, having evolved over thousands of years in a way that would suggest the survival advantage of a natural cycle of regular activity necessary to gather food, provide shelter, seek safety, and socialize. But it's also important to recognize that our ancestors used movement for much more than daily subsistence. Physical activity also played a key role in the uniquely human "wellness" profile that includes enhanced spirituality and joy in and from moving—in play, in prayer, in dramatic expression, and in community ritual.

It is a sad commentary on our "couch potato" culture that people today must be taught how to move or be coerced into becoming physically active. The good news is that when people do become active, it appears to trigger a cascade of other positive health habits. Numerous studies show that people who exercise are also likely to exhibit other positive behaviors, such as eating a nutritious diet and avoiding cigarettes and substance abuse.

This well-documented relationship, sometimes called the "granola effect" of exercise, is an important lifestyle benefit of practicing healing moves. While there is little research showing that exercise actually causes these healthy behaviors, numerous scientists speculate that exercise is a "gateway" behavior that helps people adopt other healthy lifestyle practices by:

✳ *Relieving stress.* Since exercise boosts mood, exercisers discover they can handle stress without resorting to destructive habits like smoking or drinking.

✳ *Boosting mood.* Some alcoholics report using the exercise "high" as a kind of alcohol-replacement therapy.

✳ *Enhancing self-esteem.* Studies show that kids who are physically active are less likely to get into fights, bring weapons to school, or engage in early sexual activity.

✳ *Maintaining a healthy weight.* Women often fear quitting cigarettes because they don't want to gain weight, but studies show that exercise can help female smokers quit and stay quit, in part by minimizing weight gain.

✳ *Prompting a desire for nutritious foods.* The impulse to reach for fruits and vegetables instead of chips may come from physiologic cravings triggered by an active body's desire for nutritious fuel.

✳ *Improving sleep.* Since regular exercise helps people get to sleep more easily and deepens sleep, it helps people "recharge their batteries" more effectively so that they function better and can make better health choices throughout the day.

✳ *Promoting "hardiness."* Just as your high school coach told you, exercise builds character. Research indicates that people who exercise regularly develop a characteristic called "stress hardiness," which means they are less vulnerable to the ravages of daily problems.

✳ *Enhancing self-efficacy.* Belief in your ability to accomplish a goal is one of the greatest predictors of success. People who have successfully adopted the exercise habit know that they have the discipline, strength, and willpower necessary to adopt other healthy behaviors, too.

HOW TO USE *HEALING MOVES*

We've arranged *Healing Moves* into nine chapters, each of which focuses on a specific body system or characteristic (such as being male or female). Each chapter discusses the diseases that commonly affect that system, explores how movement can prevent and/or relieve these ailments, and presents a detailed workout designed to help that system function at its peak.

There's no single "right way" to read this book or practice healing moves. Some people may want to read the entire volume cover to cover. Others may turn to a specific ailment and read only those sections they find relevant to their lives. A few might want to simply study the more than one hundred illustrated healing moves interspersed throughout the book. While we suggest that everyone read the first chapter, Exercise for Health and Fitness, the rest is up to you. But we hope you do more than just read about healing moves. Put the book down and try some, too.

It's a sad fact that, despite the overwhelming evidence of exercise's health benefits, most Americans don't exercise; it is equally disappointing that half of all adults who do start an exercise program drop out within six months. Adopting a healthy new habit can be as hard as breaking a destructive old one. As Sir Isaac Newton observed, a body at rest will tend to remain at rest. Even the promise of better health and improved appearance won't get most people to exercise regularly.

But there is one motivator that can pry even the most confirmed "spud" off the sofa. Freud called it the pleasure principle: People do things that feel good and avoid things that feel bad. That's why, throughout *Healing Moves*, we focus on the importance of fun and make our exercise prescriptions as flexible as possible, to allow each individual to choose among a wide range of options and personalize a physical-activity plan that will interest, suit, and delight. The only way to truly adopt the exercise habit is to make movement a joy.

A recurring theme in *Healing Moves* is the

idea that "when exercise is fun it will get done." Focusing on fun helps enhance compliance, but it's also a way to gain the most benefit from activity. To achieve the wide array of physical, mental, and spiritual healing that movement can provide, strive to approach this powerful therapy with a playful mind-set. Remember that exercise isn't just about strengthening your heart or building your biceps; it's also about relieving your stress, clearing your mind, lifting your spir-

its, and experiencing the beauty of the present moment.

Healing Moves can enrich your life and dramatically improve your health. All it takes is a little time and some effort. But with the right focus, information, and inspiration, exercise is as easy as child's play, yet as powerful as a "wonder" drug.

Movement heals. And you can put its curative power to work right now. Read on, and we'll show you how.

1

Exercise for Health and Fitness

OPTIMUM HEALTH AND FITNESS

Throughout civilization, humans have struggled to create devices to ease the body's burdens. From the wheel to the computer, labor-saving milestones have marked mankind's progress in gaining freedom from physical demands.

But now, health experts warn, our passion for avoiding physical activity has spiraled out of control. We've evolved a push-button, drive-through, remote-control mentality that has resulted in a sedentary, overweight society where an "epidemic of inactivity" is responsible for an estimated 250,000 deaths per year, according to a report published in the *Journal of the American Medical Association.*

Americans' inactive lifestyle and junk-food diet have prompted an alarming increase in obesity, even among children, many of whom are developing chronic illnesses (such as type II diabetes and high cholesterol) once seen only in adults. Inactivity-associated ailments, such as high blood pressure and osteoporosis, are rampant. And nursing homes are filled with seniors who are institutionalized primarily because their underused muscles and bones have diminished into decrepitude.

Despite the much-publicized fitness movement, less than one-quarter of all adults exercise regularly. The vast majority of Americans still spend the vast majority of their days on their increasingly vast butts.

And it's killing us.

Inactivity is a health hazard on par with smoking, high cholesterol, and high blood pressure. This is one of the main messages contained in the *U.S. Surgeon General's Report on Physical Activity and Health,* which was issued in 1996 in an effort to jump-start our dangerously sedentary society. The report summarized the extensive scientific literature documenting the health benefits of exercise and promoted these key findings:

1. A modest amount of regular activity confers major health benefits.
2. In general, the more exercise you do, the more benefits you get.

This would come as no surprise to the Greek physician Hippocrates, who in 400 B.C. wrote, "Eating alone will not keep a man well; he must also take exercise." Our recent fitness "revolution" is not a new concept, but a return to this basic understanding that human bodies need movement for optimum health. Up until the Industrial Revolution, physical activity was a part of daily life—not just for the labor of routine existence, but for recreational, religious, and cultural expression. Games, dances, athletic competitions, and pilgrimages—plus the work of daily living—resulted in health and fitness benefits such as endurance, agility, flexibility, and strength.

In contrast, our modern lifestyle of sitting at a desk all day, driving everywhere, and spending our leisure time in sedentary pursuits, such as watching TV or movies or playing video games, is resulting in an array of ailments related to being weak, inflexible, and overweight. For the human being, it's clear that inactivity is an unhealthy aberration.

HEALTHY EXERCISE BASICS

To understand the concept of healthy exercise, it's important to recognize this essential truth: *Health is equilibrium. A person is healthy when his or her body is in balance or harmony. When this equilibrium is disturbed, the result is disease.*

That's why two of the most common approaches to exercise both can be unhealthy:

* *Fitness fanatics:* These "fitter-than-thou zealots" work out hard every day and feel guilty if they skip even one day of exercise.
* *Sanctimonious couch potatoes:* These "exercise bashers" rarely move and boast that they get plenty of exercise serving as pallbearers for their friends who jog.

Both of these extremes are hazardous to health. The body needs both movement and rest, and finding a comfortable balance between the two is crucial to using exercise to enhance well-being. One of the best ways to achieve this healthy balance is to focus on fun. Stop thinking of exercise as a *work*out, and start recognizing that it's a chance to *play*. Unfortunately, too many people view exercise as hard, painful work—a distasteful chore they must cram into their already busy day. Yet as children we didn't feel this way about moving our bodies. Most kids see physical pursuits, like skipping and running, as exciting play to be enjoyed.

The healthiest approach to exercise adopts this playful perspective. Physical activity isn't about losing weight or flattening abs, it's about using all your body parts—bones, muscles, organs, joints—so they'll stay in good working order. And when you take care of your physical self, it boosts your emotional self, enhancing your self-image and brightening your mood. At its best, exercise transcends the mere mechanical to become a truly spiritual experience, a joyous celebration of breathing and moving and being fully alive.

You don't have to spend huge chunks of time to gain the health benefits of exercise. All you need to do is accumulate 30 minutes of movement per day. This, in essence, is the new message being touted by public health officials who are urging Americans to add a modest amount of moderate activity into their lives. No need to change into gym shorts or, heaven forbid, Lycra and sweat for an hour. Instead, the surgeon general's report offers this simple exercise prescription:

Burn 150 calories per day through physical activity such as a 30-minute walk, 15-minute run, or 45 minutes of washing and waxing a car.

In other words: Sit less, move more.

Only in our high-tech, computerized era would advice like this be necessary. In a world where pizzerias make house calls and you can mow the lawn sitting down, *good health demands that we restore some of the physical energy expenditure that technology has removed from our lives.* Experts estimate that Americans expend about 800 fewer calories per day than our parents did—the equivalent of four glazed donuts. Ironically, America's waistlines are increasing even though we've reduced our consumption of fat, primarily because we've become so sedentary.

All the "advances" that make our lives easier—like e-commerce, drive-up automatic teller machines, moving walkways, and automatic doors—have contributed to the current epidemic of obesity and related diseases. For example, think about just one "energy saver": e-mail. Over time, sending e-mail messages to people in your office instead of walking to deliver them can result in enough extra pounds to jeopardize your health, reports physiologist William L. Haskell, professor of medicine at Stanford University. "Consider the office worker . . . who exchanges just two minutes of slow walking around the office to deliver messages for two minutes of sitting at a computer sending e-mail each hour for eight hours per day, five days per week," Dr. Haskell wrote in the *Journal of the American Medical Association* (July 1996). "Over the course of a year, the reduction in energy expenditure due to this change would be equivalent to 1.1 pounds of fat. Over 10 years, a positive energy balance of this magnitude could increase a person's body weight by 11 pounds . . . which is associated with significant increases in blood pressure, plasma triglyceride concentrations and insulin resistance and lower high density cholesterol levels."

E-mail is, of course, just one of countless devices that have made our lives easier and more sedentary. The solution is not stopping e-mail, one of the best communication tools of the century. Rather, it's recognizing that exercise has been engineered out of our lives, so we must *find every possible opportunity to weave activity back into our days.*

So critical is America's need to get moving for better health that more than one hundred health-related organizations (such as the American Heart Association, the U.S. Centers for Disease Control and Prevention, and the American College of Sports

Medicine) have joined together to form the National Coalition to Promote Physical Activity. Their slogan—"It's Everywhere You Go"—highlights the health benefits of simple "lifestyle activities" like taking the stairs and parking in the farthest space. Almost any activity that gets you up and moving around, they note, is probably better for you in some ways than continuing to sit.

Lifestyle activities can provide health benefits similar to a traditional gym-based workout, according to a study done at the Cooper Institute for Aerobics Research in Dallas and published in *JAMA* (January 1999). Sedentary adults were randomly assigned to two groups: a "structured group" that used a fitness center for regular work-outs and a "lifestyle group" that learned behavioral techniques to help them fit more activity into their day. At the end of two years, both groups experienced similar health benefits, such as reduced body fat and lower blood pressure. The conclusion: Every step you take counts.

"HEALTH BENEFITS" VERSUS "FITNESS BENEFITS" OF EXERCISE

One reason most people don't exercise, experts acknowledge, is that they're con-fused about how to get fit. Fads and gim-micks promise impossible results, and fitness trends change so dramatically that many people don't know what they're supposed to do to shape up. In the 1970s, running was touted as the ticket to fitness, and people were told that exercise had to be vigorous and sustained or it didn't count. In the 1980s, aerobics classes boomed, and exercis-ers were urged to "go for the burn"—while

taking their pulse and figuring their target heart rate so they could work out at the proper intensity. In the early 1990s, exercise machines exploded in popularity and it seemed essential to hop on a treadmill or join a gym to shape up.

Today, the message is much simpler: Get a half hour of moderate activity most days of the week. As a general recommendation, public health officials are promoting moder-ate activity for two reasons:

1. Research shows that moderate exercise has major health benefits.
2. Most people won't exercise vigorously.

The sad fact is, most adults don't like to work up a sweat. Only 15 percent of American adults engage regularly in vigor-ous physical activity for at least 20 minutes three times a week. By contrast, more than 60 percent of American adults are not regu-larly physically active at any intensity and 25 percent are totally sedentary.

So from a public health perspective, it makes the most sense to encourage inactive people to move moderately.

But from a personal perspective, *if you want to achieve more than just basic good health you'll need to do more than merely accumulate 30 minutes of moderate activity.* This 30-minute, user-friendly fitness for-mula will confer **health benefits** and is great for those who want to do the minimum activity possible to maintain good health. But it may not be enough to confer **fitness benefits** to those with more ambitious phys-ical goals, such as reshaping your body or winning a gold medal in your local 10K. If you have appearance or athletic goals, chances are you'll need to do more than just "exercise lite."

This distinction between the health benefits and the fitness benefits of physical activity has been one of the major findings in the field of exercise science in recent years.

✳ **Health benefits** include a reduced risk of numerous chronic diseases—including coronary heart disease, type II diabetes, hypertension, and colon cancer—as well as improved mental health and enhanced physical functioning. In addition, most sedentary people who add 30 minutes of moderate activity to their days will lose some body fat and experience improvements in blood pressure, blood glucose, and blood cholesterol.

✳ **Fitness benefits** include increased muscle strength, greater flexibility, and improvements in body composition and heart and lung capacity. Gaining fitness benefits generally requires doing a specific kind of activity at a certain intensity, frequency, and duration. For example, achieving cardiorespiratory fitness requires doing aerobic exercise at a "moderate" to "somewhat hard" intensity (55% to 90% of maximum heart rate) for 20 to 60 minutes, three to five days a week.

"There is a dose response to exercise," notes the American College of Sports Medicine in its latest guidelines for adult fitness. "Many significant health benefits are achieved by going from a sedentary state to a minimal level of physical activity; programs involving higher intensities and/or greater frequency/durations provide additional benefits."

In other words: *More exercise is better than some, and some exercise is better than none.*

For health benefits, all you need is 30 minutes of daily **physical activity**—defined as bodily movement produced by contracting muscles that substantially increases energy expenditure. For fitness benefits, it's necessary to **exercise**—defined as planned, structured, and repetitive bodily movement done to improve or maintain one or more components of physical fitness.

How much exercise you need to do depends on your goals.

FITNESS BASICS

Despite America's preoccupation with the cultural misconception that "thin equals fit," fitness has less to do with your scale weight than with your ability to climb stairs, carry groceries, open jars, and—when necessary—run after a child or scamper across a busy street. *Exercise professionals define fitness as the ability of your heart, blood vessels, lungs, and muscles to carry out daily tasks and occasional, unexpected bodily challenges with a minimum of fatigue and discomfort.*

Physical fitness has four components:

1. Aerobic fitness: The body's ability to take in and use oxygen to produce energy. Sometimes referred to as cardiorespiratory endurance, this is the capacity of the heart and lungs to perform a sustained activity.
2. Muscular fitness: The strength and endurance of your muscles as measured by their ability to exert force and to perform repeated work over time.
3. Flexibility: The ability to bend joints and move muscles through a full range of motion.

4. Body composition: The relative amounts of body fat and lean body tissue (muscle, bone, skin, and other nonfat tissue), typically expressed as a body fat percentage.

To get fit, you need to participate in a well-rounded program that includes the three main forms of exercise: cardiovascular (aerobic), strength training, and stretching. And don't believe those TV infomercials: There is no single, "best" way to get fit. There are countless exercise options, depending on your preferences, finances, abilities, and location. The best exercise for you is the one that you'll enjoy and will do regularly.

For example, if you like going to a health club (and can afford membership), you can work out at a gym three times a week for an hour per session, doing 30 minutes on an aerobic machine, 15 to 20 minutes lifting weights, and 5 to 10 minutes stretching. If you like fitness classes you can enroll in a YMCA, recreation department, or university-based program that meets three times a week for an hour each and includes aerobic, strengthening, and stretching exercises.

Or you can get fit by yourself—or with friends and family—at home. One of the most accessible ways is by taking a brisk 30-minute walk, followed by 5 minutes of stretching, three to five days a week. Add 15 to 20 minutes of resistance exercises two or three days a week (by doing calisthenics or using dumbbells and ankle weights) and you'll be doing all you need to get fit. If you'd rather not walk, you can dance, cycle, swim, skate, jump rope, run, climb stairs, cross-country ski, or do any other continuous activity that increases your heart rate into your "training zone" for 20 to 60 minutes.

In fact, one of the major trends in the fitness industry has been the explosion in exercise options—at home and at the gym. Nearly one-third of U.S. households own exercise equipment, according to a 1997 study sponsored by the Fitness Products Council, an association of equipment manufacturers. Treadmills and free weights are among the most popular home devices.

At health clubs, you can now choose from a smorgasbord of aerobic alternatives ranging from group stationary cycling—where high-energy instructors lead a class of pedal pushers on a sweat-soaked imaginary journey—to group weight-training classes and MTV dance-inspired workouts.

There's also been a surge of interest in Eastern-influenced classes that focus on connecting the mind, body, and spirit through the breath. These include yoga, tai chi, karate, and qi gong, which are increasingly offered by recreation departments, health clubs, and private studios. Boxing-style classes are hot with the twenty-something set, who punch and kick their way through cardio-kickboxing workouts. In addition, outdoor activities have boomed in popularity—particularly those that can be done by the whole family, such as hiking and walking.

A graphic illustration of how all these options relate to health and fitness is the Physical Activity Pyramid. Modeled after the Department of Agriculture's well-known Food Guide Pyramid, the Physical Activity Pyramid helps ordinary people "understand basic physical activity concepts," write Arizona State University professors Charles Corbin and Robert Pangrazi in the American College of Sports Medicine's *Health and Fitness Journal*.

The base of the pyramid, or level 1, represents lifestyle physical activity, the accumulated 30 minutes of moderate activity (such as raking leaves or walking) promoted by the surgeon general's report. Everyone should do at least this much activity to gain health benefits.

If you want to achieve fitness benefits, such as improving body composition and gaining cardiorespiratory endurance, you

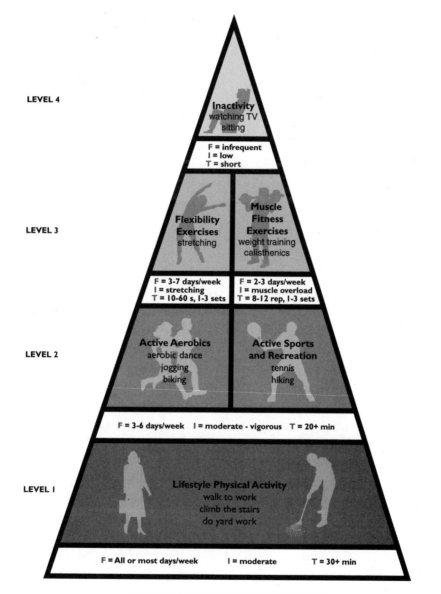

THE PHYSICAL ACTIVITY PYRAMID

Source: From Fitness for Life *by Dr. Charles Corbin, Dr. Ruth Lindsey. © 1993 by Scott Foresman and Company. Used by permission.*

need to move up to level 2 of the pyramid, which consists of sustained endurance activities and sports like aerobic dance, jogging, tennis, and hiking. Doing these more vigorous activities at least three days a week for at least 20 minutes at a time can significantly boost your fitness. (Men over age forty and women over age fifty who have been sedentary—and people of any age with risk factors for heart disease—should consult a physician before starting a program of *vigorous* activity.)

Moving up to level 3, which includes flexibility and muscle-strengthening exercises, offers even more fitness benefits. Flexibility exercises should be done three to seven days a week, while muscle-strengthening exercises need to be done only two or three days a week.

At the top of the pyramid is inactivity. "Inactivity is not necessarily bad," Corbin and Pangrazi note. "But long periods of inactivity (other than normal sleep) should be limited."

This is the bottom-line message about exercise and health: *Don't just sit there, move something.*

HOW EXERCISE HELPS

Our bodies are designed to move. Through a complex, interconnected network of chemical and nervous pathways, the body's systems communicate with one another, allowing us to perform motions as simple as getting out of bed or as complex as slugging a home run. The more you use your body, the more efficient and powerful these varied systems (musculoskeletal, cardiovascular, respiratory, immune, and endocrine) become. When your body isn't used, these systems weaken and—in the extreme—fail.

The moment you start to exercise, your body begins to adapt to the increased energy demands being placed on it. Since the muscles need more oxygen to work properly, the heart and respiration rates increase to provide an adequate supply of oxygenated blood. During one 30- to 45-minute bout of aerobic exercise, your breathing rate will increase about three times above its resting level and your heart rate may double or even triple. The volume of blood pumped out of your heart increases about fivefold, and the oxygen consumed by your working muscles climbs more than ten times above resting levels.

These changes are temporary and last only as long as you're exercising. But if you exercise aerobically on a regular basis (at least three times per week) many of these bodily functions start to change more permanently as your systems adapt to the demands of repeated exercise. For example, the heart becomes more efficient at pumping blood, so the resting heart rate slows. A sedentary person has a resting heart rate of about 70 to 90 beats per minute and pumps out about 55 to 75 milliliters of blood with each beat. A world-class endurance athlete may have a resting heart rate of less than 40 beats per minute, and pump out more than 100 milliliters of blood at each beat.

Other systems also become more proficient in response to regular exercise. As muscles grow in strength and endurance, the metabolic rate increases, allowing you to burn more calories, even at rest. Muscle cells store more fuel and burn carbohydrates and fats more efficiently. Bone cells also respond to the "loading effect" of physical activity, which "kick-starts" calcium in the system to make bones stronger and denser.

Since the body fuels exercise by taking glucose out of the blood, each bout of physical activity lowers blood glucose levels. When you exercise regularly, the body becomes better able to use glucose (blood sugar) for fuel and to transport it throughout the body. Plus, regular exercise increases the body's sensitivity to insulin.

Regular exercise also increases levels of the "good" HDL cholesterol and appears to help people break down and clear fatty substances from the blood more quickly. Even a single episode of physical activity can result in an improved blood lipid profile that persists for several days.

Exercise also affects mental health, in part by stimulating release of brain chemicals—such as endorphins, serotonin, and norephinephrine—that brighten mood, relieve anxiety, and prompt feelings of euphoria. Regular exercise enhances sleep, allowing people to "recharge their batteries" more fully. Better sleep can boost the health of both mind and body.

Physical activity may even help ward off the common cold. Exercise prompts immune cells to circulate at a greater rate, which increases the body's resistance to infection. However, excessive exercise— such as running a marathon—can stress the immune system and make an athlete more vulnerable to infection. This highlights the essential truth about healthy exercise, stated earlier:

Health is equilibrium. A person is healthy when his or her body is in balance or harmony. When this equilibrium breaks down, the result is disease.

Regular exercise is central to health, but excessive amounts of exercise—or suddenly beginning an exercise for which your body isn't conditioned—can result in injury. That's why it's important to start any exercise program slowly and progress gradually. But even though exercise can carry some risks (the most common of which is musculoskeletal injury), it's important to remember that *the overall health risks of being sedentary far outweigh those of being active.*

You don't have to be young to gain these benefits. People of any age and fitness level can experience the healthy changes that result when the body adapts to regular exercise. Research shows that even frail elderly people in their nineties can increase their muscle strength through resistance training by as much as 200 percent, allowing some to regain the ability to walk and to perform other tasks without assistance.

But these exercise-induced changes are lost when people stop exercising—a phenomenon known as "detraining." In popular terms: If you don't use it, you lose it.

EXERCISE ℞

In a culture where half the people who start an exercise program quit within six months, it's important to avoid a rigid, one-size-fits-all exercise prescription. Instead, the best exercise prescriptions are individualized, to provide you with the maximum benefit at the lowest risk and encourage you to be active all your life. To establish the right exercise prescription for you, consider your current health status and the goals you want to achieve.

Here are some guidelines for achieving the basic health and fitness goals, based on recommendations from the American College of Sports Medicine (ACSM):

Health Benefits

Burn 150 calories per day through physical activity such as walking for 30 minutes, jogging for 15 minutes, gardening for 45 minutes, or accumulating 30 minutes of "lifestyle activities" (such as climbing stairs or doing active chores). This is the least you can do to gain the health benefits of physical activity.

Cardiorespiratory Fitness

To build and maintain cardiorespiratory endurance, perform an activity that uses the large muscles of the body continuously. These kinds of activities are called "aerobic," which means "with oxygen," since they result in the heart's increased capacity to deliver oxygen to the muscles. Examples are walking, bicycling, cross-country skiing, swimming, and in-line skating. Do your chosen aerobic exercise three to six days a week, at about 55 to 90 percent of your maximum heart rate (also known as your "training zone"), for 20 to 60 minutes, either working continuously or by accumulating intermittent bouts of at least 10 minutes each. (To learn how to calculate your training zone, see Healing Moves for Health and Fitness, page 36.)

If you find checking your pulse too bothersome, another method of determining exercise intensity is "perceived exertion": Work out at a pace you perceive to be moderately hard. Listen to your body, and find an intensity where you can feel your heart rate go up some, but not so much that it's racing; you should be able to carry on a conversation without becoming breathless. On a scale of one to ten (with one being "very, very light" and ten being "extremely hard"), about four to seven is a desirable intensity range. One to three may be too light to allow you the maximum cardiovascular benefits; eight to ten is too hard for most people and increases the likelihood of orthopedic or cardiac problems.

The goal of an aerobic workout is to achieve the "training effect"—a complex constellation of physiological changes that occur as your body begins to adapt to the demands of aerobic conditioning. The more intense the workout, the less time necessary to achieve the training effect. A jog or bike ride that gets your heart rate up to 140 beats per minute will give you a training effect in just 20 minutes. By contrast, a walk that gets your heart rate slightly over 110 beats per minute would take about 45 minutes to achieve the training effect. Neither option is better than the other. They are both good choices, depending on your health status, preferences, and time.

In general, sustaining an aerobic activity at a moderately hard pace for 30 minutes three to five times a week will result in optimum heart health. Be sure to precede your activity by a five-minute warm-up and follow it with a five-minute cooldown.

To see if you're working too hard, check your pulse five minutes after you've finished your workout. It should be within 20 beats of your resting heart rate. For example, if your resting heart rate is 80, by five minutes after the end of your workout your heart rate should be 100 or less.

Muscular Strength and Endurance

To build muscle strength and endurance, do resistance exercises (such as lifting weights or using a strength-training machine) two to three days a week. Be sure you:

* Perform one to three sets of eight to ten exercises that strengthen the major muscle groups: arms, shoulders, chest, back, abdominals, hips, and legs. One set of each exercise is sufficient to boost strength and prevent loss of muscle mass in most adults, but three-set regimens, if time allows, may provide slightly greater benefits.

* Pick a weight heavy enough for you to lift at least eight but no more than twelve times. (Older and more frail people—those fifty years old and above—may find it more appropriate to choose a lighter weight they can lift at least ten but no more than fifteen times.)

Stronger muscles can help you perform everyday tasks more efficiently, boost your energy, and improve your appearance. Plus, since the muscles are the "engines of the body," having more muscle will boost your metabolic rate, which allows you to burn more fat. Without strength training, even the most dedicated aerobic exerciser will lose muscle mass with age—about one pound of muscle every two years after the age of twenty, says Boston exercise physiologist Wayne Westcott, strength-training consultant to the national YMCA. This steady loss of muscle slows the metabolism, which declines at a rate of 3 to 5 percent per decade for adults. "That's the main reason so many people add fat weight year after year," Westcott says. "With less muscle tissue, you simply burn fewer calories."

It's a good idea to get some expert help to begin strength training, since exercising incorrectly won't get you good results and, worse, might get you injured. Check with a reputable gym or university or hospital-affiliated exercise program to find an instructor who has a college degree in physical education and is certified by a respected professional group such as the National Strength and Conditioning Association, the American College of Sports Medicine, or the American Council on Exercise. You won't need a trainer to hold your hand forever. A half dozen appointments, plus a "check-in" every now and then, should suffice. (For more information, consult Healing Moves to Strengthen Muscles and Bones, page 138.)

Flexibility

To gain and maintain flexibility, the body's joints and muscles must be stretched regularly. Some of the best times to stretch are before and after aerobic activity, but be sure to warm up with some gentle movement first, since stretching a "cold" muscle can result in injury. Gentle stretching helps prepare your muscles for activity. After activity, when your muscles are engorged with blood, you're likely to find that you can stretch even more deeply.

Get in the habit of stretching tense muscles throughout the day, particularly after sitting or standing for an extended period of time. You can stretch while you talk on the phone, watch TV, read the paper, or wait in line. If you sit at a desk a lot, stretch spontaneously throughout the day to relax the "tightness triangle" of the shoulders, neck, and face.

"Stretching should be as relaxed and natural as a yawn," says flexibility guru Bob

Anderson, whose classic book *Stretching* has sold more than two million copies in seventeen languages. Stretching to a point of *mild* tension helps the muscles relax, increases your range of motion, helps prevent injuries, promotes circulation, and helps loosen the mind's control of the body.

The key is to stretch by a feeling, not by how far you can go. Instead of struggling to touch your toes or wrap your foot around your neck, simply stretch until you feel a point of slight tension—not pain. If it's painful, you've gone too far and need to back off. When you've stretched to your "tension point," hold it for about five or ten seconds, breathing naturally. Don't bounce. If the tension diminishes, you may try to stretch a bit farther before you release.

For expert inspiration, watch a dog or a cat. Animals instinctively know how to stay flexible and use stretches when making the transition from sleep to wakefulness and from sitting still to moving. And animals don't compete with each other to see who can stretch farther. *A competitive mind-set in stretching can lead to injury.*

Remember: There are no "should bes" in stretching. Everyone is unique, with his or her own muscular structure, flexibility, and tension level.

Body Composition

A high level of body fat can increase your risk of developing a variety of health problems including heart disease, high blood pressure, and diabetes. In addition, excess fat can strain your joints and contribute to orthopedic problems like back and knee pain.

But your body weight isn't necessarily a good indicator of your body composition. The scale can be deceiving because it doesn't indicate how many of your pounds are desirable "lean tissue mass" (muscle and bone) and how many of your pounds are less desirable fat. Two people of the same height and weight can have vastly different shapes—and health risks—if one person's weight is mostly lean tissue and the other person's is excessively fat. For example, a six-foot-tall sedentary man who weights 185 pounds may actually be fatter than a six-foot-tall muscular football player who weighs 220.

In other words, it's not how much you weigh that matters to your health; it's how fat you are.

Some fat is essential for the body to function properly, and it's important not to let fat levels fall too low. Excessively low body fat is linked to some health abnormalities, such as menstrual irregularities in women. Too little fat, however, isn't the problem for most Americans; too much fat is. An estimated one half of adults and one-fourth of children in the United States are currently overweight.

How much fat is too much? Opinions vary, but the generally accepted healthy range of body fat for males is about 12 to 18 percent of total body weight; for females (who naturally have more fatty tissue than males) it's about 18 to 25 percent.

There are three main ways to test body composition: hydrostatic (underwater) weighing, electrical impedance (sending a very low current of electricity through your body), and skin-fold calipers (pinching body fat at specific sites). Since all three methods are somewhat complicated to administer and have a strong potential for inaccuracy, most health professionals prefer

CALORIES BURNED DURING 30 MINUTES OF ACTIVITY

Type of Activity	130-pound adult	175-pound adult	65-pound child
Cycling	180	240	120
Swimming	210	300	140*
In-line skating	210	280	128
Softball	120	160	70*
Aerobic dance	180	240	110*
Jogging	300	400	180
Hiking (20-pound pack)	280	336	185
Tennis	180	270	110*
Martial arts	300	420	180*
Skiing	240	330	150*
Walking	130	180	80
Canoeing	80	105	45*
Bowling	170	231	90*
Weight lifting	210	240	125
Frisbee	180	240	100*

*Estimate based on adult data; no data on children exists.
Chart courtesy of Professor Robert McMurray, University of North Carolina at Chapel Hill

to use a simple measurement called body mass index (BMI), which is determined by calculating the relationship between your height and weight. (See Healing Moves for Health and Fitness, page 31.)

If you are exceptionally muscular, however, BMIs can be problematic since the number does not factor in how much of the body is fat and how much is lean tissue. For this reason, elite athletes may prefer using more sophisticated methods of determining body fat, such as underwater weighing. But since this technique relies on equipment usually available only in research laboratories, most experts consider BMI the most practical measure of fatness and associated risk for most people.

A commonsense technique also can be helpful. We call this low-tech approach the "see fat" test: Take your clothes off in front of a mirror. Move around and see if anything jiggles that nature didn't intend. Pinch yourself at trouble spots and see if you can lift skin folds thicker than your index finger. Chances are, if you look overfat, you probably are.

Not all fat is created equal. It's not just how much fat you have, but also *where it's located* that affects your health risks. Fat in the abdominal area carries a greater risk of cardiovascular disease than fat in the thighs and hips, which is why "apple-shaped" people are at greater risk than "pear-shaped" ones. But abdominal fat is typically easier to lose than fat in the lower body.

Regular aerobic exercise is the best way to burn off body fat. In addition, muscle-strengthening exercises can contribute to fat loss by increasing the amount of muscle tissue in your body. Since muscle is one of the body's most metabolically active tissues, the more muscle you have, the higher your metabolic rate and the more calories your body will burn.

To reach and maintain a healthy body composition, it's also important to eat properly, making sure to consume appropriate portions of nutritious, low-fat foods. But avoid restrictive diets, which can slow the metabolic rate. When you severely restrict calories, the body tries to conserve fat stores, so it breaks down muscle mass. This can be especially problematic for seniors, who are already dealing with an age-related loss of muscle. "For older people who are overweight, it can be very dangerous to try to lose weight in the traditional way of just cutting back on calories," says William Evans, director of the nutrition, metabolism, and exercise lab at the University of Arkansas for Medical Sciences. Caloric requirements are already low for most people over sixty, he says, so eliminating food can rob seniors of important nutrients.

For people of any age, the best way to lose fat and keep it off is through a combination of regular exercise and eating right. Be sure to:

∗ Do an aerobic activity that you enjoy that burns 250 to 500 calories a day, four to six days a week. (A 175-pound person burns about 360 calories during a brisk one-hour walk. See chart, page 23.)

∗ Pick a pace you like, since the goal is to have fun so you'll do it regularly. For most people, this means a moderate intensity, which can be as effective in losing fat as more strenuous activity but requires a longer workout to burn the same amount of calories. While high-intensity activity burns calories faster, it has a greater injury potential—especially for people who are overweight and out of shape.

∗ Do muscle-strengthening exercises two or three times a week. This is especially important for people over forty.

∗ Eat fewer calories than you burn, from a diet that is less than 30 percent fat. But be sure to eat enough to fuel your activities, which is generally at least 1,500 to 2,000 calories per day.

∗ Shun gimmicks. "Fat-melting" gizmos sold on "infomercials" are typically useless. There is no magic way to erase fat.

Remember, too, that gender and genetics affect fat storage. Some people may never get down to an arbitrary "goal weight," despite proper diet and exercise. "Too many people get hung up on reaching a number on a height-weight chart that for them, genetically and physiologically, may be unattainable," says Josephine Connolly, a nutritionist at the State University of New York at Stony Brook and a spokesperson for the American Dietetic Association. The ADA now advises people to stop focusing on weight loss alone. Instead, they recommend working toward "weight management," which they define as "achieving the best weight possible in the context of overall health."

The ADA's healthy weight-management guidelines advise people to:

∗ Change to a more healthful eating style with proportional increases in whole grains, fruits, and vegetables.

∗ Adopt a nonrestrictive approach to eating based on eating when hungry and stopping when full.

∗ Work your way up to doing at least 30 minutes of enjoyable physical activity a day.

The ADA also encourages the notion of a "healthy weight," which someone can achieve and maintain, as opposed to a cosmetic weight or ideal weight on a standardized chart. Each person's healthy weight is determined individually, based on his or her weight history and current medical conditions. Even relatively modest weight losses, such as dropping ten to sixteen pounds, can dramatically improve health. People who might never get to their goal weight on a standardized chart can still reach a weight that's healthy for them if they adopt good eating and exercise behaviors that can normalize their blood pressure, blood sugar, and blood cholesterol.

The bottom line: If you eat right and get regular exercise, your body weight will drop to the lowest level it can (and should) naturally maintain.

CAUTIONS

In general, the more exercise you do, the more benefits you get. But it *is* possible to get too much of a good thing. The body needs a chance to recover and rebuild. People who exercise hard for more than an hour and a half a day, seven days a week, face a number of risks, ranging from muscle and bone injuries to increased susceptibility to infection. In addition, excessive exercise can cause reproductive-age women to lose their menstrual cycles, which can affect bone growth and lead to the early onset of osteoporosis.

But before you burn your gym membership card, recognize that these "ultra-exercisers" who are at risk represent *less than 1 percent of the American population.* Only 15 percent of adults engage in vigorous physical activity at least three times a week for 20 minutes or more.

Remember: Exercise is much safer than inactivity in terms of health and well-being.

Most healthy people don't need to consult a physician before beginning a program of *moderate* exercise. However, you *should* see a doctor before starting to exercise if you have undiagnosed symptoms—such as chest pain or fainting spells or red, swollen knees. If you have a chronic condition that's out of control, such as high blood pressure or diabetes, you should consult a physician before exercising. And if you take prescription medications, such as those for high blood pressure, check with your doctor about how the medicine may interact with your activity.

There is a short list of grave medical conditions that might make exercise unsafe, such as severe aortic stenosis (constriction) or a serious terminal or untreatable disease. But for most chronic conditions, like heart disease and arthritis, exercise is a well-recognized and effective therapy. So if you have these conditions and you're not exercising, you're missing an important mechanism for improving your health.

People who want to start a program of *vigorous* exercise, however, may need to consult a physician first, depending on their age and health status. Men over forty and women over fifty, plus people of any age with risk factors for heart disease (such as cigarette smoking, diabetes, or obesity) should see a doctor before beginning to exercise vigorously, advises the American Heart Association. But for nonvigorous exercise—such as walking, pool aerobics, doubles tennis, or any activity you can do while carrying on a conversation—no physician's approval is generally necessary.

To avoid injury, be sure to:

✳ Start slowly and progress gradually. The most common mistake among new exercisers is doing too much too soon, which can result in injury.

✳ Stretch before and after activity, being sure to warm up gently before you stretch.

✳ Avoid working out hard every single day. Give your body time to recover from intensive exercise by alternating hard workouts with easier ones, and be sure to take a day of rest (mild to moderate activity only) one day each week.

✳ Watch out for signs of overtraining if you're exercising vigorously. These signs include poor sleep, depressed appetite, and waking up sore and/or tired every morning. If you feel these symptoms, back off from your training. Rest for several days, then ease back into exercise, being sure to give your body time to recover from hard workouts. If you feel these symptoms with just daily life activities, look for other causes. Don't stop moving.

PRESCRIPTION PAD

✳ *General health:* Accumulate 30 minutes of moderate activity most days of the week.

✳ *Heart health:* Perform 20 to 60 minutes of continuous aerobic activity, three to five days a week, at about 55 to 90 percent of your maximum heart rate.

✳ *Weight loss:* Do enough activity to burn 250 to 500 calories a day, four to six days a week.

✳ *Strong bones and muscles:* Do eight to ten strength-training exercises involving the body's major muscles groups, two to three times a week.

✳ *Flexibility:* Incorporate stretching exercises into your overall fitness program. Take all the body's muscles and joints through a full range of motion three to seven days a week.

ADDITIONAL RESOURCES

Books
✳ *American College of Sports Medicine Fitness Book*, 2nd ed. (Human Kinetics, 1998).

✳ *Getting in Shape*, by Bob Anderson, Ed Burke, and Bill Pearl (Shelter Publications, 1994).

✳ *Fresh Start: The Stanford Medical School Health & Fitness Program* (KQED Books, 1996).

✳ *Stretching*, by Bob Anderson (Shelter Publications, 1980).

✳ *Knocking at the Gate of Life and Other Healing Exercises from China*, translated by Edward C. Chang, Ph. D. (Rodale Press, 1985).

Organizations

✳ The American College of Sports Medicine, 401 West Michigan St., Indianapolis, Ind. 46202-3233; Web site: www.acsm.org.

✳ The American Council on Exercise consumer hotline, 800-234-9229; Web site: www.acefitness.org.

✳ The American Alliance for Health, Physical Education, Recreation and Dance, 1900 Association Dr., Reston, Va. 20191; Web site: www.aahperd.org.

✳ Aerobics and Fitness Association of America consumer hotline, 800-YOUR-BOD; Web site: www.afaa.com.

✳ Fitness Products Council, 200 Castlewood Dr., North Palm Beach, Fla. 33408.

✳ IDEA: The Health and Fitness Source, 800-999-IDEA; Web site: www.ideafit.com.

✳ IHRSA: The International Health, Racquet and Sports Clubs Association, 800-228-4772; Web site: www.ihrsa.org

✳ National Coalition for Promoting Physical Activity, P.O. Box 1440, Indianapolis, Ind. 46206-1440; Web site: www.ncppa.org.

✳ National Strength and Conditioning Association, P.O. Box 9908, Colorado Springs, Colo. 80932-0908; Web site: www.nsca-lift.org.

✳ The American Heart Association, 800-AHA-USA1; Web site: www.aha.org.

✳ The American Running Association, 800-776-2732; Web site: www.americanrunning.org.

✳ ✳ ✳

HEALING MOVES FOR HEALTH AND FITNESS

✳

Every other workout in this book centers on a specific aspect of health and explores how exercise can help prevent and treat ailments involving a particular bodily system. In contrast, this workout focuses on your total, overall health. It explains how exercise can get you fit, reduce your risk of illness, increase the length of your life, and—most importantly—enhance the quality of your days.

Health is much more than just the absence of disease: It is a state of physical, mental, and spiritual balance. A truly healthy person has the energy and will to perform the tasks of daily life with joy, as well as the ability to rise to the extra challenges of emergencies. Health is physiological and psychological well-being; it's social and emotional equilibrium; it's the ability to get out of bed in the morning and look forward with delight to your day.

Just as health is about much more than the physical body, so is fitness. In many ways, true fitness reflects a state of mind. That's why the foundation of our program is this two-part attitude adjustment:

1. **Bottoms up.** The typical American tries to stay seated and use as little energy as possible—parking in the closest space, picking banks and fast-food joints with

drive-through windows, clicking the remote control from the depths of the La-Z-Boy. But if you want good health, you must drop this "push-button" mentality in favor of a "bottoms-up" approach to life. Getting off your bottom and moving as much as possible throughout the day is one of the best, most practical ways to use physical activity to enhance health.

2. **Restoring recess.** The reason many people don't exercise is that they consider it hard, painful work—something "good for you" they should force themselves to endure, like tasteless tofu or nasty medicine. Yet as children we didn't feel this way. Most kids see physical pursuits—like skipping and running—as exciting play to be enjoyed. Recovering this feeling about movement is crucial to real fitness. So stop viewing exercise as a "workout," and start thinking of it as child's play—a welcome recess that frees your body from the confines of its chair. This may be difficult in our culture, which considers play frivolous. Yet "the ability to play is one of the principal criteria of mental health," wrote famed anthropologist Ashley Montague in his classic work *Growing Young*. If it helps, drop the E-word and call it physical activity or movement. Just remember that your daily "recess" isn't simply one more chore to get crossed off your list but an exhilaratingly human opportunity to move purposefully, to breathe deeply, to have fun, to be well.

If you think these attitude adjustments are merely mind games, you're right. But to gain the optimal health benefits from exercise it's crucial to connect the mind with the body and, ideally, the spirit. At its best, exercise can strengthen your body, relax your mind, and lift your spirit. When you find an activity you enjoy and do it regularly, and when you look for ways to move throughout the day, you will achieve optimum health and fitness. Of course, it's important to follow other parts of a healthy lifestyle—eating right and not smoking, for example. Just remember that the healthiest approach to getting fit is enjoying the journey as much as the destination.

Once exercise becomes a part of your life, you'll experience an amazing dividend. Not only can your mind change your body (which you'll discover by making our two attitude adjustments) but *your body can change your mind.* If you feel tense or tired, a walk in the fresh air can revive you. Depressed, discouraged, sad? A series of yoga poses and deep breathing can help restore equilibrium. Anxious, irritable, upset? Rake some leaves, ride your bike, go soak your head in a swimming pool.

When you focus on fun, exercise will become a cherished highlight of your life. Far from being a chore, it will become your daily opportunity to indulge in the gift of movement, an experience that can bring healing energy not just to the body but to the soul.

HEALING MOVES

Our program begins with:

A **Pre-Participation Checklist** to assess whether you need medical advice about getting active, plus **Five Fitness Tests** to help you determine how fit, or unfit, you are.

The workout includes four parts:

Part One: Activate Your Life

A flight of stairs here, a luxurious stretch there, and a short "walk-about" whenever possible can add up to major health benefits. This section presents twenty-five life-activating strategies to integrate more movement into your day.

Part Two: Aerobic Activity

To enhance cardiovascular fitness, body composition, and mental outlook, regular aerobic exercise is key. This section outlines a "design-it-yourself" program that lets you choose from a variety of aerobic options and pick the frequency, intensity, and duration of activity that suits you best.

Part Three: Strengthening Exercises

To build and maintain strong bones and muscles, we offer a series of resistance exercises that work all the body's major muscle groups. Not only will strong muscles help you get through your days with more energy and ease, but having more lean tissue mass will help boost your metabolic rate, so you'll burn more calories.

Part Four: Stretching

Stretching is the link between rest and movement that relaxes the mind, prepares the body for activity, helps release tension, and literally "gets the kinks out" after physical or mental stress. Our stretches are designed to keep all the body's major muscle groups flexible and supple.

Part Five: Relaxation Breathing

Also known as yoga "belly breathing," this simple technique is a powerful healing exercise that helps counter the negative effects of stress. Relaxation breathing connects the mind and the body and creates a physiologic state of calm that is the exact opposite of the typical fight-or-flight response to stress.

PRE-PARTICIPATION CHECKLIST

Before you start this, or any other exercise program, it's important to do a quick assessment to see if exercise might present any special risks to you. Most people don't need to consult a physician before doing *moderate-intensity* activity. But if you're planning to start a program of *vigorous-intensity* exercise, you should consult a physician first if you're a man over forty or a woman over fifty, or if you have any risk factors for heart disease (such as cigarette smoking, diabetes, or obesity). It's also important to see a doctor before starting to exercise if you have a chronic disease or undiagnosed symptoms—such as chest pain or fainting spells.

But remember, even though exercise can carry some risks, it's much safer than inactivity in terms of health and well-being. So look over this quick pre-activity checklist. If you answer "yes" to any of these questions, discuss your physical activity plans with your doctor before beginning this or any other exercise program:

1. Has a doctor ever told you that you have heart trouble?
2. Do you frequently experience chest pains?
3. Do you often feel dizzy or unsteady?

4. Has a doctor told you that you have high blood pressure?
5. Has a doctor told you that you have a bone or joint problem?
6. Are you taking prescription medication?
7. Is there a reason not mentioned here that might affect your ability to exercise?

FIVE FITNESS TESTS

How fit—or unfit—are you? These five simple tests will help you assess your fitness level and compare yourself with norms for your age and sex. They also can provide a baseline to compare yourself with six weeks and six months from now, to measure the results of your exercise program. (These tests and scores are based on material provided by the Cooper Institute for Aerobics Research.)

1. Push-up Test
This test measures muscular endurance of the upper body (anterior deltoids, pectoralis major, triceps).

Equipment: Watch with a second hand.
Preparation: Warm up by doing a few light jumping jacks and arm circles.

Procedure:
1. Place both hands on the floor, about shoulder width apart, with fingers pointed forward. Place a three-inch sponge or small box under your chest, or have a partner put his or her fist under your chest.
2. Lift your knees, so that your weight is supported on your palms and toes. Your legs, buttocks, and back should be in a straight line. (If this is too difficult, keep your knees on the floor and do a modified push-up, with your body in a straight line from knees to ears. Let your feet come up off the floor and cross them at the ankles or leave them slightly apart.)
3. The push-up begins in this up position. Bend your arms and keep your back straight as you lower your body to the floor until it touches the sponge or your partner's fist.
4. Push back up to the up position. This counts as one complete push-up.
5. Perform as many correct push-ups as you can in one minute. Any resting should be done in the up position.

2. Sit-up Test
This test measures abdominal muscular endurance.

Equipment: Exercise mat or padded surface, watch with a second hand.
Preparation: Warm up with easy movements such as walking in place.

Procedure:
1. Lie on your back on a padded surface with your legs together, knees bent, and heels flat on the floor; you can lace your fingers behind your head or cup your hands behind your ears.
2. Have a partner hold your feet down firmly, or secure them under a bed or a bar.
3. Contract your abdominal muscles, raising your upper body off the floor until your elbows touch your knees.
4. Go back down until your shoulder blades touch the floor. This is one sit-up.

5. Perform as many correct sit-ups as you can in one minute. Be sure to avoid pulling on your neck with your hands and breathe as normally as possible. Any resting should be done in the up position.

Note: Full sit-ups with feet secured are done for the purposes of testing abdominal strength. To strengthen the abdominal muscles, crunches are the preferred exercise. When doing crunches, don't secure your ankles; use your abdominal muscles to curl yourself up only until your shoulder blades lift off the floor.

3. Sit and Reach Test

This test measures the flexibility of the lower back and hamstrings.

Equipment: twelve-inch-high box (or step), yardstick.

Preparation: Place a yardstick on the box (or step) so that the 15-inch mark is flush with the edge of the box. Have someone hold the yardstick there or secure it with tape. Warm up with some easy movements and light stretching.

Procedure:

1. Take off your shoes and sit with your feet placed squarely against the box, straddling the yardstick with the "0" end closest to your groin. Keep your feet no wider than eight inches apart and your toes pointed directly toward the ceiling.
2. Place one hand on top of the other, with the tips of the middle fingers even, and lean forward slowly with your legs straight, reaching as far forward along the yardstick as you can. Don't bend your knees, and be sure to exhale as you lean forward.
3. Hold the position for at least one second, being sure *not to bounce, lunge, or bob.*
4. Your score is the point at which your fingertips touch the yardstick at maximum reach, recorded to the nearest quarter inch.
5. Perform the stretch three times and use the best of the three scores.

4. 12-Minute Test

This test measures aerobic power (cardiovascular endurance).

Equipment: Comfortable walking shoes, watch with second hand, indoor or outdoor track.

Preparation: Do not eat a heavy meal or smoke for at least two to three hours prior to the test. Warm up for several minutes by walking at an easy pace, then stretch gently.

Procedure:

1. Using the inside lane of the track, cover as much distance as possible in 12 minutes. You may walk, jog, or run.
2. Record the distance you covered. (Each completed lap is a quarter of a mile.)
3. Cool down by walking at a comfortable pace for several minutes.

5. Body Mass Index (BMI) Test

This test provides an approximate measure of your body composition. (No home test can perfectly measure how much of your body is fat and how much is muscle and bone. This test works only for adults and may be invalid for extremely muscular, athletic individuals.)

Equipment: Body weight scale and a measuring tape or yardstick.

Preparation: Wearing minimal clothing, measure your body weight. Then measure your height without shoes.

Procedure:

1. Multiply your weight in pounds by 703. (For example, if you weigh 149 pounds, multiply 149 × 703 to get 104,747.)
2. Multiply your height in inches by your height in inches. (If you are 65 inches tall, multiply 65 × 65 to get 4,225.)
3. Divide the answer in step 1 by the answer in step 2 to get your body mass index. (104,747 divided by 4,225 is 24.8.)

HOW TO SCORE

1. PUSH-UP TEST (BY AGE GROUP)

Men: Full-body Push-ups

	20–29	30–39	40–49	50–59	60+
Superior	62	52	40	39	28
Excellent	47	39	30	25	23
Good	37	30	24	19	18
Fair	29	24	18	13	10
Poor	22	17	11	9	6
Very Poor	13	9	5	3	2

Women: Full-body Push-ups

	20–29	30–39	40–49	
Superior	42	39	20	*Number of Push-ups*
Excellent	28	23	15	
Good	21	15	13	
Fair	15	11	9	
Poor	10	8	6	
Very Poor	3	1	0	

Women: Modified Push-ups

	20–29	30–39	40–49	50–59	60+	
Superior	45	39	33	28	20	*Number of Push-ups*
Excellent	36	31	24	21	15	
Good	30	24	18	17	12	
Fair	23	19	13	12	5	
Poor	7	11	6	6	2	
Very Poor	9	4	1	0	0	

2. SIT-UP TEST (BY AGE GROUP)

	Men						Women						
	<20	20–29	30–39	40–49	50–59	60+	<20	20–29	30–39	40–49	50–59	60+	
Superior	62	55	51	47	43	39	55	51	42	38	30	28	*Number of Sit-ups*
Excellent	51	47	43	39	35	30	46	44	35	29	24	17	
Good	47	42	39	34	28	22	36	38	29	24	20	11	
Fair	41	38	35	29	24	19	32	32	25	20	14	6	
Poor	36	33	30	24	19	15	28	24	20	14	10	3	
Very Poor	27	27	23	17	12	7	25	18	11	7	5	0	

3. SIT-AND-REACH TEST (BY AGE GROUP)

	Men						Women						
	<20	20–29	30–39	40–49	50–59	60+	<20	20–29	30–39	40–49	50–59	60+	
Superior	23.4	23	22	21.3	20.5	20	24.3	24.5	24	22.8	23	23	*Distance of Reaches in Inches*
Excellent	21.7	20.5	19.5	18.5	17.5	17.3	22.5	22.5	21.5	20.5	20.3	19	
Good	19	18.5	17.5	16.3	15.5	14.5	21.5	20.5	20	19	18.5	17	
Fair	16.5	16.5	15.5	14.3	13.3	12.5	20.5	19.3	18.3	17.3	16.8	15.5	
Poor	13.2	14.4	13	12	10.5	10	18.5	17	16.5	15	14.8	13	
Very Poor	9.4	10.5	9.3	8.3	7	5.8	14.5	14.1	12	10.5	12.3	9.2	

4. 12-MINUTE TEST (BY AGE GROUP)

	Men					Women					
	20–29	30–39	40–49	50–59	60+	20–29	30–39	40–49	50–59	60+	
Superior	1.81	1.77	1.71	1.62	1.57	1.61	1.53	1.45	1.33	1.35	*Number of Miles*
Excellent	1.65	1.61	1.54	1.45	1.37	1.45	1.38	1.32	1.21	1.18	
Good	1.54	1.49	1.42	1.33	1.24	1.33	1.27	1.21	1.13	1.07	
Fair	1.45	1.39	1.33	1.25	1.15	1.25	1.21	1.13	1.06	.99	
Poor	1.34	1.29	1.23	1.15	1.05	1.16	1.11	1.05	.98	.94	
Very Poor	1.06	1.13	.98	.92	.82	.94	.93	.89	.83	.81	

Source for charts 1–4: The Physical Fitness Specialist Manual, The Cooper Institute for Aerobics Research, Dallas, Texas, revised 1999; reprinted with permission.

5. BODY MASS INDEX TEST

Body Mass Index	21	22	23	24	25	26	27	28	29	30	31
					←	Overweight		→		Obese	
5′	107	112	118	123	128	133	138	143	148	153	158
5′1″	111	116	122	127	132	137	143	148	153	158	164
5′3″	118	124	130	135	141	146	152	158	163	169	175
5′5″	126	132	138	144	150	156	162	168	174	180	186
5′7″	134	140	146	153	159	166	172	178	185	191	198
5′9″	142	149	155	162	169	176	182	189	196	203	209
5′11″	150	157	165	172	179	186	193	200	208	215	222
6′1″	159	166	174	182	189	197	204	212	219	227	235
6′3″	168	176	184	192	200	208	216	224	232	240	248

Height in Inches (left axis) — *Body Weight in Pounds* (right axis)

Source for chart 5: The National Heart, Lung, and Blood Institute.

BMI Scoring

Less than 18.5	Underweight
18.5–24.9	Normal weight
25–29.99	Overweight
30 or higher	Obese

PART ONE: ACTIVATE YOUR LIFE

It doesn't take rocket science to conclude that we expend less energy now than did our grandparents, who had to chop wood and fetch water to survive. In fact, some experts say we expend up to 800 fewer calories per day than our parents did. Yet most people don't realize how little physical activity they actually get and how important it is for them to use every opportunity they have to move.

Fitting activity into your day can provide health benefits similar to a traditional, gym-based workout, according to studies performed at the Cooper Institute for Aerobics Research in Dallas. In a two-year study called Project Active, participants in a "lifestyle" group learned behavioral skills to help them fit more physical activity into their daily routines. By simply adding more movement into their days, they decreased their body fat by an average of about one clothing size (2.4 percent) and lowered their blood pressure by an average of 3.6 mm (systolic) and 5.4 mm (diastolic).

This is good news for people who say they don't have time to exercise. Many people think that exercise is an either-or phenomenon, where you either go to the gym and work out for 30 to 60 minutes, or you do nothing. But this is not true—every step you take counts!

In our workout, you won't be substituting lifestyle activity for aerobic exercise—you'll be doing both to optimize health and fitness benefits. But these lifestyle activities won't take big chunks of time out of your day, because they'll become an integral part of your life. We offer this starter list of twenty-five life-activating strategies. Pick ten of these to do regularly—or create some of your own. Adopt one new strategy each week, so that—in ten weeks—you'll have ten new ways of adding meaningful movement into your day.

25 WAYS TO ACTIVATE YOUR LIFE

1. Don't use the nearest bathroom. Use one that requires you to walk a bit, preferably up or down a flight or two of stairs.
2. Balance on one foot while you're brushing your teeth. Balance on the other foot while you're combing your hair.
3. Park in the farthest space.
4. Play actively with your kids. Strap on a pair of in-line skates, join in their karate class, get off your bench and swing, climb, hang, slide.
5. Hide your TV remote. Get up and walk across the room when you want to change the channel, increase the volume, or turn the TV on or off.
6. Never take the elevator when you're going fewer than three flights; take the stairs.
7. Get rid of your electric can opener and use a manual one.
8. Turn your coffee break into a walk break. Walk to a distant vending machine, cafeteria, or coffee shop to get your snack instead of using the closest one.
9. Stretch or walk while you're talking on the (cordless) phone.
10. Set an "activity" timer or program your computer to remind you to take brief walking and/or stretching breaks periodically.
11. Wait actively. If you're forced to wait for an airplane, hairdresser, dentist, doctor, or restaurant table, take a walk.
12. Walk or bike to do errands instead of driving.
13. Take a minute to stretch your arms, legs, back, shoulders, and neck whenever you get up from sitting or lying down.
14. Sweep your floors, patio, and/or front walk every day.
15. During TV commercials, get up and walk or get down and stretch.
16. Socialize actively. Instead of sitting and talking with friends and/or family, try walking and talking. Go bowling or line dancing, or play Ping-Pong, basketball, or boccie ball.
17. Put your favorite mug on a very low shelf, so you'll have to squat down to get it out and put it back.
18. Take your dog for a walk every day. If you don't have a dog, borrow your neighbor's, or just walk your "inner dog."
19. Practice "aerobic shopping" by taking a lap around the mall or grocery store before you go into a shop or put an item in your cart.
20. Avoid "drive-throughs." Park your car and walk in.
21. Practice good posture when you're forced to wait in line. Stand firmly on both feet and try to raise the top of your head to touch an imaginary hand held a quarter inch above you. Let your spine extend, shoulders relax, and arms fall at your sides.
22. Don't automatically drive. If the dry cleaner is across the parking lot from the bank, walk there. (Wear decent walking shoes or keep a good pair in your car.)
23. Install a chin-up bar in a convenient doorway, then use it often to do chin-ups, pull-ups, or simply hang.
24. Try musical housework. Put on dancing music and sweep, vacuum, or wash windows to the beat.

25. Every time you hear a bell ring (for example, a phone bell, doorbell, or church bell) take a deep breath and smile. Think of it as "mouth yoga" that relaxes hundreds of muscles in your face. And it's contagious, so pass it on.

PART TWO: AEROBIC ACTIVITY

The word *aerobic* means "living in air" or "utilizing oxygen," according to Dallas physician Kenneth H. Cooper, the man who coined the term in his 1968 best-seller by that title. Aerobic exercises are activities that require the body to use oxygen for a prolonged period of time, such as walking and swimming. When you do aerobic activities regularly, the body adapts to meet the demands of your exercise by strengthening your heart, lungs, and blood vessels. Aerobic exercise is also the top calorie-burning form of activity, which makes it essential to maintaining a healthy weight.

There is no single best aerobic exercise—*the best aerobic exercise for you is the one you like and you'll do regularly*. We're not going to tell you that you must do a specific activity, a specific number of days per week, for a specific amount of time. Instead we'll help you individualize your own program with this design-it-yourself approach:

1. *Pick an exercise* from this list of popular options: Walking, cycling, swimming, running, aerobic dancing, in-line skating, rope skipping, jogging, cross-country skiing, rowing. Depending on how you do them, some other activities may also be aerobic, such as: ashtanga (power) yoga, karate, tennis, basketball, soccer, line dancing. The important consideration in choosing an activity for cardiovascular fitness is that it keeps you moving at a moderately hard pace for 20 to 60 minutes; you can work continuously or in intermittent bouts of at least 10 minutes each. So if your tennis game is largely watching your partner run after balls, it's not aerobic. Also, feel free to pick more than one activity and then alternate. (For example, you can run one day and swim the next.) This practice, known as cross-training, has many benefits: It allows you to work different muscle groups on different days, helps avoid injury, and banishes boredom.

2. *Pick an intensity.* To gain the training effect (the beneficial changes that occur in the lungs, heart, and vascular system in response to regular aerobic exercise) it's important that you work out at 55 to 90 percent of your maximum heart rate—which is called your training zone. If you've been sedentary, you may want to exercise at the lower end of this range. If you're very fit, you can probably tolerate exercise in the higher end of this range. To find your training zone, first calculate your maximum heart rate by subtracting your age from 220. Then multiply that number by .55 to get your lower-limit heart rate and by .9 to get your upper-limit heart rate. (For example, if you're forty, subtract 40 from 220 to get 180. Multiply 180 by .55 to get 99 and by .9 to get 162. Your training zone is then 99 beats to 162 beats per minute.) Another way to think of intensity is by using your personal perception of how hard you're working. Try to move at a pace you consider "moderate" to "somewhat hard."

3. *Pick a duration*. For optimal cardiovascular conditioning, it's important that you perform your aerobic activity with your heart rate in your training zone for 20 to 60 minutes. While intermittent aerobic exercise bouts of 10 minutes each can also add up to cardiovascular benefit, we recommend doing your activity for at least the 20-minute minimum. Add on a 5-minute warm-up and 5-minute cooldown, and the shortest workout for cardiovascular fitness would be a half hour. Going longer can have additional benefits, such as burning more calories. If you choose a high-intensity activity, such as running, however, you'll burn calories faster than if you choose a moderate-intensity activity, such as walking. (A 175-pound adult burns about 180 calories in a half-hour walk, compared to about 400 in a half-hour run.) The lower the intensity of your activity, the longer the duration needed to achieve a training effect. So balance your preferences, time constraints, and health status to determine the duration and intensity that's best for you. One of the safest, most practical formulas for most people is a brisk, 30- to 45-minute walk. (For step-by-step advice on starting a walking program, see Healing Moves for Heart Health, page 214.)

4. *Pick a frequency*. Performing your aerobic exercise three to six days a week is crucial to achieving cardiovascular fitness. If you're doing an intense, high-impact activity, it's a good idea to pick a *lower frequency*—like three days a week—to allow your body to rest and repair. (You can do a low-impact activity on alternate days or use those days for your strength training.)

If losing weight is also one of your goals, it's a good idea to do a low- to moderate-impact activity at a *greater frequency*—like six days a week—to maximize calorie burning. (For more information about weight loss, see the section on obesity, page 67, and Healing Moves to Regulate Metabolism, page 77.)

Now that you've chosen your personal aerobic-fitness formula, fill in these blanks to design your own exercise contract:
I will do _____ (activity/ies) _____, at an intensity of ____ (target heart-rate range), on ____ (at least/at most) ____ days of the week, for ____ (at least/at most) ____ minutes per session.
(Example: I will do walking and/or in-line skating, at an intensity of 120 to 140 beats per minute, on three to five days of the week, for 30 to 45 minutes per session.)
Signed _____ Date _____

If you've been sedentary, it may take you several months until you're able to exercise this amount. That's fine! Just be sure you start slowly and progress gradually by following these ABCs:

✳ Always warm up by doing your chosen activity at a gentle pace for 5 minutes.

✳ Begin with as little as 5 minutes of your selected activity at a moderate pace.

✳ Continue to exercise regularly, adding an additional 5 minutes of activity per week and gradually picking up the pace until you're working at your "contract" amount.

Remember: Have fun! Don't fall into the trap of gritting your teeth as you force yourself to run on a treadmill to nowhere while you watch TV to distract yourself from the experience. This kind of exercise may burn calories, but it's not likely to nourish your soul.

PART THREE: STRENGTHENING EXERCISES

Performing resistance exercises two or three times a week will help you build muscle and bone, improve your overall fitness, and rev up your metabolism so you'll burn more calories—even at rest. Strength training is particularly important for people over forty, since sedentary people begin to lose muscle in midlife, with a dramatic drop in muscle mass after age fifty-five. But it's important to use good technique, since poor technique can make your workout ineffective or injurious.

It's a good idea to learn the basics from a qualified professional at a reputable gym or university-based wellness center. A half dozen lessons is enough to get you started, with an occasional maintenance check. And many trainers will let you share the expense (anywhere from $25 to $75 per hour) with a friend.

For optimum strengthening benefit, pick a weight you can lift at least eight, but no more than twelve, times. Older and more frail people (about 50 years old and above) may find it more appropriate to choose a lighter weight they can lift at least ten, but no more than fifteen, times.

And remember these weight-training ABCDs:

✳ Apparel. Any comfortable clothing is fine for lifting weights, from tank tops and shorts to leotards and tights, although some gyms have dress codes requiring people to wear T-shirts. But it's important to wear shoes with good support and to remove any jewelry that could catch on the equipment. Wear weight-training gloves if you want to avoid developing calluses.

✳ Breathe. Inhale as you prepare to move the weight, then exhale on exertion and inhale on release. If you find this difficult, just breathe any way that feels comfortable to you and try to exhale on effort (i.e., when lifting the weight or moving against resistance). The important point is to *never hold your breath* while you're lifting weight. This could be harmful because it increases the pressure within the chest cavity, which affects blood pressure and can result in dizziness, headache, and—in the extreme—short periods of blackout.

✳ Control. Never clang and bang weights in an uncontrolled rush. Instead, follow a slow, controlled tempo while you mentally focus on the muscles you're working. A good basic tempo is to count to two on the way up (counting one one thousand, two one thousand), then have a slight hesitation at the top and count slowly to four on the way down. Think "slow and rhythmic" and remember that the lowering phase is as important as the lifting. Be sure you resist gravity and avoid letting the weight accelerate as it descends. If you like working out to music, try rhythmic selections with a comfortable, slow to moderate beat.

✳ Don't forget to warm up first and stretch after. Do 5 to 10 minutes of easy movement, such as walking or pedaling a stationary bike, to prepare your body for strength training. Spend 5 to 10 minutes stretching out your muscles (see the flexibility exercises in this section) after your workout.

The following routine works all the major muscles groups. (When you've mastered this one, check out Healing Moves to Strengthen Muscles and Bones, page 141, and the strengthening section of Healing Moves for Women, page 275.)

1. Chair Squat (Works the Thighs and Buttocks)

Stand tall with your legs shoulder width apart, your arms crossed over your chest, and a bench, stool, or armless chair behind you. Keeping your head up and back straight, inhale while squatting slowly until your buttocks lightly touch the bench. Continue keeping tension on the thighs, and don't sit down. Exhale while returning to the starting position. Repeat 8 to 12 times.

✳ Variation 1: Perform the same exercise with your arms held straight out in front of you.

✳ Variation 2: Perform the same exercise without a chair. Squat until your upper thighs are parallel to the floor, then return to starting position.

✳ Variation 3: Perform the same exercise with a dumbbell resting on each shoulder, with your elbows forward and parallel to the floor.

2. Dumbbell Bench Press (Works the Chest Muscles)

Lie on a padded bench with your feet flat on the floor. Hold two dumbbells together at arm's length above your shoulders with your palms facing each other and elbows slightly bent. Lower the dumbbells slowly until they

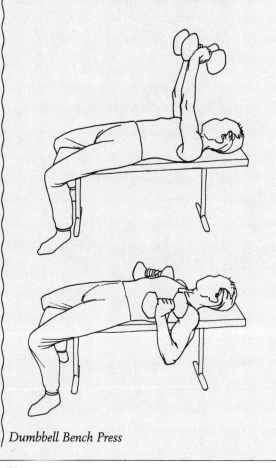

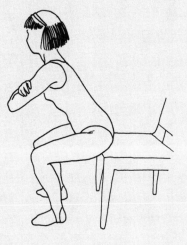

Chair Squat

Dumbbell Bench Press

are chest height, with your hands near your armpits, then return them to the starting position. Repeat 8 to 12 times.

3. Dumbbell Bent-Over Row (Works the Muscles in the Back)

Bend forward at the waist until your torso is parallel to the floor, and place your right hand and right knee on a bench. Grasp a dumbbell with your left hand, letting your arm hang straight down, palm facing in. Slowly raise the weight straight up toward the side of your chest, keeping your arm close to your side and your head and back straight. Pause, then slowly lower to the

starting position. Repeat 8 to 12 times, then switch to the other arm.

4. Dumbbell Shoulder Shrug (Works the Muscles of the Neck, Shoulders, and Upper Back)

Stand erect with a dumbbell in each hand and your arms hanging down, palms facing in. Raise your shoulders as high as possible, keeping your arms straight and your torso erect. Pause, then lower. Repeat 8 to 12 times.

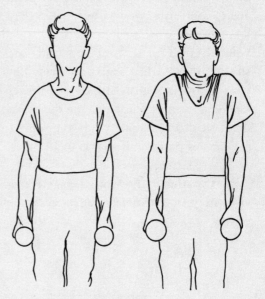

Dumbbell Shoulder Shrug

5. Seated Side Lateral Raise (Works the Muscles in the Shoulders)

Sit at the end of a bench or on a stool with your feet firmly on the floor. Hold dumbbells in each hand, palms in and arms hanging straight down at your sides. Keeping a slight bend in your elbows, slowly raise both arms out to the side until they're slightly

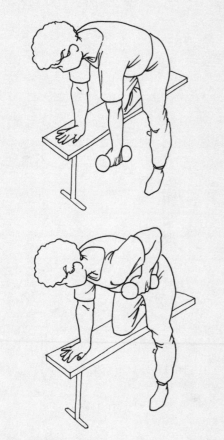

Dumbbell Bent-Over Row

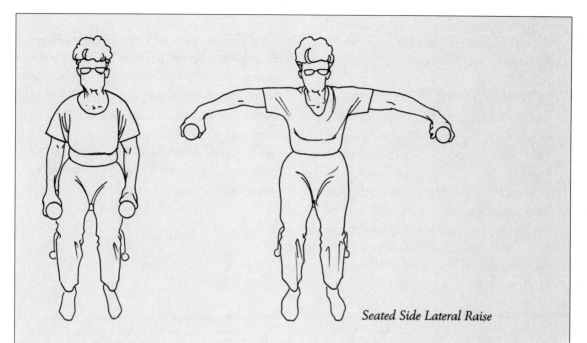

Seated Side Lateral Raise

above shoulder height, palms down. Pause, then lower back to the starting position. Repeat 8 to 12 times.

6. Seated Triceps Dumbbell Extension (Works the Muscles in the Back of the Upper Arm)

Sit on the end of a bench or stool with your feet flat on the floor, holding a dumbbell in your right hand, palm facing in. Bend over as far as possible and bring your right upper arm to your side, but leave your forearm extended down to the floor so that your elbow makes a ninety-degree angle. Push back with the dumbbell until your entire arm is parallel to the floor, then lower slowly to the starting position. Repeat 8 to 12 times, then switch to the other arm.

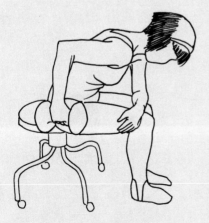
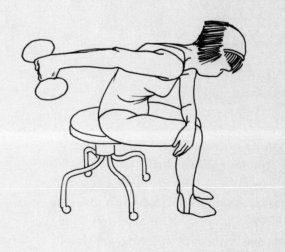

Seated Triceps Dumbbell Extension

7. Seated Biceps Curl (Works the Muscles in the Front of the Upper Arm)

Sit at the edge of a stool or bench with your feet flat on the floor, back straight, and eyes facing forward. Hold a dumbbell in each hand, arms extended down toward the floor, palms facing in. Turn the palms forward as you slowly raise both dumbbells toward your shoulders, keeping your elbows in. At the top of the curl your palms will be facing in toward your shoulders. Slowly return to starting position. Repeat 8 to 12 times.

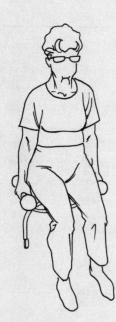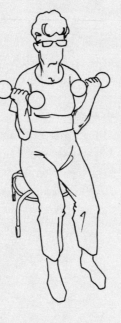

Seated Biceps Curl

8. Up-Against-the-Wall Sit-ups (Works the Abdominal Muscles)

Lie on your back with your knees bent and the soles of your feet placed firmly against a wall. Position yourself so that your shinbones and thighbones form a right angle and your feet are parallel to each other. Cross your arms over your chest and hold each elbow with the opposite hand. Exhale as you tuck your chin to your chest and contract your abdominal muscles to lift your head and upper back off the floor slowly, one vertebra at a time. Inhale as you lower back down. Repeat 10 times, working up to doing three sets of 10 sit-ups.

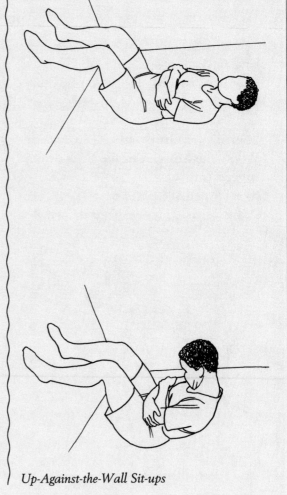

Up-Against-the-Wall Sit-ups

✳ Variation 1: Instead of crossing your arms over your chest, place both palms on the top of your head, with your elbows pointed forward and your forearms parallel. Exhale, tuck your chin, and contract your abdominals as you bring your elbows toward your thighs. Inhale as you lower back down.

✳ Oblique variation: Keeping your arms as in variation 1, exhale and bring the right elbow toward the left knee, then inhale as you lower back down. Exhale and bring the left elbow toward the right knee, then inhale and lower back down. Continue alternating knees to elbows, 20 times.

9. Yoga Upper-Body Strengthener (Works the Arms, Chest, Torso, Wrists, and Legs)

Get on your hands and knees, then straighten your legs and position your body so your weight is resting on the toes of your feet and the palms of your hands. Be sure

your shoulders are over your wrists and your legs and torso are in a straight line. This is the yoga "plank" pose. Bend your elbows and keep them as close to your body as possible as you slowly lower your chest until it's about two inches from the floor. (If this is too difficult, lower your knees to the ground first, then bend your elbows and lower your chest until it's about two inches from the floor.) This is the yoga "chaturanga dandasana" pose. Stay in this pose, breathing normally for 5 to 10 seconds, then relax. Gradually work your way up to holding this pose for 30 seconds.

10. Step-ups (Works the Thighs, Buttocks, Calves, and Lower Back)

Stand comfortably in front of a securely placed bench, step, or chair. (The higher the step, the harder the exercise, so if you have knee problems, choose a low step or skip this exercise.) Place your right foot on the

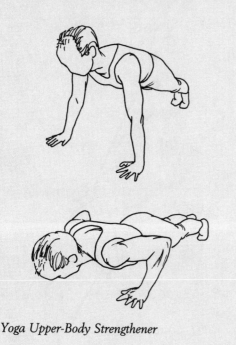

Yoga Upper-Body Strengthener

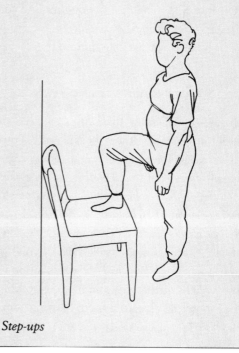

Step-ups

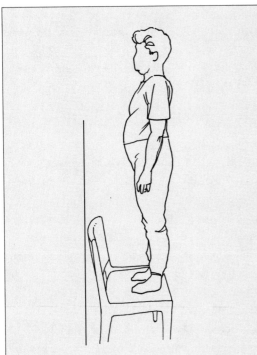

Step-ups

bench and step up onto it so that your left foot joins your right. Then step back down, right foot first. Continue for one minute (or 60 step-ups). Repeat the exercise, starting with the left foot, for one minute.

PART FOUR: STRETCHING

Most people know that stretching is an essential part of fitness because it keeps muscles and joints flexible and reduces the risk of injury. But many people aren't aware that *if you do aerobic activities and strength training **without stretching,** your muscles can become hard and short.* That's why it's essential to stretch after any activity involving continual, repetitive muscle contraction—like weight lifting or running. Stretching your muscles helps keep them long and supple. The best times to stretch are:

1. At the end of your workout.
2. After you warm up but before you start your main activity.
3. Whenever you get up from sitting or lying down for an extended period of time.
4. Any time your muscles feel tense or tight.

Remember to stretch for a *feeling*—not for a preconceived idea, like touching your head to your knee. Stretch until you feel a slight tension (if you feel pain, you've stretched too far and should back off). Do not bounce; hold the stretch at that tension point, breathing naturally. Imagine your breath "unknotting" the tension.

Here is a series of stretches for the major muscles in the body:

1. Back, Shoulders, Arms, and Hands

Sit or stand and interlace your fingers above your head, palms facing upward. Push arms

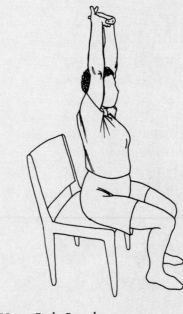

Upper-Body Stretch

slightly back and up. Breathing normally, hold the stretch for 10 to 20 seconds.

2. Shoulders

Sit or stand with your arms overhead and your elbows by your ears. Hold the elbow of your right arm with your left hand. Gently pull the elbow behind your head. Breathing normally, hold for 15 seconds, then repeat with the other arm. (To add a side stretch, do this exercise as you slowly lean to the side until you feel a mild stretch.)

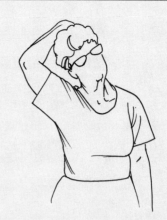

Neck Stretch

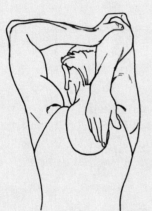

Shoulder Stretch

4. Doorknob Stretch for Backs of the Legs

Stand tall about an arm's length in front of an open door and grasp both knobs (you can also do this by grabbing a fence, countertop, sink, or any other convenient handle). Exhale, bend your elbows, and lean into the door, keeping your body straight from head to heels. Breathe naturally for 15 seconds, then relax.

3. Neck

Sit or stand with your arms hanging loosely at your sides. Place your right palm on your head, fingers slightly touching your left ear. Gently use your right hand to tilt your head so that your right ear moves toward your right shoulder. Being careful not to raise your left shoulder, focus on pressing your left shoulder down. Breathing normally, hold for 15 seconds, then repeat on the other side.

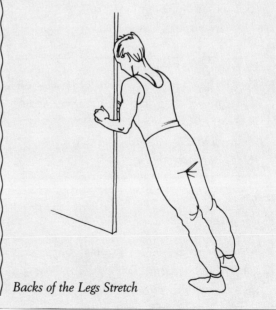

Backs of the Legs Stretch

5. Doorknob Stretch for Back and Arms

Stand tall about an arm's length in front of an open door and grasp both knobs. Exhale and bend at the hips, stretching your buttocks away from your hands. Keep your neck relaxed and in line with your spine. Breathe normally for 15 seconds, then relax.

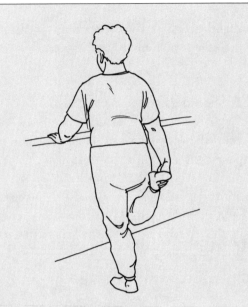

Front of Thigh Stretch

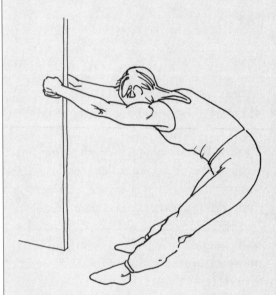

Back and Arms Stretch

6. Front of Thigh

Stand a little way from a wall and place your left hand on the wall for support. Standing straight, grasp the top of your right foot with your right hand. Pull your heel gently toward your buttocks. Hold 10 to 20 seconds, breathing normally. Repeat on the other side.

7. Calves

Stand a little way from a wall and lean on it with your forearms, resting your head on your hands. Place your right foot in front of

you with the knee bent and your left leg straight behind you. Slowly move your hips forward until you feel a mild stretch in the calf of your left leg. Keep your left heel on the floor and the toes of both feet pointed

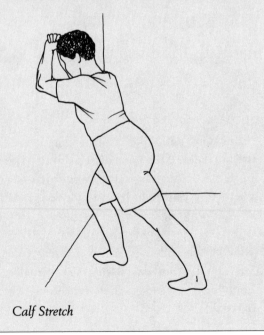

Calf Stretch

straight ahead. Hold the stretch for 10 to 20 seconds, breathing normally. Repeat on the other side.

8. Front of Hip and Lower Back

Stand tall, then step forward with your right leg until your right knee is directly over your right ankle. Lower your left knee to the floor and rest your fingertips on the floor. Lower the front of your hips directly downward until you feel a gentle stretch. Breathing normally, hold for 15 seconds. Repeat on the other side.

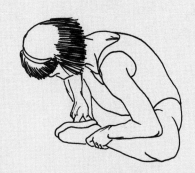

Lower Back, Hip, and Groin Stretch

it over your left leg so that the right foot is outside the left knee. Place your right hand behind your hips on the floor, rotate your upper body to the right, and place your left elbow outside your right knee. Keeping your back as straight as possible, press your left elbow against your right knee as you continue the spinal twist. Hold for 15 seconds, breathing normally. Repeat on the other side.

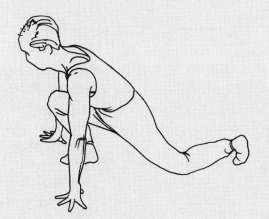

Hip and Lower Back Stretch

9. Lower Back, Hip, and Groin

Sit on the floor and place the soles of your feet together. Hold on to your toes or ankles, press your elbows down on your knees, and gently pull your upper body forward, bending from the hips. Hold for 15 seconds, breathing normally.

10. Lower Back, Side of Hip, and Neck

Sit on floor with your left leg straight out in front of you. Bend your right leg, then place

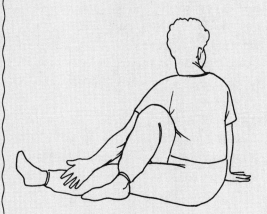

Lower Back, Hip, and Neck Stretch

11. Lower Back and Hips

Lie on the floor, legs straight or with one leg bent. Pick up your right knee, grasp it with both hands, and pull it toward your chest.

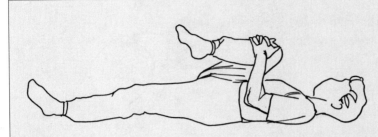

Lower Back and Hips Stretch

Try to keep your lower back flat and your head on the floor. Hold for 15 seconds, breathing normally. Repeat with the other leg.

PART FIVE: RELAXATION BREATH-ING (YOGA "BELLY BREATHING")

One of the single most important healing moves in this book is relaxation breathing, nature's perfect antidote to stress. Yogis have known for centuries—and modern studies confirm—that breathing provides a powerful link between body and mind, uniting them and helping establish a state of physiologic calm. As yoga master B. K. S. Iyengar writes in his classic guide *Light on Yoga:* "Regulate the breathing, and thereby control the mind."

Relaxation breathing can be easily integrated into your day, since all it involves is sitting quietly, focusing on the breath, and allowing air to completely fill the lungs right down to the abdomen. Many people discover that only their chest expands when they breathe. That's why the first step in learning the technique is teaching people to stop being "chest breathers" and start being "abdominal breathers." To do this:

1. Lie on your back and place a book on your belly. Relax your stomach muscles and inhale deeply into your abdomen so that the book rises. When you exhale, the book should fall. You'll still be bringing air into your upper chest, but now you're are also bringing air down into the lower portion of your lungs and expanding your entire chest cavity.

2. Sit up and place your right hand on your abdomen and your left hand on your chest. Breathe deeply so that your right, "abdominal" hand rises and falls with your breath, while your left, "chest" hand stays

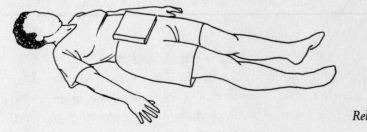

Relaxation Breathing, Lying Down

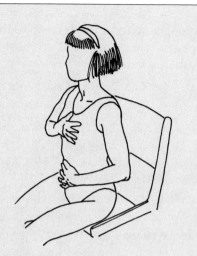

Relaxation Breathing, Seated

relatively still. Breathe in through your nose and out through your nose or mouth, and spend a few minutes enjoying the sensation of abdominal breathing.

3. Place a timer or clock with a second hand in clear view. Breathe in slowly, filling your abdomen, as the timer counts off five seconds. Then breathe out slowly to the same count of five.

Perform relaxation breathing throughout the day, such as when you awaken and before you go to sleep, in any stressful situation, or anytime you hear a bell (phone, door, or church) ring. To enhance your practice of relaxation breathing, try these variations:

✳ *Color breathing.* Sit or lie down in a comfortable position, and take a deep breath. Allow the ground or your chair to accept the weight of your body as your muscles relax and accept gravity's pull toward the earth. Visualize the earth beneath you as filled with an energizing shade of red. As you inhale slowly, visualize yourself drawing this energizing red into your body. Imagine it flowing up through your feet, legs, abdomen, torso, arms, neck, and head. Then exhale the red slowly out of your lungs, imagining it filling the air around you so that your body and the space surrounding it form a glowing, energized red ball. Try this exercise with different colors, such as calming green, peaceful silver, tranquil blue, healthy gold, cool violet, or warm orange.

✳ *Mantra breathing.* Pick a word or phrase that has special meaning to you and mentally recite the phrase in synchrony with your breathing. For example, Zen master Thich Nhat Hahn suggests this phrase: *Breathing in I calm myself, breathing out I smile,* or simply, *In calm, out smile.* You might try a religious phrase that has meaning to you, such as *Hail Mary, full of Grace* for Catholics, *Sh'ma Yisroel* for Jews, *Insha'Allah* for Moslems, or *Om* for Hindus. Or you might make up a phrase to suit the situation, such as "In energy, out fatigue" or "In peace, out anger."

✳ *Restorative breathing.* Before you begin your breathing, set yourself up in this yoga posture that allows for total relaxation: Lie on your back on the floor with your arms comfortably out to your sides, palms up. Place a bolster, pillow, or rolled blanket under your knees and a folded blanket under your head. Place an eyebag over your eyes if you have one, or wrap your forehead and eyes gently in an Ace bandage (a great headache remedy!). Cover yourself with a light blanket, if desired. Relax your eyes and forehead, let your tongue drop from the roof of your mouth, and let the weight of your body melt into the floor. Focus on your deep abdominal breathing, keeping it slow and steady. If your mind wanders, gently lead it back to your breath without judgment. Continue this practice for 10 to 20 minutes. (For more information on breathing, see Healing Moves to Breathe Easy, page 298.)

PERSONALIZED PLAN IDEAS

Now that you know what it takes to achieve optimum health and fitness, the way you put it together in a personalized program is up to you. Here are some options:

Gym-Based Plan (Three 1-Hour Sessions per Week)

At each exercise session, warm up for 5 minutes, do an aerobic activity for 30 minutes, strength-train for 20 minutes, then stretch for 5 minutes. Option: Only strength-train twice a week and use that extra 20 minutes of your third session for additional stretching or aerobics.

Time-Crunched Plan (Five 30-Minute Sessions per Week)

Three days a week, take a brisk, 30-minute walk. Two days a week do a 5-minute warm-up, then 15 minutes of strengthening exercises, followed by 10 minutes of stretching.

Maximum Weight-Loss Plan (Six 1-Hour Sessions per Week)

Four days a week, do your chosen aerobic activity or activities for an hour, being sure to incorporate a short warm-up and cool-down, followed by stretching. Two days a week, take a brisk 30-minute walk (or do some other aerobic activity for 30 minutes), then do 20 minutes of strengthening exercises, followed by 10 minutes of stretching.

In all these plans—and any individualized one you devise—remember to be as active as possible throughout the day and to integrate relaxation breathing into your daily routine.

2

Metabolic Disorders

DIABETES

Diabetes is the most rapidly growing chronic disease in America, and its alarming rise is linked to our expanding waistlines, junk-food diet, and inactivity. The number of Americans diagnosed with diabetes has increased sixfold since 1958, to a record high of ten million people, which includes a worrisome and growing number of overweight children developing the type of diabetes normally found only in adults. In addition, nearly six million more people have diabetes but don't know it, according to the Centers for Disease Control and Prevention in Atlanta (CDC).

A metabolic disorder in which the body doesn't produce or properly use insulin, diabetes often progresses undetected for years. In its early stages, symptoms may be nonex-

istent, hard to recognize, or easy to ignore. Early-warning signs of diabetes include: frequent urination, excessive thirst, blurred vision, very dry skin, more infections than usual, sores that are slow to heal, and tingling or loss of feeling in the hands or feet.

If left untreated, chronic effects of the disease can include damage to blood vessels, nerves, and other tissues. Many people first become aware they have diabetes only after developing one of its serious complications, such as cardiovascular disease, kidney disease, blindness, or nerve disease.

Diabetes itself is the seventh-leading cause of death in the United States, but it contributes to many more deaths since sufferers most often die of its complications—particularly heart disease and stroke. It is a major risk factor for cardiovascular disease, and people with diabetes frequently have other risk factors for that condition too, such as high blood pressure and high blood cholesterol. Diabetes is the nation's leading cause of kidney failure and adult blindness and is a major cause of amputations of the toes, feet, and legs.

Genetics and aging play important roles in diabetes, but the condition is also strongly affected by lifestyle. This is why, as America's junk-food diet and sedentary habits spread across the globe, so has a skyrocketing rate of diabetes. The World Health Organization (WHO) predicts that diabetes will increase dramatically around the planet during the first quarter of the century, with the biggest increase hitting developing countries. WHO predicts that 228 million adults will suffer from the disease in developing nations by 2025—a staggering 170 percent increase from 1995. In industrialized areas, a 41 percent increase is expected, rising from 51 million diagnosed in 1995 up to 71 million by 2025.

While heredity and environment strongly influence the development of diabetes, its cause is unknown. Since there is no current cure, U.S. public health officials have launched campaigns to encourage healthy lifestyle strategies—like exercise and eating right—to help people both prevent and manage the condition. Some experts feel that *the most common form of diabetes (type II) is preventable with a proper diet and regular exercise.* Even people with a strong genetic predisposition may be able to avoid the disease if they perform regular physical activity, eat sensibly, and maintain a healthy weight.

One theory suggests that diabetes may have evolved as a survival advantage in populations that live with cycles of feast and famine—as did many of our ancestors. In times of food scarcity, genes that cause people to store fat and become obese could mean the difference between life and death. But these same genes may become a health hazard when food is present in abundance all the time and people overeat continually. Studies of the Native American tribe of Pima Indians support this notion. Most Pima Indians now live a sedentary lifestyle on a reservation in Arizona, where 50 to 60 percent of adults are obese and 60 percent become diabetic. A small group of Pima Indians moved to rural Mexico a generation ago, however, and began a more vigorous farming lifestyle. These physically active Mexican Pimas have a significantly lower rate of obesity and very few cases of diabetes.

Research with other indigenous populations, such as Australian Aboriginals, show similar findings. Before European contact, Aboriginals were nomadic hunter-gatherers with active lifestyles and low-fat diets. But when they adopted Western lifestyles, they became especially vulnerable to obesity and diabetes. Research reported in the journal *Ethnicity and Disease* revealed that when a group of ten diabetic Aboriginals reverted to traditional lifestyles for seven weeks (eating foods such as kangaroo meat, which is lean, and exercising daily) they lost an average of 2.2 pounds per week and their fasting glucose and insulin levels decreased by about 50 percent. Also, they had substantial decreases in blood triglycerides and blood pressure. Findings such as these lead some researchers to speculate that *diabetes may be an alternative, genetically determined metabolism that becomes a disease only when people are inactive and obese*. Reducing the alarming increase in diabetes may depend less on miracle cures than on helping people in industrialized countries embrace healthy elements of traditional lifestyles such as regular exercise and sensible eating.

DIABETES BASICS

Diabetes has been recognized since antiquity. The full name for the condition, *diabetes mellitus*, comes from Greek and Latin words for *siphon* and *honey*. *Siphon* is used because people with the condition drink and urinate frequently; *honey* describes the sweet taste of the patient's urine (due to the presence of sugar)—the ancient means of diagnosing the disease.

Diabetes is actually a group of disorders with one thing in common—a problem with insulin. Either the body doesn't make any insulin, it doesn't make enough insulin, or it doesn't use insulin properly.

Insulin is a hormone secreted by the pancreas that helps maintain the proper level of a sugar—called glucose—in the blood. Glucose is the body's fuel, and it's used by cells to produce energy to grow and function. During digestion, enzymes in the intestine break down most of the food you eat into glucose. The glucose is then absorbed into the bloodstream, which circulates the fuel to cells throughout the body. Insulin serves as a sort of "glucose escort," orchestrating the transport of glucose from the blood into the cells and promoting its storage in muscles, fat, the liver, and other tissues.

But in people with diabetes, the glucose either has no escort or an inadequate escort, which prevents the right amount of the fuel from entering your cells. Without the proper escort—holding the "keys" to unlock the doors to the cells—the glucose can't fuel the cells adequately. Unused glucose builds up in your blood, a condition called *hyperglycemia*, which, over time, can have a toxic effect on blood vessels, nerves, and other tissues. Unused glucose also is dumped into the urine by the kidneys, which accounts for the sweet taste. The sugar draws water along with it, which results in excessive urination.

There are several type of diabetes, which are essentially different disorders with different causes. The two most common kinds are:

1. Type I Diabetes

Previously called insulin-dependent diabetes mellitus (IDDM) or juvenile-onset diabetes (because it was thought to begin only in childhood), type I diabetes accounts for just 5 to 10 percent of diabetes. It is an autoimmune disease, which means that the body's infection-fighting mechanism (the immune system) turns on itself and destroys its own insulin-producing cells. Since people with type I diabetes produce little or no insulin, they must take daily insulin injections to stay alive. Type I diabetes usually starts in childhood or adolescence, but it can begin at any age.

2. Type II Diabetes

Previously called non-insulin-dependent diabetes mellitus (NIDDM) or adult-onset diabetes, type II diabetes accounts for the vast majority—about 90 to 95 percent—of all diagnosed cases of diabetes. A metabolic disorder resulting from the body's inability to make enough, or properly use, insulin, type II diabetes typically occurs after age forty, and the risk increases with advancing age. Currently, there is an alarming trend toward type II diabetes in obese, sedentary children. Type II diabetes is linked with inactivity and an expanding waistline because when people are overweight and sedentary their tissues may become less sensitive to the influence of insulin. This condition, known as insulin resistance, forces the pancreas to produce more of the hormone to handle the glucose load that enters the blood after meals. Insulin resistance, in turn, triggers other hormonal changes that appear to contribute to high blood pressure and an increased risk of heart disease.

For a few years, even decades, obese people can make the extra insulin they need. But over time, the insulin-producing cells in the pancreas may slow down, which means insulin levels fall and glucose starts to build up in the blood. Diabetes results and gets worse as obesity worsens. So it's no wonder that, in our aging, inactive, and overweight society, the incidence of type II diabetes is nearing epidemic proportions.

In addition to these two main types of diabetes, another common form is **gestational diabetes.** This condition occurs in 2 to 5 percent of all pregnancies, but it usually disappears when the pregnancy is over. Women at increased risk of gestational diabetes include those who are overweight, who have a family history of diabetes, and who are African American, Hispanic or Latino American, or Native American. Women who have gestational diabetes are at increased risk of developing type II diabetes, and some studies indicate that nearly 40 per-

cent of women with a history of gestational diabetes develop type II diabetes in the future.

A very small proportion of diabetes—1 to 2 percent of cases—results from certain genetic syndromes, surgery, drugs, malnutrition, infections, and other illnesses. These forms are classified as "**other specific types of diabetes.**"

In all forms of diabetes, early diagnosis is critical, because the longer it's left untreated, the greater the risk of serious complications. For that reason, the American Diabetes Association in 1997 revised its screening guidelines to help increase early detection. The association now recommends that all adults have a fasting plasma glucose test at age forty-five. If test results are normal, the test should be repeated every three years. However, if you're at high risk for diabetes or have symptoms, the ADA recommends that you be tested at a younger age and more frequently. In fact, some public health officials advocate screening for diabetes at age twenty-five to save people from blindness, kidney failure, and amputations. In a report published in the *Journal of the American Medical Association* in 1998, CDC researchers recommended screening all adults at age twenty-five and up to decrease the average age of diagnosis by nearly six years, which would help avoid serious complications. *Without such screening, type II diabetes typically exists nine to twelve years before diagnosis.*

The test requires that you fast overnight (or for eight to twelve hours) and have a blood sample drawn and its glucose level measured. Most people have a level between 70 and 100 milligrams of glucose per deciliter of blood (mg/dL). A level of 126 mg/dL or higher on two tests confirms a diagnosis of diabetes. (Previously, a level of 140 or higher was used to diagnose diabetes, but these numbers were revised in 1997.)

RISK FACTORS

The international Expert Committee on the Diagnosis and Classification of Diabetes Mellitus, working under the sponsorship of the ADA, published a report in 1997 (in the journal *Diabetes Care*) citing the following characteristics as putting people at "high risk" for diabetes:

* Obesity
* A family member with diabetes
* Belonging to high-risk ethnic groups, such as African Americans, Hispanics, or American Indians
* Delivering a baby weighing nine pounds or more or being diagnosed with gestational diabetes
* High blood pressure
* Blood lipid abnormality

Age also is a risk factor for type II diabetes, which usually develops after age forty and whose incidence increases sharply after age fifty-five. (However, it's increasingly being found in obese children as young as ten.) Taking certain medications, such as some diuretics and steroids, may contribute to the development of type II diabetes. For type I diabetes, there is some speculation that environmental triggers may be involved. These include certain types of viruses, cold weather, and lack of breast feeding.

Not every person at risk will develop the illness. For example, research on identical twins (who have identical sets of genes) reveals that when one twin has type II diabetes, the other twin has a 50 to 75 percent chance of also developing the disease. Many studies have shown that people with a family history of diabetes can reduce their risk of getting the disease if they stay thin. And regular exercise can dramatically reduce the risk of getting type II diabetes, with substantial research showing that the more physically active people are, the less likely they are to develop the condition. Evidence indicates that, for every 500 calories burned each week in physical activity, the risk of type II diabetes drops by 6 percent.

HOW EXERCISE HELPS

Exercise was recognized as an important therapy for diabetes as far back as the Sui dynasty (about A.D. 600), when a famous Chinese doctor of that period, Ch'ao Yuen Fan, advised patients suffering from diabetes-related diseases to "walk one hundred and twenty steps or more, not to exceed one thousand steps," before each meal.

Walking and other forms of exercise help prevent and manage diabetes because they affect the very thing that needs to be controlled in this condition—blood glucose levels. When people exercise, the body fuels the activity by taking glucose out of their blood to use for energy. This lowers blood glucose levels, which can be extremely therapeutic in a disease characterized by elevated blood sugar.

But lowering blood sugar is just one mechanism by which exercise helps. Regular exercise also has important metabolic effects that influence the condition, including:

Improving the body's ability to use glucose. This means that when people exercise regularly, the amount of insulin they need decreases.

Increasing the body's sensitivity to insulin. This can help reverse the insulin resistance that often occurs when people become overweight.

Aiding glucose transport. Contracting muscles help stimulate the movement of glucose throughout the body.

Helping people control their weight. Weight loss reduces blood glucose levels, improves insulin sensitivity, and helps reduce risk of heart disease. Yet *when people try to lose weight by diet alone, the body often reacts by slowing the metabolic rate to conserve energy.* Not only does this mean that they burn fewer calories, but when they do lose weight, much of it comes from lean tissue— which means muscle and bone. When people begin to exercise regularly—and embark on a healthy diet—the weight they lose typically comes from fat. In particular, *physical activity promotes fat release and utilization and helps people reduce the amount of abdominal fat (a.k.a. the "spare tire" or "beer belly") that is associated with diabetes.*

Exercise also boosts the health of people with diabetes because it:

Helps prevent cardiovascular disease, which is the leading killer of people with diabetes (see the section on coronary artery disease, page 190).

Relieves stress and enhances mood. Stressful events can prompt a release of adrenaline, which can raise glucose levels in the blood. Physical activity exerts a calming effect and relieves symptoms of depression and anxiety. Regular exercise also prompts a sense of mastery and control that can be particularly helpful to people forced to cope with a chronic disease.

Exercise may reduce—or eliminate—the need for diabetes medication. Since exercise makes blood glucose levels fall, some people with type II diabetes who take drugs to manage their condition find that after they start exercising regularly, they no longer need the pills. People with type I diabetes, whose bodies don't produce insulin, typically require a lower dose of injectable insulin when they exercise.

Exercise alone will not improve glucose control in people with type I diabetes, although it can be important in managing the condition and avoiding complications. Since people with type I diabetes are at risk for low glucose levels (called hypoglycemia), they must be careful to monitor their blood glucose before and after exercise to avoid low blood sugar, also known as an "insulin reaction." Low glucose levels can be dangerous for people with type I diabetes because it can cause confusion, irritability, lack of coordination, and, in extreme cases, unconsciousness or convulsions.

Finding a healthy balance between food (which makes blood glucose levels rise) and exercise and insulin (which make blood glucose levels fall) can be a delicate juggling act for people with type I diabetes. In fact, before home blood glucose monitors were developed in recent years, physicians typically discouraged people with type I diabetes from engaging in excessive endurance exercise to avoid dangerous low-blood-sugar reactions. This was extremely frustrating for many athletically inclined people with type I diabetes.

For example, back in the late 1970s doctors warned Paula Harper not to run a marathon because she had type I diabetes, but the nurse and mother of three from Phoenix chose to ignore them. "I noticed right away that the more activity I did, the less insulin I needed," says Harper, who in 1985 founded the International Diabetic Athletes Association (see Resources at the end of this chapter for information). Racing with a T-shirt that proclaimed, "I run on insulin," Harper has completed more than thirty marathons, a fifty-mile ultramarathon, five triathlons, and six bicycle races over a hundred miles long. "In retrospect, what I did seems scary," she admits. "But I knew that running made me feel better and helped me cope with my diabetes."

Today, people with diabetes participate in virtually every sport—from scuba diving to sky diving—and at all levels of competition. Many world-class athletes have the disease, and famous competitors with the condition included Arthur Ashe, Ty Cobb, Sugar Ray Robinson, and Jackie Robinson. Over the last decade, physicians have increasingly recommended exercise as one of the most effective ways to prevent diabetes among people who don't have it and to help those people who do have it lead normal lives and reduce their risk of serious complications.

EXERCISE ℞

It's essential that people with diabetes develop an individualized exercise program with the guidance of their physician, because each person's metabolism reacts differently to the balance of activity, food, and insulin. Also, exercise can have special risks for diabetics, including hyperglycemia and the exacerbation of existing diabetes-related complications such as heart arrhythmias, eye problems, and lower-extremity injury. That's why it's important that a physician examine you for underlying cardiovascular disease or related complications. Be sure to discuss all the specifics of your exercise regimen with your doctor, including:

1. Frequency, duration, and intensity of exercise.
2. Time of exercise in relation to insulin administration. (Many experts recommend testing blood glucose before and after exercise.)
3. Time of exercise in relation to meals.
4. Kind of exercise and its impact on specifics of your condition.
5. How to avoid problems.

Exercise is especially beneficial for people with diabetes, notes the American Diabetes Association, which recommends regular physical activity as an essential part of good diabetes control. They offers these **general guidelines:**

1. Use proper footwear and protective equipment.
2. Avoid exercise in extreme heat or cold.
3. Inspect your feet daily and after exercise.
4. Avoid exercising during periods of poor blood glucose control.

Specifically for Those with Type I Diabetes:

1. Monitor your blood glucose yourself so that necessary adjustments can be made in diet or insulin dosage. It's always a good idea to check your level before you start exercising; if you are low (under 70 mg/dL), have a snack to avoid having low blood sugar while you exercise.
2. If you're exercising more than 1 hour after eating, you may want to eat a high-carbohydrate snack, such as six ounces of fruit juice or half a plain bagel before moderate exercise such as walking. If you plan on doing heavier exercise, such as running or aerobics, you may need to eat a little more, such as half of a meat sandwich and a cup of low-fat milk.

Specifically for Those with Type II Diabetes:

1. Get an exercise stress test if you are over thirty-five years of age.
2. Be sure to monitor your blood glucose level if you take oral hypoglycemic medications or insulin. Check your blood sugar level before you start exercising, and if you are low, have a snack.
3. Perform moderate aerobic exercise for 20 to 45 minutes, at least three days per week. Remember, exercise must be done regularly for maximum benefit in controlling diabetes.
4. Be sure to find a form of exercise you enjoy, start slowly, and progress gradually. Walking is highly recommended.
5. Always do low-intensity warm-up and cool-down exercises.
6. Add activity into your daily life with simple strategies, such as parking in the farthest space and taking the stairs.

Specifically for Women with Gestational Diabetes

1. Work with your health-care practitioner to design an individualized meal plan and physical activity schedule.
2. If you've been active, you may continue a program of moderate activity with your physician's approval. (See the section on pregnancy, page 252.)

CAUTIONS

People with type I diabetes must be extremely careful to minimize the risk of low-blood-sugar reactions. This is particularly important if your exercise would present a life-threatening danger should you become confused, dizzy, faint, or unconscious with symptoms of hypoglycemia— such as if you are swimming or mountain climbing.

*Exercisers with **type I diabetes** should be sure to:*

✽ Carry along food that is high in carbohydrates, in case you need a quick source of energy. Glucose tablets, hard candy, raisins, fruit juice, and some sports nutrition bars may be good choices.

✽ Exercise with a partner.

✽ Wear an ID bracelet indicating your diabetic condition.

✽ Consume plenty of fluids before, during, and after exercise.

✽ Consider checking blood glucose levels before exercise, during prolonged exercise, and after exercise.

✴ **STOP IMMEDIATELY if you feel an insulin reaction coming on while exercising, and have a snack,** such as half a cup of orange juice, a nondiet soft drink, or three glucose tablets. It's vital to treat an insulin reaction as soon as you feel it, or it can get worse.

People with type I diabetes also should see a health-care provider regularly to minimize the onset of diabetic complications. If you do have complications, it's important to discuss the effect of your exercise intensity and type. For example, people with severe retinopathy (diabetic eye disease) may need to avoid activities that jar the head, such as karate, or that lower the head, such as certain yoga poses.

As stated earlier, anyone with diabetes should consult a physician before embarking on an exercise program, to identify any underlying cardiovascular disease or related complications. This is likely to include a stress test for anyone who wants to start a program of vigorous exercise. Be sure a qualified health-care professional individualizes an exercise program for you that takes into account your abilities, interests, and health status.

Exercisers with **type II diabetes** *should:*
✴ Wear appropriate, well-fitted footwear and clean, well-fitting socks. People with diabetes are particularly prone to nerve disease that may decrease sensations in the feet and legs. This creates the risk of traumatic injury and ulceration of the feet. Also, overweight people run the risk of developing foot injuries due to added stress placed on these joints by weight-bearing activity.

So it may be advisable to avoid high-impact activity. It's also critical that you wear proper footwear and inspect your feet after every exercise session.
✴ Avoid high-intensity or isometric exercise that involves a sustained increase in systolic blood pressure (such as heavy weight lifting) if you have diabetes complications involving blood-vessel disease of the eye or kidney.
✴ Check with your doctor about timing your exercise with meals and medications if you take drugs to control your diabetes. (For example, if you are susceptible to hypoglycemia, a small carbohydrate snack before moderate activity is often sufficient to prevent a risky drop in blood glucose.)

PRESCRIPTION PAD

1. Consult a physician before embarking on an exercise program to identify any underlying cardiovascular disease or related complications.
2. Ask your health-care provider to help you develop an individualized exercise plan that takes into account the specifics of your diabetes, your personal preferences, and your abilities.
3. In general, a moderate aerobic exercise program, such as walking for 20 to 45 minutes at least three days per week, is recommended. Remember, frequency is essential and exercising every day or nearly every day will confer maximum benefit.
4. Be sure to start slowly and progress gradually.
5. Wear good footwear and inspect your feet after exercise.

6. Add activity to your daily life, such as parking in the farthest space and taking the stairs instead of the elevator.

ADDITIONAL RESOURCES

✳ The American Diabetes Association, 1600 Duke St., Alexandria, Va. 22314, is the nation's leading organization for people with diabetes, supporting research and helping people with diabetes live better. The ADA offers numerous resources for people with diabetes and their families, such as a monthly magazine and guide to diabetes supplies. Call 800-232-3472 or 800-DIABETES. To order publications, such as *The Fitness Book for People with Diabetes* ($18.95 plus shipping), call 800-ADA-ORDER. Visit the Web site: diabetes.org.

✳ The National Diabetes Information Clearinghouse of the National Institutes of Health (NIH) offers fact sheets, booklets, and information packets. Call 301-654-3327 or visit the Web site at www.niddk.nih.gov.

✳ The International Diabetic Athletes Association, 1647 West Bethany Home Road #B, Phoenix, Ariz. 85015, is a non-profit organization that educates and encourages individuals with diabetes about regular physical activity and its benefits. Call 800-898-IDAA or visit the Web site at www.diabetes-exercise/org.

✳ The American Dietetic Association, 216 West Jackson Blvd., Suite 800, Chicago, Ill. 60606, is an association of professional dietitians who can provide information and referrals to member dietitians in your area. Call 800-877-1600 or visit their Web site at www.eatright.org.

HIGH CHOLESTEROL (HYPERLIPIDEMIA)

Amid all the hoopla over oat bran and fish oil, synthetic fats and selected prescription drugs, one of the simplest, safest, least expensive, and most effective strategies for improving cholesterol is frequently neglected. Regular exercise has a particularly positive effect on your cholesterol ratio, raising the level of "good" HDL cholesterol and lowering the level of "bad" LDL cholesterol. Yet the important contribution exercise can make to cholesterol status is often overlooked when people focus solely on diet and drugs.

In recent years, however, experts have begun to recognize that *diet alone is an inadequate means of combating America's cholesterol crisis and must be combined with regular exercise to exert optimum benefit.* A major study, reported in the *New England Journal of Medicine* in July 1998, revealed that people who were on a low-fat, low-cholesterol diet for a year did not show a reduction in "bad" LDL levels. *However, those who followed that same diet and walked or jogged the equivalent of about ten miles per week experienced a 15-point reduction in LDL levels among the women and a 20-point reduction among the men.*

"This finding highlights the importance of physical activity in the treatment of elevated LDL cholesterol levels," concluded the study by Marcia Stefanick, associate professor of medicine, and her colleagues at Stanford University School of Medicine in California. "Diet alone doesn't do what people think it will," Stefanick says. *In fact, in some overweight people, a low-fat diet alone may actually adversely affect levels of HDL (good) cholesterol.*

"But when you adopt a healthy diet and exercise program together," Stefanick says, "you get this tremendous benefit."

CHOLESTEROL BASICS

Despite its "negative press," cholesterol is essential to survival. The body uses the soft, waxy substance to build some hormones, cell membranes, brain and nerve tissues, and vitamin D. Cholesterol also aids digestion as an ingredient in the bile acids. Actually, it's only when excess cholesterol is deposited like "sludge" in the blood vessels that this basic body building block becomes a mediator of disease.

Cholesterol comes from two sources: your body and the foods you eat. Blood cholesterol is made in the liver, and most people produce enough cholesterol naturally to meet their needs. Dietary cholesterol enters the body when you eat cholesterol-rich foods, like meats, whole-milk products, and egg yolks. Chronic consumption of too much dietary cholesterol can make blood cholesterol levels rise. When there is more cholesterol in the blood than the body needs to function, some of the excess builds up on the walls of the arteries that carry blood to the heart—a process called *atherosclerosis*. This buildup of fatty material, or plaque, can narrow the arteries and slow down or block blood flow to the heart, brain, or other organs. When the heart doesn't get enough oxygen-rich blood, for example, a person may experience chest pain. If a blood clot becomes trapped in the narrowed artery, the result can be a heart attack. One and a half

million Americans have heart attacks each year, and one-third of them die. A similar kind of process involving the blood vessels in the brain may lead to stroke; in the arteries of the kidneys it may lead to high blood pressure, and in the arteries of the legs to claudication.

Cholesterol buildup is the most common cause of cardiovascular disease, which is the number one killer of men and women in the United States. (See Coronary Artery Disease, page 190.) Yet the buildup process happens so slowly—often over decades—that people usually aren't aware of this "internal time bomb" ticking away in their arteries. Children as young as six have been found to have "fatty streaks," or early cholesterol deposits, in their arteries, showing that the process of *atherosclerosis can begin in youth*. For many people, the first symptom of atherosclerosis is a heart attack or stroke, which is why it's important to try to prevent the condition by controlling cholesterol.

A fatty, oily material, cholesterol travels in the bloodstream. Blood is mostly water, however, and, like oil and water, cholesterol and blood do not mix. The body coats cholesterol with a layer of protein so it can be transported through the bloodstream as a minute particle called a lipoprotein. Two types of lipoproteins affect your risk of heart disease:

✳ *Low-density lipoprotein (LDLs), the so-called "bad" cholesterol*, carries most of the cholesterol in the blood. The cholesterol and fat from LDLs are the main source of dangerous buildup and blockages in arteries. The more LDL cholesterol you have in your blood, the greater your risk of cardiovascular disease.

✳ *High-density lipoprotein (HDLs), the so-called "good" cholesterol*, carries some of the cholesterol in the blood and is believed to act like a "lipid scavenger," which means it's a kind of cholesterol garbage truck. HDL cholesterol helps clear blood vessels by picking up excess cholesterol and hauling it back to the liver for excretion. HDLs help keep cholesterol from building up in the walls of your arteries, which is why it's considered "good." If your level of HDL cholesterol is too low, you have a higher risk of cardiovascular disease.

The National Heart, Lung, and Blood Institute advises all adults age twenty and over to have their blood cholesterol checked at least once every five years. Both total cholesterol and HDL cholesterol can be measured from a blood sample taken from your finger or arm. Generally, a total blood cholesterol level of under 200 mg/dL is considered desirable and puts you at a lower risk for cardiovascular disease.

When it comes to HDL cholesterol levels, higher numbers are healthier. Since HDL is the "good" cholesterol that helps prevent fatty buildup, the higher your HDL level, the lower your risk for cardiovascular disease. An HDL level of less than 35 mg/dL puts you at an increased risk of cardiovascular disease, while an HDL level of 60 or higher is associated with lower risk.

Some people may need to get their LDL-cholesterol levels checked, too, because this measurement can be a better predictor of heart-disease risk than total cholesterol. (You should probably get your LDL-cholesterol level checked if your total cholesterol level is 240 mg/dL or greater, if your HDL-cholesterol level is less than 35 mg/dL, or if your total cholesterol level is 200 to 239 mg/dL *and* you have two or more other risk factors for heart disease, such as smoking, high blood pressure, family history of heart disease, inactivity, diabetes, or obesity.) Before this test, it is necessary that you fast, having nothing to eat or drink except water for nine to twelve hours before your blood is drawn.

The NHLBI has set these cholesterol risk categories for adults over twenty:

Total Cholesterol

Less than 200 mg/dL	Desirable
200 to 239 mg/dL	Borderline high
240 mg/dL or greater	High

HDL Cholesterol

Less than 35 mg/dL	Undesirable, increased risk

LDL Cholesterol

Less than 130 mg/dL	Desirable
130 to 159 mg/dL	Borderline high
160 mg/dL and above	High

If you have a high LDL cholesterol level or a borderline-high LDL-cholesterol level plus other risk factors for heart disease, it is essential that you consult a physician for help in starting a program to lower your risk.

Many physicians calculate a ratio of total cholesterol to HDL cholesterol, considering this ratio to be an important predictor of cardiovascular-disease risk. The cholesterol ratio is obtained by dividing the HDL cholesterol level into the total cholesterol. For example, if you have a total cholesterol of 200 mg/dL and an HDL cholesterol level of 50 mg/dL, the ratio would be stated as 4:1. While experts still disagree on what the optimum ratio should be, most recommend that at least 25 percent of your total blood cholesterol should be HDL. Because exercise tends to boost HDL, active people often have a high percent of this good cholesterol. Their total cholesterol may be higher than that of a sedentary person, but as long as 25 percent of it is HDL, these individuals have a lower risk of heart problems. In general, the higher the HDL percent, the better.

Over the last few decades, as the role excess total cholesterol plays in cardiovascular disease has become clear, many Americans have successfully lowered their own blood cholesterol levels. From 1978 to 1990, the average blood cholesterol level in the United States dropped from 213 mg/dL to 205 mg/dL, according to the NHLBI. *This means the average American is in the borderline-high total cholesterol range, which leaves them at significant risk of heart disease.* Fifty-two million American adults have such high total blood cholesterol that it needs to be lowered under a doctor's care. One in five has a total blood cholesterol level in the high range—240 mg/dL or greater. A person with this high a level of total cholesterol has more than twice the risk of heart disease than someone whose total cholesterol is 200 mg/dL.

Regular exercise and eating a nutritious diet low in saturated fat and cholesterol are the foundations of treatment to improve your cholesterol profile, and can be expected to lower total cholesterol by about 15 per-

cent and raise HDL levels equivalently. For some people, in whom these changes are not enough, medications may also be advised. But even for people on medications, exercise and diet still remain the foundation of therapy.

It's never too late to start healthy habits to help manage your cholesterol. Even for people who have both high cholesterol and established heart disease, lowering blood cholesterol levels significantly reduces the risk of future heart attacks. For every 1 percent reduction in blood cholesterol, the occurrence of coronary heart disease is reduced by 2 or 3 percent. Some studies suggest that a comprehensive program of exercise, diet, and stress reduction can *reverse already established cholesterol buildup* in the arteries to some degree.

RISK FACTORS

Certain characteristics put you at greater risk of having high cholesterol. Those you can't influence include:

✳ *Heredity.* Your genes influence how your body makes and handles cholesterol. The tendency to have high cholesterol can run in families.

✳ *Sex.* Males are at higher risk of cardiovascular disease and typically have higher total blood cholesterol levels than women the same age, until women reach menopause. After menopause, women often have an increase in their LDL cholesterol levels, which means their risk of heart disease increases. Postmenopausal women who take estrogen generally find that it improves their cholesterol profile: LDL levels decrease and

HDL levels increase. In some women, pregnancy is accompanied by a temporary rise in blood cholesterol levels; levels typically return to normal about twenty weeks after delivery.

✳ *Age.* Blood cholesterol levels tend to rise with age, typically increasing in both men and women around age 20. However, women's blood cholesterol levels tend to be lower than men's until menopause, when women's cholesterol levels—and heart-disease risk—catches up to men's.

✳ *Other diseases.* Some chronic illnesses, such as diabetes, can affect how your body handles lipids. Also, long-term use of certain medications, such as steroids, may affect your cholesterol metabolism. If you have a chronic medical condition, the beneficial effect of regular exercise may be particularly important to your cholesterol management. In this setting, consultation with your doctor about comprehensive cholesterol control with exercise, diet, and medical management is prudent.

Other factors that help determine your blood cholesterol level can be influenced by your behavior. These include:

✳ *Diet.* Two kinds of nutrients in the foods you eat can make your cholesterol levels rise: *saturated fat*, which is found mostly in foods that come from animals, and *cholesterol*, which is found exclusively in animal products. Saturated fat is the major culprit in elevated blood cholesterol levels and is found in fatty cuts of meat, poultry with skin, whole-milk dairy products, lard, and some vegetable oils, including coconut, palm kernel, and palm oils. Although Americans have

cut back on their consumption of dietary fats, they still eat higher amounts than are recommended for good health, consuming an average of 12 percent of their calories from saturated fat and 34 percent of their total calories from fat. The National Cholesterol Education Program advises healthy Americans over two years of age to get less than 10 percent of their calories from saturated fat and less than 30 percent of their total calories from fat.

✳ *Physical activity levels.* Inactivity puts people at greater risk of having unhealthy total and LDL cholesterol levels. Regular physical activity can improve your blood cholesterol profile by lowering "bad" LDL-cholesterol levels, increasing "good" HDL-cholesterol levels, and helping your body become more efficient at utilizing and breaking down fats. Regular aerobic exercise also is associated with weight loss, which in itself can lower total cholesterol levels. Physical activity also affects other physiological characteristics that can further reduce your risk of heart disease, including lowering blood pressure, reducing stress, and improving the fitness of your heart and blood vessels.

✳ *Obesity.* Excess weight tends to increase total blood cholesterol levels, and being overweight can make your LDL-cholesterol levels go up and your HDL-cholesterol levels go down.

✳ *Smoking.* Quitting cigarettes can help increase your level of "good" HDL cholesterol.

HOW EXERCISE HELPS

People who exercise regularly have higher levels of the "good," HDL cholesterol, which helps scavenge and transport excess cholesterol from blood vessels to the liver for elimination. Some research indicates that the more exercise you do, the higher your levels of "good" HDL cholesterol may be. For example, a study by cardiologist Arthur Leon of the University of Minnesota School of Public Health revealed that the HDL levels of endurance-trained male and female athletes were generally 20 to 30 percent higher than those of healthy, age-matched sedentary people.

"Even a single episode of physical activity can result in an improved blood lipid profile that persists for several days," notes the *U.S. Surgeon General's Report on Physical Activity and Health* (1996). Exercise also reduces elevated levels of triglycerides, another blood lipid associated with heart disease. And it appears to increase the activity of certain enzymes that remove cholesterol and fatty acids from the blood.

In addition to these direct, positive effects on blood cholesterol, regular exercise may result in weight loss and increased metabolism, which has a dramatic effect on the cholesterol profile. Excess fat puts people at increased risk of having unhealthy cholesterol levels, particularly if the fat is stored in the abdomen. Overweight adults with an "apple" shape (potbelly) tend to have a higher risk for heart disease than those with a "pear shape" (bigger hips and thighs).

When overweight people lose weight, their total cholesterol typically drops about 1 mg/dL for every pound lost. So an overweight person who sheds twenty pounds can expect a 20-point drop in total blood cholesterol levels.

While any weight loss typically results in an improved cholesterol profile, some experts speculate that exercise-induced weight loss may be particularly beneficial. *Since exercise promotes fat release and utilization, the weight people lose from exercise tends to be mostly from fat.* The weight people lose from diet alone, however, tends to contain more than just fat; it also includes a significant amount of lean mass (muscle and bone). That's because when you severely restrict calories, your body tries to conserve fat stores, so it breaks down lean tissue mass, robbing your body of muscle and bone. Then, when you go off your strict diet, the weight you'll gain back is typically fat.

Also, when people exercise regularly for at least three months, many beneficial physiological changes kick in, including an improved ability to burn fat. The exact mechanisms by which these positive changes occur is still unclear, but it appears that becoming fit may allow people to break down and clear fatty substances from the blood more quickly.

EXERCISE (AND DIET) ℞

In the Stanford University study cited on page 60, participants walked or jogged the equivalent of about ten miles per week. This is becoming the standard exercise prescription for improving your cholesterol profile. If neither walking nor jogging appeals to you and you prefer another form of aerobic activity (such as cycling or in-line skating), think of the exercise prescription this way: *Do some form of moderate to hard aerobic exercise, five days per week, for at least 30 minutes per session.* Or try to burn at least 1,000 calories per week (the equivalent of walking or running eight to ten miles) through aerobic activity.

If you don't have 30 minutes a day, try doing two 15-minute exercise bouts. Although moderate- to hard-intensity activity appears to be most beneficial for your cholesterol status, even light- to moderate-intensity activity—such as gardening or strolling—can be beneficial if done daily.

While 30 minutes of moderate activity, most days, should be enough exercise to produce favorable changes in your HDL cholesterol level and to result in some weight loss, people who want to lose even more weight (and further lower their total cholesterol) may need to exercise moderately for a longer duration. For example, walk for an hour a day, six days a week. Increasing the intensity of exercise also may boost weight loss. (For more details on weight loss, see the section on obesity, page 67.)

Although exercise will improve your cholesterol profile, you can't run away from a bad diet. So for maximum benefit, it's important that you eat properly too. Studies show that *it is the combination of good eating habits and regular exercise that exerts the optimal effects on cholesterol status.*

Don't make the all-too-common mistake of simply focusing on eating low-fat foods. *Just because a food is low in fat doesn't mean it's low in calories or nutritious.* Instead, follow these simple guidelines:

✳ Eat five servings of fruits and vegetables and six servings of grains each day.
✳ Choose fish, skinless poultry, and lean cuts of meat. Eat moderate portions—no more than about six ounces per day (a three-ounce portion is the size of a deck of cards).

✳ Choose low-fat or non-fat dairy products.
✳ Eat only enough calories to achieve and maintain a healthy weight.

Remember that all adults age twenty and over are advised to have their total blood cholesterol levels and HDL-cholesterol levels checked at least once every five years. People at high risk of heart disease may need to have their cholesterol checked annually.

CAUTIONS

If you've been sedentary, be sure to start your exercise program slowly and progress gradually. Begin with as little as a daily 5-minute walk, and add on 5 more minutes per week until—over the course of about six weeks—you've built up to walking 30 minutes per day. (For guidelines on starting a walking program, see Healing Moves for Heart Health, page 214.) If you've been sedentary and you plan to start a program of *vigorous* activity—and you're a man over forty or a woman over fifty, or if you have risk factors for heart disease or other medical conditions for which you take medication—check with your physician first.

PRESCRIPTION PAD

✳ Do some form of moderate to hard aerobic activity for at least 30 minutes, most days of the week.
✳ Eat a nutritious, well-balanced diet that includes five servings of fruits and vegetables and six servings of grains each day. Avoid foods that are high in saturated fat.

✳ *The American Heart Association* has numerous brochures and fact sheets about cholesterol and heart disease. Call 800-AHA-USA1 or visit the Web site: www. americanheart.org.

✳ *The National Heart, Lung, and Blood Institute's Information Line* offers free material about cholesterol and heart disease to consumers and health professionals. Call 800-575-9355 or write the National Cholesterol Education Program, NHLBI, P.O. Box 30105, Bethesda, Md. 20824-0105. Check the Web site at www.nhlbi.nih.gov/nhlbi/nhlbi.htm

✳ *Healthfinder*, an Internet site for health-related government agencies, such as the National Institutes of Health and the Department of Health and Human Services, can provide a wealth of information about controlling cholesterol. Access the Web site at www.healthfinder.gov, then follow the "search" cues to access material about cholesterol and heart disease.

✳ *The Rockport Fitness Walking Test* is a free brochure to gauge your fitness level and start you on an individualized walking program. Call 800-ROCKPORT.

✳ The American Volkssport Association has more than five hundred clubs nationwide that run noncompetitive walking events in the outdoors. For information, call 800-830-WALK.

OBESITY

Right now, tens of millions of Americans are dieting to lose weight, and countless others are struggling to maintain their current weight. In our bulge-battling society—where obesity has risen to epidemic proportions—nearly everyone wants to shed fat to look better, feel better, and boost their health.

But the sad fact is, most people's efforts to lose weight and keep it off fail. Americans spend more than $33 billion a year on weight-loss pills, potions, and paraphernalia—some of which has dangerous medical side effects. Yet most of this money is wasted, since only a fraction of those who try to lose weight actually drop pounds and keep them off.

Those rare individuals who successfully shed pounds and maintain their lower weight tend to have one thing in common: dedication to physical activity. "Regular exercise is the single best predictor of whether an overweight person will lose weight and keep it off," says Yale University psychology professor Kelly Brownell, an expert on obesity and eating disorders. Dieting alone doesn't work, since caloric restriction slows the metabolism and is difficult—and often unhealthy—to maintain. But when people combine sensible eating habits with regular exercise, their body weight will drop to the lowest level it can naturally maintain.

This weight may not be as "skinny" as our thin-obsessed culture might dictate, however. According to an increasing number of researchers who contend that fit and healthy bodies come in all shapes and sizes, some people are genetically and physiologically unable to meet societal standards of thinness. That's why experts are taking a new approach to combating America's obesity epidemic. *Instead of trying to get overweight people to become thin, which is aimed primarily at appearance, they're trying to get overweight people to become healthy, which is aimed at normalizing blood pressure, blood glucose, and blood cholesterol levels.*

To achieve these health goals, it's important to concentrate on *behaviors* people can control (eating right and exercising regularly) rather than *outcomes* people can't control (weight loss). And it means looking beyond just the number on the scale to consider other significant measures of health, such as heart rate, cholesterol levels, and psychological status.

This is difficult for some people to comprehend because, over the last few decades, our society has confused health with thinness. In a culture that glorifies anorexic models and the emaciated look known as heroin chic, we've been ignoring the fact that some people's bodies will never measure "down" to societal notions of "ideal" weight. Overweight people who successfully lose ten to twenty pounds (which can significantly decrease health risks) still feel like failures because their bodies aren't "skinny enough." All too often, failure to reach these unrealistic weight goals results in a "bad scale day," which can be physically and psychologically devastating. Already damaged self-esteems take a nosedive. Stress mounts. Depression deepens. People consider themselves failures and abandon healthy habits. The frequent result: more weight gain.

So instead of striving to reach an arbitrary goal weight, health experts now say people should focus on adopting the positive lifestyle behaviors that will result in better health—as evidenced by some weight loss and improved blood pressure, blood sugar, and blood cholesterol profiles. Chief among these behaviors is exercise, which many experts consider the single best "medicine" to counter obesity. That's because physical activity does much more than simply burn calories (although that's one of its most powerful effects). Exercise also counters many factors that contribute to overeating: it relieves stress, boosts mood, enhances self-esteem, and lifts depression.

And in an age when technology has engineered activity out of our lives, putting exercise back in is the single best way to keep weight gain from becoming inevitable. The only cost is some time, and the only side effect is improved fitness.

OBESITY BASICS

On the beaches, flesh bulges over bathing suits. In the malls, widening waistlines have spawned a booming market for plus-size clothes. In the schools, kids are fatter and less fit than previous generations.

We are a nation gone to potbelly.

Obesity is Public Enemy Number Two, say health officials, who call it the second major cause of preventable death, right after smoking. It's responsible for 300,000 deaths in the United States each year and is increasing at an alarming rate. These figures highlight the problem:

✷ The percentage of obese adults ballooned from 14.5 percent in 1976 to 1980 to 22.5 percent in 1988 to 1994, according to data from the National Health and Nutrition Examination Surveys.

✷ Women and people in low-income

ethnic populations are more likely to be obese, with African American women showing the highest incidence of all.

✳ The number of overweight children has increased by almost 50 percent over the last two decades, and the number of extremely overweight children has nearly doubled.

If current trends continue, scientists estimate that 100 percent of adults in the United States will be obese in two centuries!

"The cause is not gluttony," says epidemiologist Claude Bouchard, a professor at Laval University in Quebec. "We're actually eating a bit less." The cause isn't fat intake either, since our diets are 33 to 34 percent fat now and used to be 40 percent fat.

Instead, Bouchard and other health professionals say that the driving force behind our growing girth is the dramatic decline in physical activity. "No need to do rocket science to conclude that we are expending less energy than did our grandparents, who had to chop wood and fetch water to survive," he says. Some experts estimate that adults today expend 800 fewer calories per day than did previous generations, largely because technology has engineered much of the physical activity out of our lives.

Labor-saving devices make it possible to do housework and yardwork at the push of a button, and computers let people correspond electronically without even licking a stamp and walking to the mailbox. Virtually anything can be purchased with a telephone and credit card, and nearly any topic researched on the Internet. Plus, our society often places obstacles in the way of activity. Complex highway systems make it difficult

to bicycle or walk in many areas, elevators and escalators are usually easier to find than stairwells, and fear of crime keeps some people from strolling through their own neighborhoods. Some golf courses won't let players walk, but require them to drive carts.

One result of this "forced sedentariness" is the alarming rise in obesity. That's why public health experts are urging Americans to get off their rear ends. Since exercise has been engineered out of our lives, we must find ways to schedule it back in.

"The best approach to combating obesity is through physical activity," says U.S. Surgeon General David Satcher. Yet the 1996 *U.S. Surgeon General's Report on Physical Activity and Health* showed that the vast majority of Americans get little or no exercise, and it advocated modest amounts of moderate physical activity to improve health.

The new advice: Burn 150 calories per day in physical activity such as walking for 30 minutes, climbing stairs for 15 minutes, or washing and waxing a car for 45 minutes.

The new message: Exercise isn't about painfully sweating to reach an elusive—and sometimes impossible—cosmetic goal like rock-hard abs or a model-thin silhouette. Instead, exercise is simply spending some time off your behind, doing moderate physical activity that is essential to maintaining good health and preventing disease—including obesity.

HOW EXERCISE HELPS

A major reason why exercise helps combat obesity is that physical activity burns calories. But regular exercise also boosts weight loss because it:

* **Builds muscle.** Muscle tissue is one of the most metabolically active tissues in the body, so people with more muscle burn more calories, even at rest.

* **Revs up the metabolism.** The metabolic rate rises during physical activity and stays elevated for a significant period of time after the exercise is finished.

* **Affects psychology.** Exercise helps boost self-esteem and body image, reduce depression, and relieve stress. "This can give people more psychic strength to adhere to a diet," says Yale professor Kelly Brownell, who believes that the psychological benefits of exercise may be at least as important as the physical effects in explaining why people lose weight through regular exercise.

Unlike other methods of weight loss, such as pills or surgery, the side effects of exercise are nearly all positive. In addition to helping prevent and manage obesity, exercise reduces the risk of numerous other chronic diseases, boosts mood, and reduces tension.

"If we could get 25 percent of the people who are sedentary up and moving," Surgeon General Satcher says, "we could save $4 billion a year in medical costs."

But while exercise is essential in countering the ill effects of obesity, physical activity will not make all fat people thin. It can, however, help them become healthier, since even those who don't lose enough weight to appear slender are still likely to shed enough fat to significantly reduce their risk of disease.

Some researchers contend that obesity itself isn't hazardous to health; they say it's the inactivity that leads to excess weight that's responsible for disease. This controversial viewpoint holds that inactivity itself is the main cause of disease and obesity is merely a marker of the unhealthy lifestyle that leads to medical problems.

Despite our culture's misconception that "thinner is healthier," *an active heavy person is likely to be fitter than an inactive thin one,* notes Dallas epidemiologist Steven N. Blair, who served as senior scientific editor of the *Surgeon General's Report.* Blair's research, following more than 25,000 men over nearly twenty years, found that fit men had a lower risk of early death than sedentary ones, regardless of weight. More important than just the number on the scale are the numbers indicating what some experts call "metabolic fitness": heart rate, blood pressure, cholesterol profile, and glucose tolerance. Regular exercise can make a dramatic difference in these measures of metabolic fitness, even when people lose as few as five pounds. Plus, it helps people improve "functional fitness," which means exercisers have more energy, more endurance, a better outlook, and fewer aches and pains.

But in our "you can't be too rich or too thin" culture, it's important not to confuse the aesthetic desire for cosmetic thinness with the health imperatives of achieving metabolic fitness. Many unhealthy behaviors—such as smoking, fad diets, and eating disorders—stem from societal pressures to be thin. That's why more and more obesity experts are shifting their focus from trying to get fat people thin to trying to get fat people healthy.

"I tell patients to forget the idea that

achieving an ideal body size is the cure-all," says Wayne Miller, director of the Healthy Weight Management program at George Washington University Medical Center. "Live a healthy lifestyle, eat right, and exercise regularly. Then your weight will settle somewhere that's healthy for you."

GENETICS LOADS THE GUN, ENVIRONMENT PULLS THE TRIGGER

Obesity is more than merely a problem of eating more calories than we burn.

"There are genetic differences in the susceptibility to weight gain and in the way our bodies build fat deposits," says Claude Bouchard, who, along with other scientists, is studying the genetic components of obesity in an effort to create a "human obesity gene map" that would identify the genes that put people at greater risk.

Still, environment has a strong impact on obesity, as demonstrated by studies of the Native American Pima Indian tribe, described on page 52. "Genes are important," Bouchard says. "But what we do in terms of energy expenditure is also crucial."

Or as Judith Stern, professor of nutrition and internal medicine at the University of California at Davis, puts it: "Genetics loads the gun, but environment pulls the trigger. For some people it's a hair trigger and for others it's not."

One indication that genetics is just part of the obesity picture is that "fat people have fat dogs," says Stern, who chaired an Institute of Medicine committee charged with evaluating weight-management programs.

"Obesity is . . . a complex, multi-factorial disease of appetite regulation and energy metabolism involving genetics, physiology, biochemistry and the neurosciences, as well as environmental, psychosocial and cultural factors," sums up *Weighing the Options*, the book Stern's committee wrote to offer people guidance in selecting weight-management programs. "Unfortunately, the lay public and health-care providers, as well as insurance companies, often view it simply as a problem of willful misconduct—eating too much and exercising too little."

The grim reality about obesity, Stern says, is that it's "a chronic disease with many causes, including inactivity. We can't cure it, but we can manage it, which means losing some of the weight and keeping it off."

Typically, weight loss is slow and regain is common. And any treatment, whether drugs or exercise, doesn't work once it's stopped.

The millions of Americans who are struggling to lose weight often have great expectations based on outrageous claims made by some weight-loss programs. But studies show that those who complete weight-loss programs lose approximately 10 percent of their body weight, only to regain two-thirds of it back within one year and almost all of it back within five years.

The best result most obese people can achieve, Stern says, is to lose 15 percent of their body weight and keep it off. For a 200-pound, five-foot-seven person, this would mean losing and keeping off 30 pounds, for a maintenance weight of 170. Although this isn't likely to satisfy our culture's cosmetic "thin" ideal, this amount of weight loss can dramatically improve the person's health. Even small weight losses (5 to 10 percent reductions in body fat) are associated with a decrease in cardiovascular risk; improved glucose tolerance, blood pressure, and cholesterol profile; reduced symptoms of degenerative joint disease; and improved gynecological symptoms.

Yet a person who experiences this great success may still feel like a failure. That's because, at 170 pounds and five feet seven inches, he or she won't appear thin. Obesity experts have recognized this problem and have changed their approach to focus on health, not thinness.

"Instead of having the goal of weight loss, which is aimed primarily at appearance," Stern says, "the new goal is weight management, which is achieving the best weight possible in context of overall health."

NO MORE "BAD SCALE DAYS"

Forget the notion of an ideal weight or a diet that considers some foods "good" and others "bad," says the American Dietetic Association, which in 1997 issued a new position statement on weight management.

"Too many people get hung up on reaching a number on a height-weight chart that for them may be unattainable," says ADA spokeswoman Josephine Connolly, who's also a nutritionist at the State University of New York at Stony Brook. So the ADA has "redefined success," she says, to focus on healthy behaviors people *can* control. These include:

* *Gradual change to a more healthful eating style* with proportional increases in whole grains, fruits, and vegetables.

* *A nonrestrictive approach to eating* based on eating when hungry and stopping when full.

* *Gradual increase to at least 30 minutes of enjoyable physical activity* each day.

In addition, Connolly says, "we're encouraging the notion of a healthy weight, which someone can achieve and maintain, as opposed to a cosmetic weight or ideal weight on a standardized chart." Each person's healthy weight is determined individually, based on his or her weight history and current medical condition.

An essential part of this new approach is to consider how someone *feels* as opposed to how someone *looks*. This means recognizing that becoming thin may be impossible for some people.

Becoming healthier, however, is well within virtually anyone's reach. Instead of looking to the scale to measure success, individuals look to their ability to maintain healthy habits that allow them to move through their days with energy and ease.

As with most health issues, it's a question of finding the right balance

* between activity and rest;
* between eating enough and eating too much; and
* between our desire to reshape our bodies and to accept our genetic limitations.

Yet in America, weight is an emotional issue. While most people understand and accept the fact that they can't become as tall as Shaquille O'Neal, many can't understand and accept the fact they can't become as thin as Ally McBeal.

Some physicians still shame, blame, and alienate the obese. Many primary-care doctors and health insurance companies continue to rely on scale weight as an indicator of body fatness, even though obesity experts prefer using the body mass index, or BMI, a number determined by a formula that uses both height and weight. (See chart, page 34.)

Americans consider a BMI of 27 or more an indication of health-endangering excess weight, Stern says, while Europeans consider a BMI of 25 and above problematic. Shape Up America!, a national initiative to promote healthy weight and increase physical activity, classifies BMI this way:

BMI Category	Health Risk Based Solely on BMI	Risk Adjusted for Comorbid Conditions
<25	Minimal	Low
25–<27	Low	Moderate
27–<30	Moderate	High
30–<35	High	Very High
35–<40	Very High	Extremely High
+40	Extremely High	Extremely High

While BMI measurements are considered better than the old-fashioned height-weight charts with their so-called ideal weights, BMIs can be problematic. When people are exceptionally muscular, their BMIs don't accurately reflect their health risk, since the number does not factor in how much of the body is fat and how much is lean tissue. For example, the Baltimore Orioles star third baseman Cal Ripken is six foot four and 220 pounds, which gives him a BMI of 27. That puts him in the "moderate to high" health-risk category for obesity, even though Ripken's weight clearly doesn't come from excess body fat.

The most accurate determination of body composition is done by underwater weighing, which requires sophisticated equipment available only in research laboratories. So, for now, obesity experts consider BMI the most practical measure of fatness and associated health risk. For most people, as BMI increases, so does health risk.

Government health goals for the year 2000 call for no more than 20 percent of adults and 15 percent of adolescents to be obese. Yet the nation is moving further away from, rather than closer toward, this goal.

"One remarkable feature of obesity is that its management requires a great deal of effort from the individual," according to *Weighing the Options.* "And there are few diseases in which health-care providers can offer so little for those who struggle so much."

Surgical treatments have been suggested over the years for some extremely obese individuals, and some drug treatments may also be beneficial when combined with healthy eating and exercise habits. "The problem now is the abuse by physicians who are prescribing drugs without lifestyle changes," Stern says. "I'm convinced that until we actually understand more about the disease, we're not going to make any progress until we can get people physically active."

The inactivity trend is particularly disturbing among children, who typically are driven to and from school, lack daily physical education classes, and remain indoors and sedentary after school. Not only are the growing numbers of obese children likely to become obese adults, but they are subject to numerous psychological stresses, such as depression and lowered self-esteem from the discrimination obese people face in our society.

For adults, the best advice comes from Shape Up America!: Eat sensibly, exercise regularly, drop a few pounds.

"Exercise should be made an honorary vitamin," asserts Shape Up America!'s chairman, C. Everett Koop, who says if he had been able to do one more thing during his tenure as U.S. surgeon general, it would have been to launch a campaign against obesity. "If you don't have it daily, then you're deficient."

EXERCISE ℞

The general rule of thumb for weight loss is to create a 300- to 500-calorie deficit each day. This means consuming 300 to 500 fewer calories than you expend through a combination of eating less and exercising more. (See "Calories Burned" chart, page 23.)

Yet many "exercise-phobes" try to create the calorie deficit solely through extremely low-calorie diets, which is a dangerous mistake that can harm health and is unlikely to result in permanent weight loss.

"People who are overweight want to lose fat," notes exercise physiologist Steve Farrell of the Cooper Institute for Aerobics Research in Dallas. "But many don't realize that about half of the weight lost on extremely low-calorie diets isn't from fat, it's from lean tissue." It's important to eat enough to fuel your body, notes Farrell, who warns men not to eat less than 1,200 calories

per day and women not to eat less than 1,000. Farrell recommends that half of the 300- to 500-calorie deficit come from eating less and half from exercising more.

"We generally advise people who want to lose weight to expend at least 250 calories more each day than they have in the past," he says. "Additionally, they should eat 250 fewer calories than they've been eating."

The best calorie burner is **aerobic exercise,** which is any physical activity that demands large quantities of oxygen for prolonged periods of time. Regularly performing aerobic exercise not only burns calories but ultimately forces the body to improve those systems responsible for transportation of oxygen. This typically means improvements in measures of metabolic fitness— blood pressure, blood cholesterol, and blood sugar.

Examples of popular aerobic exercises are walking, running, bicycling, in-line skating, dancing, swimming, and aerobic dance. Which is best? The one you like and will do regularly.

For most people, walking is the easiest, safest, and most convenient form of exercise. In general, a three-mile walk five days a week, combined with good eating habits, is enough to result in significant weight loss and fitness gain. (Remember: Focus on what you have to gain from being active, not what you have to lose to feel successful.)

In addition, **strength-training exercises** can help you build muscle, which will improve your functional fitness and boost your metabolic rate. Do eight to ten resistance exercises for the large muscle groups of your body two to three times a week.

Be sure to:

* Pick a workout pace you like, since the goal is to have fun so you'll stick with your program. For most people, this means a moderate intensity, which can be as effective for losing fat as more strenuous activity. While high-intensity activity burns calories faster, it also has greater injury potential.

* Add as much activity to your day as possible. Park in the farthest space, take the stairs, bike to the store. Every step you take counts.

* Exchange labor-saving devices for calorie-burning activity. Get rid of the blower and rake your leaves, wash your car by hand, and get up and change the channel or turn off the TV entirely.

* Shun gimmicks. There is no magic potion or product to melt fat.

* Stop looking only to the scale to note your progress. Consider, too, how your clothes fit, how you feel, and how you're able to meet the physical challenges of daily life.

* Refuse to engage in any self-abusing internal dialogue. Remember that no matter what your size, you deserve the pleasure of movement.

EATING

Since this book is about exercise, we'll leave the extensive dietary details to others. To maximize weight loss, however, exercise should be combined with healthy eating, which means:

* Eating a sensible, well-balanced diet with emphasis on fresh fruits, vegetables, and whole grains.

* Striving to reduce your intake of fats, so that they make up less than 30 percent of your diet.

* Not "supersizing" it. In America, portions are often excessive, and many people don't realize that one serving of meat is two to three ounces (about the size of a deck of cards) and one serving of a bagel is one-half of a small one. (An entire bagel is two to four servings, depending on the size.)

* There are no "good foods" and "bad foods." What you love, you can have in moderation.

* Eat when you're hungry. Stop when you're full. Eat slowly enough to know the difference.

CAUTIONS

Preventing injury is extremely important, since ailments like a sprained ankle or wrenched back are major reasons why people quit exercising. To minimize stress on the joints, people who are very large should consider non-weight-bearing or low-impact activities such as water aerobics, walking, stationary cycling, or line dancing. Also, it's important to wear good, supportive athletic shoes designed for the activity you're doing. Be sure to buy shoes at the end of the day, when your feet are at their largest, and choose a pair that is snug in the heel but has "wiggle room" at the toe. There should be a thumb's width distance between the end of your big toe and the shoe.

If you've been sedentary, *start slowly and progress gradually* to avoid injury. Begin with as little as three minutes a day and add three more minutes a week until you can stay active for 30 to 60 minutes. Start with an easy warm-up, stretch gently, then do your activity and finish with a cooldown.

You probably don't need to consult a doctor to go for a walk or do other, moderate exercise. (See Pre-Participation Checklist, page 29.) But be sure to check with a physician before starting a *vigorous* exercise program if you're a male over forty or a woman over fifty or if you have risk factors for heart disease, such as smoking or obesity.

Remember, too, that large people may be especially sensitive to heat. So when it's hot outside, be sure to exercise during the cool times of the day or in a cool room, pool, health club or mall, drink plenty of water, and wear comfortable clothing.

PRESCRIPTION PAD

✳ Avoid injury by starting exercise slowly, progressing gradually, staying hydrated, and wearing good, supportive athletic shoes.

✳ Burn about 250 to 500 calories doing an aerobic activity, four to six days a week. Examples are 30 minutes of swimming, 45 to 60 minutes of walking, 45 minutes of cycling, or 30 to 45 minutes of in-line skating.

✳ Perform eight to ten of the muscle-strengthening exercises, two to three times a week.

✳ Increase daily-life activities. Climb stairs, walk to the store, stand up and stretch.

✳ Eat appropriate portions of food from a sensible, well-balanced diet that is made up of less than 30 percent fat.

ADDITIONAL RESOURCES

Print

✳ *Great Shape: The First Fitness Guide for Large Women*, by Pat Lyons and Debby Burgard (Bull Publishing, 1990).

✳ *The Black Health Library Guide to Obesity*, by Mavis Thompson, M.D., with Kirk A. Johnson (Henry Holt, 1993).

✳ *Big Fat Lies*, by Glenn Gaesser (Fawcett Columbine, 1996).

✳ *Radiance: The Magazine for Large Women*, P.O. Box 30246, Oakland, Calif. 94604; (510) 482-0680. Web site: www.radiancemagazine.com.

Video

✳ *Idrea: The Larger Women's Workout*, 47 minutes; $19.95 plus $4.50 shipping and handling from Collage Video, 800-433-6769.

✳ *Yoga for Round Bodies I & II*. Each 90-minute video includes three 30-minute yoga sessions; $29.95 each, plus $1.75 shipping and handling, from PLUS Publications, 800-793-0666.

✳ *Chair Dancing*. Series includes *Sit Down and Tone UP*, $14.95, and *Chair Dancing Around the World*; $19.95, plus shipping from Collage Video, 800-433-6769. Web site: www.chairdancing.com.

✳ *Women at Large Breakout*, 50 minutes; $19.95 plus $4.50 shipping and handling from Collage Video, 800-433-6769.

Organizations

✳ WIN: The Weight-Control Information Network, run by the National Institute of Diabetes and Digestive and Kidney Diseases. Call 800-WIN-8098, visit the Web site (www.niddk.nih.gov/NutritionDocs.html), or write WIN at One WIN Way, Bethesda, Md. 20892-3662.

✳ Shape Up America!, a not-for-profit coalition of industry, medical-health, nutrition, physical fitness, and related organizations chaired by former U.S. surgeon general C. Everett Koop. Calculate your body mass index and visit their Cyberkitchen on their Web site: www.shapeup.org. Or write for a list of publications, many of them free: Shape Up America!, 6707 Democracy Blvd., Suite 306, Bethesda, Md. 20817.

✳ The American Dietetic Association's Consumer Nutrition Hotline features recorded messages about healthy eating and offers a referral service to registered dieticians: 800-366-1655 (weekdays). For free brochures on weight management, send a business-sized self-addressed, stamped envelope to ADA's National Center for Nutrition and Dietetics, Attn: Weight Control, 216 West Jackson Blvd., Chicago, Ill. 60606. Or visit the Web site: www. eatright.org.

✳ The National Coalition for Promoting Physical Activity offers fact sheets and information for new and continuing exercisers: P.O. Box 1440, Indianapolis, Ind. 46206. Web site: www.ncppa.org.

✳ ✳ ✳

HEALING MOVES TO REGULATE METABOLISM

✳

One of the most persistent myths about shaping up is that people who have trouble losing weight are simply cursed with a slow metabolism. But while it's easy to blame excess fat on a "sluggish metabolism," only rarely is a medical problem—such as a thyroid disorder—responsible.

Instead, the metabolic slowdown that occurs over the years in most Americans results primarily from the physical slowdown of becoming increasingly sedentary with age. Inactivity leads to excess fat, muscle loss, and dieting—all of which decrease the metabolic rate. But by exercising regularly and eating right, you can rev up your metabolism, so that your body will burn more calories, even at rest. Regular exercise also enhances lipid and insulin metabolism, which helps your body process sugars and fats in your blood. For people with metabolic disorders, such as diabetes and high cholesterol, this can be extremely therapeutic.

The metabolic rate is a measure of how many calories your body needs to function. A variety of factors affect that rate, some of which you can't influence (age, gender, height, genetic makeup) and some of which you can (body composition, activity level, food consumption). One of the most important factors in determining your metabolic rate is the amount of lean tissue (muscle, bone, organs) you have. The more lean tissue, the higher your metabolic rate. Muscle mass boosts metabolism because muscle is active tissue that requires nourishment.

Your muscles contain calorie-burning structures called mitochondria, which help convert food into water, heat, and energy. In contrast, fat is more passive tissue that acts primarily as a storage form of body energy. So when your body is deciding what to do with the food you've eaten, the more muscle you have, the more calories it can send to muscle cells to be burned. This leaves fewer calories to go to fat cells to be stored.

Or think of it this way: *Muscle burns calories, fat stores calories.* The more muscle you have, the greater your calorie-burning engine.

Many people assume that age itself causes the metabolism to slow, and it's true that growing older does exert some reduction in metabolic rate. Yet many experts feel that *the primary reason metabolism declines with age is that most people's activity level and muscle mass decrease as they get older.* Typically, caloric requirements peak in adolescence, when activity levels are high and growth is rapid. Then, from about age twenty on, lifestyles and behaviors begin to change. As adults move toward middle age, physical activity generally declines, muscle mass begins to shrink, and body fat grows. Muscle mass in sedentary individuals declines by about 15 percent between the third and eighth decade of life. Caloric requirements—and metabolic rate—decline accordingly. This is why an active, muscular twenty-five-year-old can eat much more than a sedentary, potbellied fifty-five-year-old, without gaining weight.

In fact, an average seventy-year-old needs 500 fewer calories per day to maintain his or her body weight than an average twenty-five-year-old, according to William Evans, an expert on nutrition and aging and director of the Nutrition, Metabolism, and Exercise Lab at the University of Arkansas for Medical Sciences. The average eighty-year-old needs 600 fewer calories. In short, says Evans, from around age twenty onward, you need to take in about 100 calories less per day each decade to maintain the status quo. Yet most of us eat the same way we did when we were younger, and then we wonder where that potbelly came from.

Dieting is another behavior that can slow the metabolic rate. When you restrict calories, your body senses starvation and switches into a "conservation mode," which slows the metabolism. When you *severely* restrict calories, your body tries to conserve fat stores, so it breaks down muscle mass for energy. This means that *instead of losing fat, people who try to lose weight exclusively through extreme diets actually rob their own bodies of muscle and bone.* Then, when they go off their diets and gain the weight back (which is what typically happens), the regained weight is usually fat. It's not uncommon for people to starve themselves to lose ten pounds, which will contain a great deal of muscle and bone, then gain back ten pounds of pure fat. Dieting often results in this unhealthy spiral of muscle lost and fat gained, which further slows the metabolic rate. That's why it's important to properly fuel your body by eating a sensible, nutritious diet, which should contain at least 1,200 calories per day for men and 1,000 calories per day for women. Eating less is likely to slow your metabolism.

The good news is that the typical metabolic decline—and the "creeping obesity" or "middle-age spread" that results—aren't inevitable. Over time, regular exercise can rev up (or at least maintain) your metabolic rate as your activity burns fat and builds muscle. The metabolic rate rises during physical activity and stays elevated for several hours afterward. So not only are you burning calories at a higher rate during exercise, but you continue to burn extra calories during the immediate postworkout period.

Three kinds of exercise are important in boosting your metabolism: daily (or near daily) aerobic workouts, lifestyle activity, and strength-training workouts. In addition, relaxation exercises can be extremely helpful in combating the stress that can exacerbate metabolic disorders and lead to overeating. That's why our Metabolism Regulating Workout includes three basic components and one optional add-on:

Part One: Daily Aerobic Activity

Exercising aerobically every day—or almost every day—for 30 to 60 minutes is essential to powering up your metabolism, thereby enhancing your body's ability to burn calories and effectively process sugars and fats.

Part Two: Activate Your Life

Every step you take counts toward burning calories and building muscle. Studies show that fitting activity into your day can provide health benefits similar to those of a traditional gym-based workout. This section presents a five-step life "activation" plan to help you integrate more movement into your day.

Part Three: Relaxation Exercises

Having a disordered metabolism can be stressful—especially when it's associated with excess pounds in a culture that bombards us with pressure to be thin, from a media that glorifies anorexic women to insurance companies that charge obese clients higher rates. Relaxation exercises are an essential part of this workout because they can help reduce tension, establish emotional equilibrium, and create a sense of clarity and control.

Part Four: Strength Training

Building muscle is an important means of boosting your metabolic rate. However, since many people who are struggling with excess fat are very deconditioned and out of shape, it's prudent to start slowly and progress gradually. Also, if you have certain complications from diabetes, lifting heavy weights may be inadvisable. For these reasons, we've included an easy-does-it strength-training section that you may decide to add on down the road, after you've been doing the other three parts of the program for several months.

Remember: Before beginning this or any other exercise program, people with chronic medical conditions (or risk factors for them) should consult their physicians. If you have diabetes, bring this workout to your doctor so he or she can help you individualize it to suit the specifics of your condition. (See Pre-Participation Checklist, page 29.)

PART ONE: DAILY AEROBIC ACTIVITY

Aerobic exercises are any activities that increase your heart rate and breathing for an extended period of time. The options are vast: walking, cycling, dancing, swimming, running, rowing, skating, aerobic dancing, stair stepping, and hiking, to name a few. If you are overweight or out of shape, it's a good idea to pick a low-impact activity such as walking, water exercise, or riding a stationary bicycle. It's helpful, too, to pick a primary activity, which you enjoy and will do most days, and one or two alternate activities for variety.

Your goal will be to perform your selected activity at a pace you consider "moderate" to "somewhat hard" for 30 to 60 continuous minutes, most days of the week. If you've been sedentary, it may take you months to reach this goal, and that's fine. Start with as little as five minutes of your chosen activity, then add two more minutes each week until—fourteen weeks later— you'll be exercising continuously for 31 minutes. (For a step-by-step guide to starting a walking program, see Healing Moves for Heart Health, page 214.) The longer you exercise, the more calories you'll burn. So if your goal is weight loss, exercising aerobically for 60 minutes five or six days a week will get you maximum benefits. Be sure to start slowly and progress gradually so that you safely ease your body into activity. If you pick an activity that stresses a particular body part—such as jogging, which may be hard on the knees and ankles—alternate it with an activity that is easy on the stressed part—in this case swimming, which is easy on the joints—to help prevent overuse injuries.

Also, the greater the intensity of your exercise, the more calories you'll burn. For example, a 175-pound adult will burn 180 calories in a half-hour walk and 400 calories in a half-hour run. But higher-intensity activities may have a greater risk of injury, espe-cially if they are high impact. And if you're obese, activities that pound your joints, such as running or high-impact aerobics, may be inadvisable. That's why, in general, if you're overweight and have been sedentary, it's better to begin an exercise program with a moderate-intensity, low-impact activity. After your body has become accustomed to exercise and you build up your strength and endurance, you can progress to a higher-intensity activity if you want. (Men over forty and women over fifty, as well as those of any age with risk factors for heart disease, should consult a physician before starting a program of vigorous exercise.)

Frequency is the key to improving meta-bolic disorders, and aerobic exercise needs to occur daily—or close to it—to have a long-lasting effect on your metabolism. For example, the improvements in insulin sensi-tivity that occur because of exercise last, at most, only two or three days, so it's essential for people with diabetes to exercise regu-larly. Remember, regularly performing aero-bic activity not only burns calories but ultimately forces the body to enhance those systems responsible for transportation of oxygen. This typically means improvements in measures of metabolic fitness, such as blood sugar and blood cholesterol.

Many experts recommend that you do your aerobic exercise first thing in the morn-ing for several reasons:

* *Morning exercisers are most likely to be compliant.* That is, they are less likely to make excuses for skipping activity, which are more common later in the day when you're tired, busy, running late, or stuck at work.

✳ *Putting your exercise first, literally, makes a statement to yourself and to the world* about the importance you place on your daily physical activity and its contribution to your health.

✳ *Exercising in the morning revs up your metabolism early* and can give you a physical and psychological boost that lasts the day. (By contrast, exercising intensely too close to bedtime can interfere with sleep.)

✳ *Morning exercise can help you focus on your day's goals* and mentally prepare for the challenges ahead.

If you're not a morning person and you'd rather exercise before dinner or in the middle of the day, that's fine, too. The important thing is that you exercise aerobically five or six days a week. No excuses.

In general, a three-mile walk five days a week, combined with good eating habits, is enough to result in significant weight loss, metabolic improvements, and fitness gains. To maximize results be sure that with each exercise session you:

A. Warm up by doing a "light and easy" version of your primary activity for about five minutes. For example, if your activity is lap swimming, warm up with several minutes of easy strokes and kicks. If your activity is riding a stationary bicycle, pedal slowly for a few minutes to warm up.

B. Stretch gently. Do easy stretches for each of the major muscle groups—front and back of the legs, arms and shoulders, back and hips. (See Healing Moves for Health and Fitness, page 44, and Healing Moves to Strengthen Muscles and Bones, page 149, for good stretch routines.)

C. Exercise in your "moderate to somewhat hard" zone for 30 to 60 minutes. This is a subjective measure that will change as you get more fit. For example, when you start out exercising, 5 minutes of walking at a pace you consider moderate may barely get you once around the track. But over time, you may find that you can go around the track twice in five minutes as you get fitter and your idea of what's moderate changes. While even easy strolling exerts some health benefits, for maximum metabolic benefits you need to pick up the pace to a point where your breathing is deep but you can still carry on a conversation. (If you can sing, however, you're probably not exercising hard enough.) At this point, you should consider your intensity moderate to somewhat hard—only you know how this feels for you. You'll burn more calories at a somewhat hard pace than at a moderate one, but both intensities will get you good results, so it's a matter of personal preference.

As your body adapts to activity and you get more and more fit, you may want to challenge yourself to stay in this "moderate to somewhat hard" zone. For example, if you've been walking on flat surfaces, you could start to walk hills. Or you can pick up your pace, add some stairs, or wear a backpack with a few pounds of books inside. But once you reach this "maximum results" zone, it's not necessary to push yourself to go faster. It's better to exercise at a pace you enjoy and will maintain than to push yourself into a stressful, sweat-and-strain pace that could result in injury or burnout.

D. Cool down for five minutes. Never abruptly stop doing an aerobic activity. Ease down by slowing your movements and performing your activity in a light and easy manner.

E. Stretch. The best time to stretch is now, after your workout, when your muscles are warm and pliable.

Remember, too, you can't run away from a bad diet. Since this book is about exercise, we'll leave the extensive dietary details to others. (For a summary of weight-loss eating strategies, see page 75.) To optimize weight loss, create a 500-calorie deficit each day by burning at least 250 calories through exercise and cutting 250 calories from your diet. Be sure to eat enough to fuel your activity and avoid the metabolic slow-down that comes from starvation diets. Bottom line: Eat modest portions from a sensible, well-balanced diet with emphasis on fresh fruits, vegetables, and whole grains. Exercise aerobically every day.

PART TWO: ACTIVATE YOUR LIFE

It's not easy to be active and eat right in our push-button, "Super-Size it" culture. Our society exerts enormous environmental pressure to be sedentary and eat junk food, says Yale University obesity expert Kelly Brownell, who contends that our environment is becoming increasingly "toxic" by encouraging consumption of high-fat foods and discouraging physical activity. He points to these examples:

Toxic Food Environment

Fast food is everywhere, from schools and gas stations to airplanes and hospitals. "Voodoo advertising" allows potato chips to trumpet the fact that they're "cholesterol-free" even though they're loaded with saturated fat. Food commercials bombard us—the average child sees ten thousand a year.

Toxic Physical Activity Environment

Moving walkways, automatic doors, remote controls, drive-through windows, and other conveniences make it less necessary—or possible—to move during the day. Walking or biking is difficult in towns without pedestrian or bike lanes, and fear of crime keeps many people from exercising outside. Computers make it possible to communicate, shop, play games, and socialize without lifting more than your fingers.

That's why this portion of our workout, where you learn to integrate more movement into your daily routine, is the true foundation of using exercise to enhance health. Studies show that daily lifestyle activity can make a dramatic difference to your health and fitness level. So follow our five-step plan to help you activate your life:

1. *Stop viewing exercise as something you can do only at the gym.* There's something terribly wrong with our approach to exercise when we sit on our bottoms pushing buttons all day, then drive to the health club—and fight for the closest parking space—so we can walk on a treadmill for 20 minutes. Or we ride the elevator all day at work, then go to the gym to use the stair-climber. Be aware that *every step you take counts.* Whenever you're faced with an activity "choice point"—like an escalator beside a staircase at the mall—choose to move.

2. *Brainstorm ways you can add movement to your life.* If you usually sit on the sidelines during your child's soccer practice, how about walking laps around the field instead? If you usually telephone co-workers in your building, how about walking to their offices when you need to talk? Be creative and write down a list of as many "moving ideas" as you can.

3. *Every day, for one week, write down how many hours you spend sitting.* You may be surprised to find that you spend most of your waking hours on your behind. List some creative ways to spend some of your "sit time" moving, or at least vertical. For example, "When talking on the phone in my office, I'll stand up." Or, "Instead of watching two hours of TV each night, I'll watch for ninety minutes and play catch with my kids for thirty minutes."

4. *List your top 10 "activation strategies" and 5 "sit less" tactics.* Start integrating them into your life. But recognize that adopting a positive habit like getting active can be as difficult as breaking a bad habit like smoking. So provide some added motivation by giving yourself a point every time you do one of your moving techniques. When you've collected 100 points, give yourself a healthy reward—like a massage, some flowers, a sea-salt bath, or tickets to hear live music or see a play.

5. *Consider using a "step counter."* (They cost about $20 and are available from New Life Styles, at 888-SIT-LESS, and Accusplit, at 800-935-1996.) Clip it on your belt and set a goal to walk ten thousand steps per day. (A sedentary person takes about three thousand.) Check the step counter at midday, and if you haven't taken five thousand steps, plan the rest of your day accordingly.

(For added inspiration, see "25 Ways to Activate Your Life," in Healing Moves for Health and Fitness, page 35.)

PART THREE: RELAXATION EXERCISES

In our stressful society, many people are desperate for a quick fix to their problems. Yet most health conditions defy simplistic answers. Obesity is a complex, multifactorial disease that involves genetics, physiology, and biochemistry as well as environmental, psychosocial, and cultural factors. So an important part of a complete program is taking 5 to 15 minutes each day to do a relaxation exercise geared to helping you center yourself, ease stress, and tune in to the "inner voice" of your body's own wisdom. Overeating—and underexercising—are often related to stress, depression, anxiety, low self-esteem, and unresolved emotions such as grief, anger, and sadness. Exercises that relax body and mind can help you become calmer and better able to adopt new, healthy behaviors. Making a daily ritual out of one or both of these relaxation exercises can help you change negative thoughts, eliminate unhealthy behaviors, assert your needs, and create a sense of clarity and control.

(*Enhancement option:* Turn these exercises into sacred meditation moments by lighting a scented candle or some fragrant incense and/or playing soothing music. Turn off your phone, shut your door, and put out a

"Do Not Disturb" sign. Make sure family members respect your need for 15 minutes of privacy.)

1. Body-Scan Breathing

Lie comfortably on the floor, with a pillow under your head, knees, and/or neck if you want. Place both hands lightly on your abdomen, thumbs resting near your navel. (You may also do this exercise seated, if you wish.) Pay attention to your breathing. Feel your hands rise on each inhalation and fall on each exhalation.

Bring your attention to your forehead and become aware of any muscle tension you feel there. As you breathe in, imagine that you are inhaling golden healing light. As you breathe out, imagine that you're directing this golden healing light to your forehead, where it will erase any tension in the muscles there. Continue this process for several breaths.

When you are ready, move your attention down to your eyes and repeat this process. Imagine that you are inhaling a golden healing light. As you exhale, direct this golden healing light to your eyes, where it will erase any tension in the muscles there. Continue for several breaths, then move your attention to the following body parts and repeat the process in each area:

Mouth and jaw
Neck and shoulders
Spine—from base of skull to tailbone
Right arm, from shoulder to hand
Left arm, from shoulder to hand
Chest
Stomach
Pelvis and buttocks
Right leg, from thigh to ankle
Right foot
Left leg, from thigh to ankle
Left foot
Entire body, from top of the head to the toes

Variations: Try this imagining different colors (instead of the golden healing light)—for example, cool soothing blue, warm strengthening red, soft relaxing green, vibrant energizing orange, or lush nourishing purple. Or try the exercise without imagining colors, just using your breath to smooth out tension.

2. Relaxation Response

Developed by physician Herbert Benson, president of the Mind/Body Medical Institute at Harvard Medical School, this simple, two-step technique prompts a physiologic calming effect that is the opposite of the body's fight-or-flight response to stress. It can be elicited by doing two things:

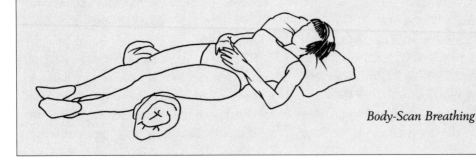

Body-Scan Breathing

1. Repeating a word, sound, or prayer (or doing a repetitive physical activity like walking or running).
2. Gently brushing aside any distracting thoughts to return to your repetition.

You can elicit the relaxation response nearly any time or any place, sitting still or moving. (See the guide to walking meditation, page 101.) But here is a simple, straightforward way to begin practicing it:

1. Pick a focus word or phrase that conforms to your belief system. For example, Catholics might use *Hail Mary, full of grace*, Protestants might use *The Lord is my shepherd*, Jews *Sh'ma Yisrael*, Muslims *Insha'Allah*, Hindus *Om*, and nonbelievers *Nature heals*.
2. Sit quietly in a comfortable position.
3. Close your eyes.
4. Relax your muscles.
5. Breathe slowly and naturally.
6. Mentally repeat your focus word, phrase, or prayer as you exhale.
7. Assume a passive attitude. Don't worry if you're doing this "right."
8. If other thoughts come into your mind, say to yourself, "Oh well," and return to your repetition.
9. Continue for 10 minutes. (Set a timer beforehand, so that you don't have to check a clock.)
10. Open your eyes slowly. Sit quietly for another minute or two, breathing naturally and allowing your normal thoughts to return. (For information on Dr. Benson's two books, see the listings on page 98.)

Building muscle is an important means of boosting your metabolic rate. But if you've been sedentary, it's prudent to wait to begin this muscle-strengthening section until you've been doing the aerobic, lifestyle, and relaxation activities regularly for about three months. (Remember, if you have complications from diabetes, check with your physician before you begin.)

This is an "easy-does-it" strengthening program using relatively light weights; it should be done two or three times a week, with forty-eight hours between workouts. Once you've mastered this workout, you can "graduate" to the more challenging strength-training exercises presented in Healing Moves for Health and Fitness (page 38) and Healing Moves to Strengthen Muscles and Bones (page 141).

1. Shoulder Strengthener

Sit in a chair with your back straight and your feet flat on the floor, about shoulder width apart. Grasp a dumbbell (or a soup can or a sock filled with pennies) in each hand, and hold your hands straight down at your sides, palms facing inward. Slowly lift your arms straight out to the side—to a slow count of 3—until they are parallel to the ground. Hold for one second, then lower your arms to the slow count of 3 until they are straight down by your sides again. Pause for one second, then repeat 10 to 15 times.

2. Biceps Curl

Sit on a bench, stool, or armless chair with your back straight and your feet flat on the floor, shoulder width apart. Hold your hand

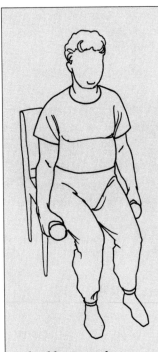
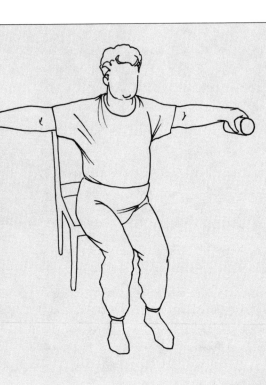

Shoulder Strengthener

weights with your arms down by your side, palms facing in toward your body. Bend your left elbow and lift your hand weight slowly toward your chest to the count of 1, 2, 3, turning your palm so that it faces your chest. Hold for one second, then slowly return to your starting position to the count of 3. Pause for one second, then repeat with your right arm. Alternate until you've done the exercise 10 to 15 times on each side.

3. Toe Raises (Strengthens Calves and Ankles)

Stand tall, with both feet flat on the floor, and lightly rest your fingers on a chair or countertop for balance. Slowly rise up on your toes, counting 1, 2, 3 as you rise up. Hold for one second, then slowly lower yourself down to the count of 3. When this

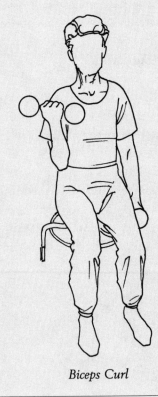

Biceps Curl

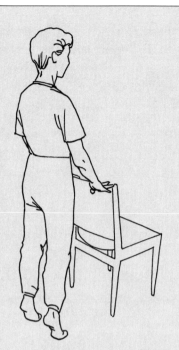

Toe Raises

becomes easy, try it on your right leg only, then your left leg only. When that's easy, try it without holding on to anything for balance.

4. Knee Extension (Strengthens Muscles in the Front of the Leg)

Sit tall in a chair, with your feet flat on the floor, about shoulder-width apart, hands resting lightly on your thighs. Slowly raise your right leg in front of you, to the count of 3, until it's parallel to the floor with your knee straight. Hold your foot in this position to the count of 3, then slowly lower it back to the count of 3. Repeat with your left leg, then alternate legs until you've done the exercise 10 to 15 times with each leg. When this is easy, try the same exercise with a light ankle weight.

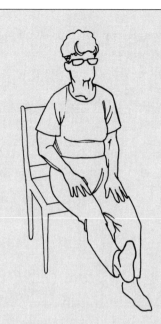

Knee Extension

5. Hip Extension (Strengthens Muscles in the Buttocks and Lower Back)

Stand tall, about an arm's distance away from a chair or countertop, feet about shoulder-width apart. Bend forward from your hips and lightly rest your forearms on the

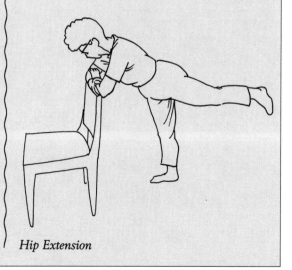

Hip Extension

chair or countertop for balance. From this position, slowly raise your right leg straight behind you—without bending your knee or pointing your toes—to the count of 3. Hold the position for the count of 3, then slowly lower back to the starting position to the count of 3. Repeat with the left leg, then alternate until you've done the exercise 10 to 15 times with each leg. When this becomes easy, try it with a light ankle weight.

3

Mental Health Conditions

STRESS, DEPRESSION, AND ANXIETY

When *Sports Illustrated* magazine asked world-class endurance swimmer Julie Ridge why she started swimming laps during her freshman year at Boston University, she replied: "It was a sanity thing." Like Ridge, most regular exercisers are intimately acquainted with this link between physical activity and psychological well-being. While sedentary people may assume that working out is about *looking good*, habitual exercisers know that working out is largely about *feeling good*. They rely on their physical-activity "fix" not just to strengthen their bodies but also to enhance their minds.

The mood boost of exercise is clear to anyone who has lifted his or her spirits with a simple walk in the fresh air, a dip in the pool, or a game of catch. Children know this instinctively. They run and jump and swing, not because it's good for their heart or lowers their cholesterol but because it's *fun*. Moving your body—the process we've labeled "exercise"—is not merely a mechanical chore. It's a sensual experience of feeling arms and legs surge with energy as they slice through wind and water, and it's a confidence builder that provides the heady thrills of mastery, accomplishment, and control. On a deep, psychological level, exercise can physically connect people with the fundamental joy of being alive. It's a form of "active play" that nourishes the soul.

Grandma knew about this mind-body link when she advised taking out your anger on the woodpile. And in our high-stress society, we've come to sanction slamming tennis balls, shooting hoops, or stepping out for a walk as socially acceptable ways to relieve tension and adjust attitude. Now scientific evidence indicates that telling someone under stress to "take a hike" or "go soak their head" in the swimming pool might actually be good medicine.

A growing body of research shows that physical activity does, indeed, exert a powerful "feel-good" effect that can reduce stress and enhance mental health. "There is some evidence that physical activity may protect against the development of depression," notes the 1996 *U.S. Surgeon General's Report on Physical Activity and Health*. "In general, persons who are inactive are twice as likely to have symptoms of depression than are more active persons."

Exercise also may indirectly enhance mental health by controlling weight, which impacts on self-esteem, and by helping regulate biorhythms, which improves sleep and boosts energy levels, vigor, and cognitive functioning.

Evidence indicates that exercise may be therapeutic for people with more advanced symptoms of depression and anxiety. In a society where clinical depression affects an estimated 10 percent of the population—and carries a $43 billion annual price tag—many experts are embracing the idea of "sweat therapy" as a powerful adjunct to standard treatment—which is typically antidepressant medication and/or psychotherapy. Some research even suggests that, in cases of mild to moderate depression, exercise may be as effective as standard therapies—without the costs or risks.

For many people, exercise may be more acceptable than traditional treatments. Unlike drugs and therapy, exercise is free (or inexpensive), has few side effects, and carries no stigma. And you don't need health insurance to go for a walk or crank up the music and dance.

Easy to administer, readily available, low cost, and low risk, exercise holds great promise as a powerful means of regulating your moods and coping with stress. Studies show that after every aerobic exercise bout, there is at least a temporary period of calm lasting from two to four hours—which means that a workout can literally quiet the storm of a rough day. All this, and the primary side effect is improved fitness!

MENTAL HEALTH BASICS

In our high-speed, high-pressure culture, stress has reached epidemic proportions. Almost 75 percent of Americans say they feel great stress one day a week, and one out of three indicate they feel this way more than twice a week, according to *Prevention* magazine's 1996 "Prevention Index Survey." In contrast, back in 1983, only 55 percent said they felt under great stress on a weekly basis. More than three-quarters of Americans say they live with "a notable amount of stress," reports the American Institute of Stress (AIS) in Yonkers, New York, while 26 percent say they have "a lot of stress" in their lives.

Chronic stress can have a devastating effect on mental and physical health and can lead to life-threatening conditions, such as heart attack, hypertension, and cancer. "Stress has a much more profound effect on cholesterol levels than diet," notes physician Paul J. Rosch, president of the AIS, who offers these distressing stress statistics:

* A 1992 United Nations Report called job stress *the* twentieth-century disease. Today's workers are putting in longer hours and dealing with increased job insecurity and workplace ailments, such as repetitive stress syndrome. Just one in four American workers deemed themselves "extremely satisfied" at work, compared to four in ten in 1973.

* 75 to 90 percent of all visits to primary-care physicians are for stress-related complaints, including headache, backache, insomnia, anxiety, depression, arthritis, herpes, gastrointestinal and skin problems, obesity, alcoholism, and drug abuse.

* An estimated one million people are absent from work on an average workday because of stress-related disorders.

The ability to handle stress is critical to physical *and mental* health, since failure to cope with mental stress can lead to clinical depression. Unlike the occasional lows or "blue moods" that virtually everyone experiences from time to time, clinical depression is a biologically based illness, characterized by extremes in intensity and duration. Clinical depression indicates an imbalance in the brain chemicals called neurotransmitters, and its symptoms include:

* Prolonged sadness or unexplained crying spells
* Significant changes in appetite and/or sleep patterns
* Irritability, anger, worry, agitation, anxiety
* Pessimism, indifference
* Loss of energy, persistent lethargy
* Feelings of guilt, worthlessness
* Inability to concentrate, indecisiveness
* Inability to take pleasure in former interests, social withdrawal
* Unexplained aches, pains
* Recurring thoughts of death or suicide.

Anyone experiencing four or more of these symptoms, persisting for longer than two weeks, should seek help from a medical professional, says the National Depressive and Manic Depressive Association. There is no simple tool, such as a blood test, to confirm clinical depression. However, your doctor may want to conduct tests to rule out other possible causes, such as a thyroid problem, chronic fatigue syndrome, or a brain injury.

Clinical depression is also known as an affective disorder, because it affects a person's mood. Affective conditions, such as depression and anxiety disorder, are among the most frequently reported mental illnesses. More than one in ten adults suffers from a depressive disorder in a given year; between 13 and 17 percent suffer from an anxiety disorder. Depression is associated with suicide, which is the ninth-leading cause of death among Americans.

Genetic, biochemical, and environmental factors can contribute to the onset and progression of depression. Body chemistry can trigger a depressive disorder, as the result of physical changes caused by an illness, altered health habits, substance abuse, or hormonal fluctuations. For example, an estimated 3 to 5 percent of reproductive-age women experience a disabling depressive condition called premenstrual dysphoric disorder, only during the two-week period prior to menstruation. (See section on PMS, page 259.)

Depression also can be triggered by distressing life events, such as the death of a loved one, resulting in an ailment called reactive depression. If these symptoms continue or increase in intensity for more than two weeks, reactive depression may evolve into clinical depression.

Currently, depression is being "seriously undertreated," according to a consensus statement published in the *Journal of the American Medical Association*. Only 20 to 25 percent of people with depression get diagnosed and treated, for a variety of reasons, including the stigma associated with mental illness, failure to recognize the symptoms, and lack of health insurance. Fifteen percent of patients with depression who aren't treated kill themselves. And even among those who do seek treatment, not everyone responds to standard therapies.

This is one reason why an increasing number of health professionals are prescribing exercise as an effective, inexpensive, socially acceptable, safe, and enjoyable way to enhance the mental health of the general population and of people with certain psychiatric conditions, including depression and anxiety disorders. Exercise, however, is not a panacea, and people with mental illnesses should consider physical activity as just one part of their care.

Current research has shown physical activity to have the strongest positive effects on people with affective conditions, such as depression, anxiety, and panic disorders. Less is known about the effects of exercise on severe mental illnesses, such as schizophrenia, dementia, and personality disorders.

RISK FACTORS

In addition to a sedentary lifestyle, sex, age, and genetics may affect your chances of getting a mental illness. Women are twice as likely as men to experience clinical depression, while manic depression affects the sexes equally. Affective disorders are often triggered between the ages of twenty-five and forty-four, although they can occur at any age.

Genetic predisposition to mental health disorders also may play a role, although just because a family member has had a mental illness does not guarantee that you will develop it, too. However, with certain conditions, such as depression, there is an increased likelihood of experiencing the illness when a family member is known to be affected. For this reason, many experts advise individuals with a family history of mental illness to engage in prevention strategies such as regular exercise.

HOW EXERCISE HELPS

While the link between physical activity and psychological well-being is firmly established, the mechanisms by which exercise exerts its feel-good effects are still the subject of intense debate. Popular theories point to exercise's impact on brain chemicals, on body temperature, and on psychosocial factors, such as being with other people or getting away from problems.

One of the most well-known theories is the "endorphin hypothesis." This concept attracted public attention in the mid-1980s, when researchers found that long-lasting aerobic exercise appears to activate the body's natural opioid systems, stimulating the release of morphinelike substances called endorphins that trigger feelings of euphoria and tension relief. This became known as the "runner's high." Since that time, however, research has shown that other brain chemicals also may be involved in the physical-activity feel-good effect, including serotonin and norephinephrine.

Another theory is the "thermogenic hypothesis," which suggests that the temperature elevation caused by exercise relaxes muscles and lowers the level of arousal. Raising body temperature is a centuries-old method of producing a feeling of calm; in Europe, aristocrats "took the cure" by traveling to spas where they soaked in hot mineral waters. The modern equivalent, the five-minute hot shower, is also associated with a significant decrease in anxiety, report researchers from Indiana University. At present, however, the merits of the thermogenic hypothesis are still open to debate.

Some researchers speculate that repetitive, rhythmic physical activity—such as swimming laps or running—may exert a tranquilizing effect on the brain stem and nervous system in a manner similar to rocking a baby. Others note that exercise enhances sleep, allowing people to "recharge their batteries" more fully. In our sleep-deprived society, in which 40 million people suffer from sleep disorders, physical activity can be a welcome sleeping "pill," since studies show that regular exercise helps people go to sleep more easily and also deepens sleep. Fit people typically take less time to fall asleep, awaken less often during sleep, and experience more delta sleep, which is the "deepest sleep of the night, the non-

dreaming sleep that promotes the greatest amount of body recovery," according to Peter Hauri, administrative director of the Mayo Clinic Sleep Disorders Center and author of the book *No More Sleepless Nights*. Since disturbed sleep is both a symptom of depression and an aggravating factor, exercise's beneficial effect on sleep may be important in helping stabilize mood.

In addition to these physiological mechanisms, exercise also has numerous psychological components. The "distraction theory" holds that exercise simply helps people escape temporarily from their problems. Accomplishing a goal, mastering a new skill, interacting socially, or getting away alone are all psychologically based theories about why exercise improves mood. Exercise is generally something people can control, which boosts self-confidence and feelings of competence.

Other factors may also play a role in exercise's mood-elevating effect. People who exercise outdoors may experience the additional lift—and perspective shift—of being surrounded by nature. Exposure to sunlight may be particularly helpful during winter months for people prone to seasonal affective disorder, a condition characterized by depressive symptoms triggered by shorter hours of daylight. And people who exercise to music, which in itself can "soothe the savage breast," may further boost activity's mood-elevating effect.

Some experts propose another intriguing theory, known as the "anthropological hypothesis," to explain both the feel-good effect of exercise and the high incidence of depression in our sedentary society. "Thousands of years ago, our ancestors had to depend on physical activity to survive," says Norwegian psychiatrist Egil Martinsen, who is considered by many to be the world's foremost authority on exercise and depression. "It's only in the last twenty to forty years that we've been able to survive without being active. We know inactivity isn't good for the heart. Perhaps it's not good for the soul, either."

Research into how the brain responds to stress lends support to this hypothesis. Exercise is a stimulus to the body's fight-or-flight system—releasing hormones, raising blood sugar and blood pressure, increasing cardiovascular contractions, and making people feel more alert. Studies at the National Institute of Mental Health show that, in certain kinds of depression that are characterized by lethargy and fatigue, this system appears to be "turned off." Exercising may be a way of voluntarily activating a fight-or-flight system that has become blunted, which may explain why exercise makes people with this condition feel better. Conversely, in another kind of depression, known as melancholic depression, this system is turned up abnormally high. For these people, who are in a state of hyperarousal, exercise may not be as effective.

Some experts speculate that in ordinary, sedentary people, this fight-or-flight mechanism—also known as the "stress system"—may be set too low, possibly because of an exercise deficiency. Our bodies and minds may have evolved to expect a certain stimulus to the stress system conferred by voluntary physical activity. Without adequate exercise, this system—and people's moods—may become depressed. We may need to experience a regular release of these hormones to feel optimally well.

Animal studies show that rats who exercise are more resistant to stress. This leads some researchers to suggest that, since regular exercise is a type of physiologic stress, it may help people develop a more efficient biochemical mechanism for handling life's pressures. Over time, exercisers may develop a kind of "stress hardiness" that protects them from depression.

Turning to exercise to help relieve stress can provide a positive alternative to unhealthy stress relievers like excessive eating, alcohol, cigarettes, or drugs. This is one reason why many drug and alcohol treatment facilities incorporate regular physical activity into their programs, to improve their patients' physical and mental health and offer a practical, life-enhancing means of relieving tension, handling anger, lifting depressing, and getting control of their lives.

Many therapists encourage patients experiencing a variety of mental health problems to get regular exercise, and some have gone one step further by routinely taking patients outdoors to "walk and talk" during sessions. Free of the constraints imposed by sitting formally in a therapist's office and moving together in the fresh air, "people are less defensive and more open," says Keith W. Johnsgard, a therapist in private practice in San Jose, California, and a retired emeritus professor of psychology at San Jose State University. "Exercise is a very powerful in terms of people opening up. They're more likely to express emotions, particularly anger and grief."

A marathon runner and founder of the Fifty-Plus Runner's Association, Johnsgard has been researching and writing about the link between exercise and mood for four decades and believes that physical activity can help a variety of psychological ailments, including addictions, obsessive-compulsive behavior, and phobias. He teaches a class at San Jose State on exercise and mental health and has written a book on the topic.

"There are times when unrelenting depression will not yield to medication, psychotherapy, the support of good friends, or prayer," he writes in *The Exercise Prescription for Depression and Anxiety*. "At these times some of us, as a last resort, turn to sneakers."

The complexity of the exercise-mood connection presents a challenge for researchers, who are studying a broad array of topics in the field, including finding definitive proof that exercise actually *causes* these mood-elevating effects. Although the connection between exercise and psychological well-being is firmly established, conservative scientists caution that further research is needed to prove a cause-and-effect relationship. "Persons who have good mental health may simply be more likely to be active," the surgeon general's report notes.

That people feel better after exercise seems logically simple, yet it's actually a very complex dynamic involving a wide array of factors, including a person's current level of physical conditioning, their mental health status, and their personality traits. For example, if an activity is not tailored to the specific preferences and fitness level of an individual, it may actually *produce* stress rather than relieve it. But people who are allowed to choose exercise forms that they find appealing and meaningful may reap extensive benefits.

In fact, those who come to rely on the mood boost of exercise can find it extremely stressful to go without their regular workout. One study showed that habitual exercisers who were deprived of their regular workout for three days reported a variety of mood disturbances, including tension, depression, anger, fatigue, and confusion.

The wide array of variables affecting people's psychological response to exercise ties into one of the most perplexing questions in the field: "If exercise makes people feel good, why do so many people remain sedentary?" Typically, humans tend to do things that feel good and avoid things that feel bad—an observation Freud called "the pleasure principle." Yet despite exercise's well-documented feel-good effect, the majority of Americans get little or no regular physical activity. And half of all people who start a new exercise program quit within six months.

The reason, suggest some experts, is that *exercise must be purposeful, as opposed to getting on a treadmill to nowhere*. Too many people view exercise as a distasteful chore—especially when it involves monotonous exercise machines and irrelevant activities that aren't likely to sustain their interest. When people's lives were filled with purposeful physical activity—such as splitting wood or raking leaves or walking into town—they didn't have to worry about carving out time to squeeze in a step aerobics class at the health club. This is one reason why public health officials are now encouraging Americans to find physical activities that have meaning in their lives, such as walking with family members or doing yard work, so that exercise comes with a sense of accomplishment that can enhance the health of both body and mind.

EXERCISE ℞

Scientists are still researching the specifics of an exercise prescription for improved mental health, and it appears that rigid guidelines will not play a role. Instead, the most important consideration in prescribing exercise to combat mental stress, enhance mood, and counter feelings of anxiety and depression is this: *Individualize a program that is feasible, flexible, and pleasurable.*

Some people with mental health disorders experience feelings of hopelessness and fatigue that can make exercise seem daunting, and others may be prone to self-blame and guilt if they fail to follow a regimen. That's why it's essential to brainstorm for appealing exercise suggestions and set up a realistic, flexible plan that focuses on making physical activity fun.

Research indicates that intensity may not be an important factor for psychological benefits, and that individuals with clinical depression don't need to exercise hard enough for fitness benefits to experience mental health benefits. This means that virtually any activity that gets someone moving—even slowly—can provide benefits. Both aerobic activities (like walking, running, swimming, and biking) and nonaerobic activities (stretching and weight training) are helpful.

The activity most people find easiest and most pleasurable is walking. Those who need and want social support can arrange to walk with a friend or family member or join a walking group. Those who want solitude can walk alone. Others may wish to get the benefits of companionship without the "human hassles" by walking with a dog. A good goal is to walk for 30 minutes, most days of the week. Start slowly if you've been sedentary, with as little as a 3-minute walk, and gradually work your way up to a half hour. It's critical to hang in there, since greater antidepressant effects are seen when training continues beyond 15 weeks. For mental health, the main work is commitment, not exertion. Make the time, find the time, and the benefits will follow.

Mind-body exercises such as tai chi and yoga can also be extremely helpful for relieving stress. Not only do these activities help unite mind and body, restoring emotional and physiologic balance, but specific yoga poses and tai chi forms are even designed to enhance mental health. (See Healing Moves for Mind-Body-Spirit, page 98.) Consider commiting to a class in these disciplines, or learn some mind-body routines with a personal trainer or an exercise video.

If these ideas aren't appealing—or if you want to vary your program—look for any enjoyable physical activity that you can make a lifestyle habit. Think back to activities you liked as a child and try them: dance, run, skip rope, skate, play Ping-Pong, swing, work in the garden, play basketball, bicycle, or take an active class such as karate, aerobics, line dancing, or group indoor cycling or rowing. People who do an intense workout need not exercise daily. If you're taking a one-hour karate or aerobics class, three times a week is sufficient.

Consider maximizing the "fun factor" by exercising outdoors in the fresh air and sunshine. And, if possible, put on your favorite music while you work out at home, or wear a personal stereo if you exercise in the gym or outside. *But more important than where or when or how you exercise is simply the quality of the experience. Strive for a daily "play break," where you move your body continuously for at least half an hour, doing something you enjoy.*

Be sure to start gently and keep on with it. *Remember: Doing something is better than doing nothing.* Even just being upright, in a vertical position, is preferable to always sitting or lying down.

CAUTIONS

Despite the upbeat effect of exercise, too much of a good thing can have a downside. While regular physical activity appears to boost mental health, excessive exercise can lead to mood disturbances such as loss of libido and appetite, fatigue, and lethargy. Known as overtraining, excessive exercise can be a problem for some competitive athletes, who must learn to walk the fine line between commitment and compulsion.

In addition, a small proportion of recreational athletes take their healthful habit to an unhealthy extreme, becoming "exerholics" who use sport as a way of escaping from their lives. Signs of exercise dependency are continuing with a regular workout despite injury or illness, exercising in risky conditions to avoid missing a workout, and frequently getting complaints from friends or family members about the effect your workout has on them.

For these conditions, cutting back on physical activity can relieve symptoms and restore health. Compulsive exercisers may also find therapy helpful in examining whether they are running *toward* health or running *away* from problems. The key is to find a healthy balance in the ways your physical and emotional needs are met.

PRESCRIPTION PAD

✳ Find an activity you enjoy and will commit the time to do, avoiding excuses.

✳ Start slowly and progress gradually, working toward the goal of being active for 30 minutes a day, most days of the week. (If you pick an intense, longer activity—like a one-hour aerobics class—three days a week is sufficient.)

✳ Create a positive exercise environment. Work out with people if you want company, or alone if you want solitude. Consider exercising outdoors when possible. Add music if you like.

✳ Focus on fun. Don't worry about taking your pulse or working toward some target heart rate. Just enjoy the sensations of moving your body. Breathe deeply and have a good time.

ADDITIONAL RESOURCES

✳ The National Mental Health Association offers referrals to local mental health professionals and information about mental disorders. Call 800-969-NMHA or visit www.nmha.org.

✳ The National Alliance for the Mentally Ill (NAMI) offers help and support for families of those diagnosed with mental illness. Write NAMI, 200 North Glebe Road, #1015, Arlington, Va., call 800-950-NAMI, or visit www.NAMI.org.

✳ The National Depressive and Manic-Depressive Association provides information and services for people with these conditions and their families. Write 730 North Franklin St., Suite 501, Chicago, Ill. 60610-3526, call 800-826-3632, or visit www.ndmda.org.

✳ *The Exercise Prescription for Depression and Anxiety*, by Keith W. Johnsgard, Ph.D. (Plenum Press, 1989).

✳ *The Relaxation Response*, by Herbert Benson, M.D. (Avon, 1976).

✳ *Timeless Healing*, by Herbert Benson, M.D. (Fireside, 1997).

✳ *Relax and Renew: Restful Yoga for Stressful Times*, by Judith Lasater, Ph.D., P.T. (Rodmell Press, 1995).

✳ ✳ ✳

HEALING MOVES FOR MIND-BODY-SPIRIT

✳

Forget about building muscles, strengthening bones, or burning calories. You'll get these *physical* benefits from our mind-body-spirit workout, but consider them merely side effects. The main goal of these healing moves is to enhance your *mental* health, which means that the focus is on building energy, strengthening optimism, burning off stress, and increasing joy.

In fact, forget about "working out" entirely. Instead, think of this as a "play break"—a special, *just-for-you time*, where you move your body doing something you enjoy. The very best way to enhance your mental and spiritual fitness (with the physical fitness side effects) is to *focus on fun*.

This play break is divided into three parts:

Part One: Recess
Consider this a personalized play time where you participate in any form of physical activity that you enjoy.

Part Two: Walking Meditation
Turn an ordinary stroll into a spiritual journey that can enhance body and soul.

Part Three: Mind-Body Practices
These focused breathing exercises drawn from Eastern healing practices are designed to promote a state of mental quietness and physical calm.

These options for inner-directed, holistic exercises all use movement to help integrate body, mind, and spirit and enhance psychological well-being. But more important than the specifics of any exercise you do is *the quality of the experience*. While it's important to develop the discipline to get started and maintain your exercise habit, if you are forcing yourself to exercise, you are missing the point. Grinding your teeth, rushing to get it over with, or pushing yourself harder and harder can defeat the whole purpose. Instead, strive to keep a happy mind-set while you move by focusing not on thin thighs or rock-hard abs but on the sunlight filtering through the trees, the breeze blowing against your face, or your breath moving in and out of your body. Avoid negative, critical "self-talk" about your size, shape, or fitness level, and instead, have an *attitude of gratitude* about your body and all that it does for you. Relish this chance to "actively relax," and let movement help you reconnect with the sacred. As Indian yoga master B. K. S. Iyengar says, "The body is the surface of the mind, and the mind is the surface of the soul."

PART ONE: RECESS

Remember the feeling, as a child, when the school bell rang and joyously released you onto the playground to swing, hang by your knees, kick a ball, or do whatever your little heart—and body—desired? Today, and every day, give yourself permission to have this kind of active recess: 30 to 60 minutes where you can enjoy the sensations of moving your body, breathing deeply, and feeling connected to the world.

This is *your* play break, so pick any activity you enjoy. Start gently and build gradually in an environment you find appealing. Indoors or outdoors, alone or with company, in a class or solo, with music or in silence—it's your choice. Feel free to vary what you do each day, depending on your mood, the weather, and any other factors you find relevant.

A good goal is to work your way up to doing something active for 30 minutes on most days of the week. If you pick an intense activity, such as running, or a longer activity, such as a one-hour aerobics class, three or four times a week is sufficient. *But you must make a commitment to being physically active for a specific amount of time per week, no matter what.* For example, your commitment could be: "I will walk or work in the garden for 30 minutes, every day except Sunday."

Or it could be: "I will take a tai chi class on Tuesdays and Thursdays and ride my bike on the other days of the week."

Activities with repetitive motion, such as swimming, walking, and running, can be particularly effective in enhancing mental health since their rhythmic quality prompts a meditative effect. Activities that focus on breathing, such as tai chi and yoga, can connect body and mind and enhance feelings of calm. If you're not sure what activity you'd like to do during your recess, here's a rundown of popular choices:

1. **Walking.** The most popular physical activity in the nation, walking is an effective, flexible, and fun activity. You can walk outdoors in the fresh air or indoors on a treadmill, alone or with a pet or a friend. You can move as slowly or as quickly as you want, join a walking club, or strut solo. (For step-by-step instructions on starting a walking program, see Healing Moves for Heart Health, page 214.)

2. **Gardening.** People enjoy gardening so much that they often don't think of it as exercise. But raking, planting, pitching mulch, weeding, and all the other varied activities you do in the garden are a wonderful way to work your body. Plus, the close contact with nature's beauty "works" your spirit and provides a therapeutic value all its own.

3. **Swimming.** One of swimming's main attractions is its Zen of quiet, meditative tranquillity—back and forth, back and forth—that lets your mind float off to peaceful levels of creativity and well-being. Released from 90 percent of your

body weight and sometimes freed from physical limitations that make land movement difficult, you may find water exercise uniquely calming and refreshing. Add interest with "pool toys" for grown-ups, such as swim fins, flotation belts for water walking, webbed gloves, or foam "water weights."

4. **Cycling.** It's impossible to feel old while pedaling a bicycle, and it's a great way to rediscover the wind-in-your-face thrill of the sport you enjoyed as a child. A non-weight-bearing activity, cycling is kinder to the knees and ankles than high-impact activities like running. You can also cycle indoors on a stationary bicycle.

5. **Group fitness classes.** Aerobics class is just one option in the booming fitness world, where exercise professionals prefer the name "group fitness classes" to avoid the old-fashioned stereotype of leotard-clad ladies prancing to peppy music. At most health clubs and YMCAs you can choose from a broad array of diverse classes, such as cardio-kickboxing, group weight training, body sculpting, and a host of aerobic-style classes done to specialized music ranging from gospel to funk.

6. **Dance.** Swing dance, square dance, line dance, ballet, tap, hula, belly dance, folk dance, African dance. Take lessons at a local studio, go to clubs or rec centers that sponsor dances, or simply turn on the music and dance in the privacy of your own home—with or without a partner.

7. **Martial arts,** such as karate and tae kwon do, are excellent ways to heighten self-esteem and build confidence, which can enhance peace of mind. In particular, **tai chi chuan,** one of the "soft" martial arts, is especially helpful for people with mental health conditions because it emphasizes emotional tranquillity. Proponents of this two-thousand-year-old art say it conditions the nervous system and encourages feelings of calm and serenity. Tai chi is best learned under the guidance of a qualified instructor. To find one, check the telephone directory under tai chi or martial arts, or contact area health clubs, martial arts studios, yoga studios, senior centers, or university Asian studies departments.

8. **Yoga.** Over the last decade, a growing number of Americans have begun stretching their bodies and their minds with this more than five-thousand-year-old Indian art. *Yoga* means union, and the discipline's ultimate goal is to unify one's being with the cosmos. The physical form of yoga known as hatha yoga was created to squeeze all the tension out of the body so that practitioners could sit still to meditate. Disciplined breathing creates a bridge between body and mind, calms our constant mental "chatter," and enhances feelings of well-being and energy. Like tai chi, yoga is best learned from a qualified instructor. To find one, consult the phone directory for yoga studios or contact health clubs or university-based wellness centers.

9. **Strength training.** Nearly 40 million Americans exercise with weights, at home or in a club. If you choose to use a club, try several to find one where you feel comfortable. Get expert guidance to start, since proper technique can help you

enhance effectiveness and avoid injury. Once you learn proper technique, which usually takes only a few sessions, you'll be able to "pump iron" on your own.

10. **In-line skating.** One of the reasons why in-line skating is among America's fastest-growing sports is that flying along on skates is incredibly fun. It's easy, too, if you stay on level ground, such as an empty parking lot or school track. Beginners might want to take a few lessons—for referral to a certified instructor call the International In-Line Skate Association (800-56-SKATE).

There are countless other choices for "recess" activities, including tennis, racquetball, basketball, volleyball, running, skiing, rowing, hiking, rock climbing, skipping rope, fencing, golf, ice skating, trampolining, and handball—to name a few. To ensure that your recess stays fun, remember to:

1. Start slowly, progress gradually, and don't overdo it. (See Pre-Participation Checklist, page 29.)
2. Be committed. Don't expect your play break to "just happen"—you must schedule it into your day. Plan your recess for a time that works best for you: first thing in the morning to start your day off right, at lunchtime as a welcome break from work, or after work as a tension reliever. If your days are extremely busy, don't try to squeeze exercise in without taking something else out. For example, instead of taking an hour lunch, take a half-hour lunch and a half-hour walk.
3. Be aware of what competition means for you. If you find a meditative atmosphere

more enjoyable, pick noncompetitive activities, such as yoga, cycling, or gardening. If you love a competitive activity but experience anxiety and stress about winning, do the activity without keeping score. If you love the camaraderie of competition, join a league or organized group in your favorite sport.
4. Pick times when you won't be crowded. Sharing a lap lane with five other people can interfere with swimming's mood-enhancing effect.
5. Choose a positive exercise environment. Just as fresh air and music can enhance your activity, mirrors may detract from your experience if you tend to be self-critical. If so, enjoy your recess in a mirror-free room.
6. Consider taking a few sessions with a personal trainer if you need some help getting started. (For a referral to a trainer certified by the American Council on Exercise, call the consumer hotline at 800-529-8227.)
7. Keep it regular. Once you get in the habit, skipping recess can become stressful.
8. If you need the support of another person to ensure that you take your daily recess get a buddy. Enlist the aid of a friend or family member to help.
9. Don't rush from recess back to routine. Take at least a few minutes to enjoy feeling relaxed. Allow time for a cool drink and, if possible, a warm shower.

PART TWO: WALKING MEDITATION

We walk all day—in our homes, along city streets and country roads, around our offices. Yet most of the time when we are walking, we're lost in the past or worried about the future. But when we focus our thoughts on simply walking, staying mindful of being in the present moment, an extraordinary "antistress" effect occurs. Harvard Medical School cardiologist Herbert Benson calls it the "relaxation response," a term he coined more than twenty years ago to describe a state of bodily calm in which blood pressure is lowered and heart rate, breathing rate, and metabolic rate are all decreased. The relaxation response is the physiologic opposite of the stress response, in which the body "revs up" for fight or flight. During the relaxation response, the body "calms down," which yields many immediate and long-term health benefits. (For information about Dr. Benson's books see Additional Resources, page 98.)

At Harvard's Mind/Body Medical Institute, where Benson is president, patients learn to elicit the relaxation response with simple mental focusing or meditation techniques, such as walking meditation. Benson's research shows that performing a focused exercise activates the relaxation response: When you exercise and simultaneously focus your mind, your exercise becomes more efficient—that is, you require less energy to do physical work. In addition, his studies show that focused walking is associated with reduced anxiety and diminished negative thoughts. Joggers who use relaxation-response techniques may achieve in the first mile the "runner's high" that otherwise occurs in the third or fourth mile.

While music may be an enhancement to exercise, watching TV or reading a magazine while walking on a treadmill distracts you from the total mind-body experience of the movement. Try replacing these distractions with a meaningful word or phrase whose repetition can be tied to the inhalation-exhalation cycle of your breathing, like a mantra used during meditation. To elicit the relaxation response as you walk, pick a focus word that has meaning to you. You might want to pick a secular word like *ocean*, *love*, *peace*, *calm*, or *thanks*. Or you might prefer a religious phrase, such as *The Lord is my shepherd* (Protestant), *Sh'ma Yisrael* (Jewish), *Hail Mary, full of grace* (Catholic), *Insha'Allah* (Islamic), or *Om* (Hindu).

As you walk, repeat your focus word or phrase to yourself in a rhythmic cadence that fits comfortably with your breathing and movement. For example, every time you step with your left foot, you can say the word *calm* to yourself. Or you can mentally recite *The Lord is* when you step with your left foot and *my shepherd* when you step with your right foot. Experiment with phrases, words, and pace until you find a rhythm that's comfortable for you. If other thoughts come into your head while you're walking, let them pass through and return to your word or phrase.

Another way to perform a walking meditation is to simply focus on your breathing. Pay attention to its rhythm and adjust your pace to the flow of air in and out of your body. For example, breathe in during your first four steps and breathe out during your next four steps, continuing on so that you're inhaling for four steps and exhaling for four steps. On each step say "in, in, in, in," to yourself, then "out, out, out, out." Or count, "One, two, three, four. One, two, three, four," or repeat your personal phrase in rhythm with your inhalation and exhalation. If you walk uphill or downhill and need to inhale more or exhale more, do so. *Don't try to control your breathing; simply notice it as you continue to walk.* If you want to take three steps on your inhalation and four steps on your exhalation, that's fine, too.

The purpose of walking meditation "is to enjoy each step," writes Vietnamese Zen master Thich Nhat Hahn in his classic guide to mindful meditation *Peace Is Every Step.* "Walking meditation is really to enjoy the walking—walking not in order to arrive, but just to walk."

In his pocket guide to walking meditation, *The Long Road Turns to Joy*, he writes: "Walking meditation is like eating. With each step, we nourish our body and our spirit. When we walk with anxiety and sorrow, it is a kind of junk food. The food of walking meditation should be of a higher quality. Just walk slowly and enjoy a banquet of peace."

You can practice walking meditation anywhere—between meetings, on your way to the car, going up the stairs. Every path can be a walking meditation path as long as you give yourself some time to practice. This means that instead of allotting yourself the three minutes it takes to rush from your car to your office, give yourself ten minutes and enjoy the process. Try to do a walking meditation each day, even if it's just from your front door to the mailbox and back. Before a big meeting, giving yourself five minutes to take some mindful steps may clear your mind and help you relax and focus on the subject at hand.

Here are some ideas to enhance your walking meditation:

1. *Smile*. It doesn't have to be a big grin—just a small, effortless Mona Lisa smile. Smiling relaxes the muscles of your face, refreshes you, and transmits joy to those you meet. Although it sounds simple, or even silly, mindfully adding a smile to the end of a breath has profound effects.
2. *Keep your mind in the present*. If past anxieties or future worries pop into your head, gently dismiss them and return your mind to the present moment.
3. *Feel free to stop to look at something beautiful*—leaves changing color, a bird flying, children playing. But as you look, continue to follow your breathing.
4. *Imagine that in every one of your footsteps, a flower blooms*. Remember, each step is a miracle.
5. *Carry yourself with dignity*, an upright posture, and an expression of calm joy—as if you were royalty—because you are.
6. *Don't worry if you're doing your walking meditation "right."* If you feel peace and joy while you're walking, you're practicing properly.

Walking isn't the only form of physical activity that you can turn into a moving meditation. Exercise in any form can help you enter a meditative state, particularly if it's a rhythmic exercise like running, swimming, or cycling. Just as some Native American cultures use dance to commune with the spirit world and some Islamic sects have dervishes whirl to experience the divine, you can use nearly any physical activity as a powerful spiritual tool if you *focus on the experience of movement* and *stay in the present moment*. The key is to concentrate on your breathing and being present in your body—not allowing your mind to wander off to dinner plans or worrying about the oil light in your car.

Qi Gong. In the early-morning darkness, millions of people gather in parks throughout China to practice an ancient self-healing art called qi gong. As the first rays of sun lighten the sky, men and women of all ages begin moving in graceful patterns. Sometimes alone and sometimes in groups, they perform rhythmic, symmetrical motions, accompanied by deep controlled breathing, to center and balance their bodies, connect with their vital energy, and direct this energy to achieve maximum health. A form of traditional Chinese medicine, which recognizes the healing power of movement, qi gong is used in China to treat a variety of illnesses, including depression. Tai chi is a form of qi gong and was the one branch of the art not banned during China's cultural revolution.

The following qi gong invigorated-breathing technique, called *ch'iang chuang kung*, can be helpful for people with depression because it "turns off" anxious thoughts and helps people achieve a state of mental quietness known as *ju ching*.

Ch'iang Chuang Kung: Invigorated Breathing

1. Sit straight on a stool or chair with both feet firmly on the ground shoulder width apart. Your knees should form a ninety-degree angle and your thighs and trunk should also form a ninety-degree angle.

2. Rest your hands, palms down, gently on your legs, letting your elbows bend naturally. Relax your shoulders. Let your chin drop slightly inward. Keep your eyes partially closed. Let your lips come together naturally and your tongue lightly touch the roof of your mouth.

3. Begin to breathe naturally, in and out, through your nose. Try to make your breath soundless, smooth, and steady, letting the inhalation and exhalation be the same length. You may find it helpful to mentally count to five when you inhale, then to five again when you exhale. If your thoughts stray from your breathing, gently call them back to your breath.

4. Continue breathing and, without forcing, invite your consciousness to focus on your body's energy center in your lower abdomen. Called the *tan tien*, it is approximately three inches below your navel.

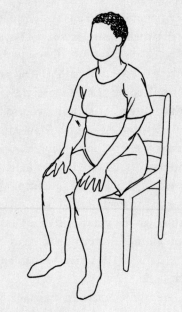

Ch'iang Chuang Kung

5. Let your breathing become longer and deeper, keeping your inhalations and exhalations the same length. Gradually work toward reducing the number of your breathing cycles (inhalations and exhalations) to six to eight per minute.

6. When you feel ready, instead of counting silently, recite a word or phrase that has meaning to you. For example, you could think of the word *slow* on the inhalation and *relax* on the exhalation, or mentally recite words from a prayer or poem you find nourishing.

7. Practice *ch'iang chuang kung* anytime you feel stressed, and build it into your daily routine. For example, do this invigorated breathing when you first sit down at your desk each morning or as the last thing you do before you go home. With practice, even a single, mindful breath may become a powerful tool of relaxation and joy.

Yoga. As described in the earlier section on "recess," yoga can be an effective antidote to the stress of modern life because it is designed to unify mind, body, and spirit and help the individual connect with the life force of the universe. Central to yoga practice is the relaxation pose called *savasana*, or the corpse pose. While it seems simple, it is among the most difficult poses to master because it requires you to let go of physical tension, quiet your mind, and be present in the moment.

Savasana: The Corpse Pose

1. Lie down on the floor on your back as if you were dead. Keep your heels together, but let your toes fall gently apart. Rest your arms by your sides a little away from your thighs, with your palms up. If you like, place a rolled blanket or towel under your knees to ease your back. You may also place a folded blanket under your head and eyebags on your eyes.

2. Mentally scan your body for tension, from head to toe, and release any muscles that are gripping or tight. Be sure to relax your jaw and teeth, shoulders, neck and back, arms and hands, legs and feet, eyes and brain. Allow your muscles to become heavy and drop away from your bones, where their weight will be accepted by the floor. Let your face be soft and open as that of a child.

3. When you begin to feel relaxed, observe your breathing. Are the inhalations and exhalations the same length? Are you breathing through both nostrils? Is your breathing quiet or noisy?

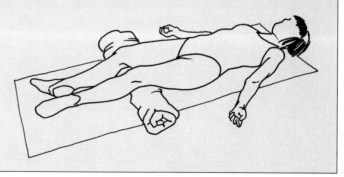

Savasana

4. As you focus on your breath, don't lose the awareness of your relaxation. Avoid the temptation to tighten any muscles or be self-critical. Merely observe your breath and be aware of keeping your muscles relaxed. (If you find it difficult to focus on your breath, try focusing on the beating of your heart.)

5. Stay in the moment. If thoughts intrude, observe them without judgment "at a distance" and bring your mind back to its focus on your breath.

6. If you want, take a long, slow inhalation that is quiet and smooth. Follow this with a long, slow exhalation, then several normal breaths. Repeat this cycle as you relax.

7. Remain in this pose for 5 to 20 minutes. When you are ready to come out, roll onto one side. Gradually open your eyes and rest in this position. Then push against the floor with your arms and hands to get into a sitting position. Stay there for a few breaths before standing up and returning to "reality."

8. Practice this pose in times of stress, and at the end of exercise sessions. Try scheduling a "savasana break" into your day—or week—at a time you find convenient, such as right after lunch, when you get home from work, or on Sunday afternoons.

4

Orthopedic Disorders

ARTHRITIS

When people have arthritis, it often hurts them to move, so many people with the disease stop moving. But inactivity can be crippling—literally—for people with any form of this common disease. Inactivity sets off a vicious cycle: unused muscles and joints become weak, leading to increased pain, immobility, and joint damage. This makes it even harder to move, and the muscles get even weaker. Sedentary living also leads to other health problems, including depression, osteoporosis, and increased risk of heart disease. And reduced mobility often prompts weight gain, which can worsen the symptoms of osteoarthritis, a degenerative joint condition that is the most common form of the disease.

A generation ago, people suffering from arthritis were sent to bed—sometimes for as long as six months—in an effort to "save their joints." Unfortunately, that practice did more harm than good, since, as we now know, inactivity causes arthritic joints to stiffen and unused muscles to atrophy. When sedentary people became weak and disabled, they assumed it was an inevitable result of their disease.

In the mid-1980s, scientists began challenging the assumption that arthritis itself caused most of the disability suffered by people with the disease. Researchers began studying the effects of exercise on people with arthritis to determine how much of their loss in function actually came from inactivity and deconditioning.

The results have been stunning. Study and after study shows that people with arthritis who exercise regularly report less pain and joint swelling, improved functioning, and increased strength, endurance, and flexibility—without harming their joints. The psychological benefits are also dramatic, with exercisers experiencing less depression and anxiety and greater feelings of control.

That's why, in recent years, there's been a dramatic turnaround in the recommendations about exercise for people with arthritis. "We've come from thinking that physical fitness was impossible for people with arthritis to knowing that exercise is one of the best ways to help most people control their disease and improve their health," says pioneering researcher Marian Minor, an associate professor of physical therapy at the University of Missouri and co-director of the university's Arthritis Rehabilitation Research and Training Center.

Today, numerous public health groups have launched campaigns to encourage people with arthritis to get moving. The Centers for Disease Control and Prevention (CDC) issued a report in May 1997 to quash the "mistaken belief that persons with arthritis should not exercise." Exercise strengthens muscles to better support and protect joints affected by arthritis, says the CDC, which notes that exercise also can "reduce the risk of premature death, heart disease, diabetes, high blood pressure, colon cancer, overweight, depression and anxiety." The *U.S. Surgeon General's 1996 Report on Physical Activity and Health* also urges people with arthritis to exercise because "regular physical activity can help control joint swelling and pain." And the American Academy of Orthopedic Surgeons, in its "Keep Moving for Life" campaign, says, "Exercise is very important for people with arthritis. Exercise keeps the joints flexible, the muscles around

the joints strong, bone and cartilage tissue strong and healthy and reduces pain." The benefits are so dramatic that the Arthritis Foundation's theme for 1998, its fiftieth-anniversary year, was "Make this the year you become active."

ARTHRITIS BASICS

Arthritis, which literally means joint inflammation, refers to more than one hundred different diseases that affect the joints and the tissues around the joints, such as muscles and bones. Nearly 40 million Americans, or one in seven, have arthritis, says the Arthritis Foundation, a national nonprofit agency that supports research and provides community-based programs for people with the disease.

The prevalence of arthritis increases rapidly after age forty-five, and nearly half of all people with the disease are sixty-five or older. As baby boomers age, the number of Americans with arthritis is expected to swell to 59.4 million—nearly one in five—by the year 2020. The main cause of disability in America, it frequently limits people's everyday activities, such as dressing, climbing stairs, and walking. And half of those who suffer from the disease don't think anything can be done to help them.

Yet regular exercise is one of the best ways to keep the joints in working order, boost overall health, and, in some cases, prevent further damage. For example, results of the Fitness Arthritis and Seniors Trial, published in the *Journal of the American Medical Association* in January 1997, concluded that "exercise is a safe and effective nonpharmacological therapy that improves both pain and function in older people with osteoarthritis of the knee." The eighteen-month study of 365 senior adults with osteoarthritis of the knee found that participants who exercised showed significant improvements in tests of physical performance (such as climbing stairs, getting in and out of a car, and lifting and carrying ten pounds) compared with seniors in a health-education group who did not exercise. Seniors in the exercise groups also scored better on assessments of physical disability and self-reported knee pain.

"In general, exercise is good for virtually all kinds of arthritis," says rheumatologist Rowland Chang, a professor at Northwestern University Medical School and co-director of the Arthritis Center at the Rehabilitation Institute of Chicago. "We know now that most people with arthritis can achieve substantial reduction in pain and increase in functioning by participating in a regular exercise program."

But since people with arthritis often hurt so much that getting out of bed in the morning is a challenge, the prospect of starting an exercise program typically seems daunting. "The trick," Chang admits, "is trying to convince people that exercise will help."

HOW EXERCISE HELPS

One of the strongest motivators in getting people with arthritis up and moving is explaining the dire consequences of inactivity. "Use it or lose it" is true for virtually all human functions, but that principle can be forgiving when people are young and healthy. When people have arthritis, however, they can lose functioning extremely rapidly if they don't exercise. Muscles can atrophy very quickly, and joints that aren't used can become "frozen," sometimes within days or weeks.

This weakening of muscles and bones is the single biggest determinant of who winds up in nursing homes, according to research done at the Thurston Arthritis Research Center at the University of North Carolina at Chapel Hill. It's not Alzheimer's disease or a heart attack or stroke that lands most people in institutions. It's bones and joints and letting your muscles get nonfunctional.

Yet many people—including some physicians—still haven't heard the new message that exercise can keep people with arthritis from spiraling into decrepitude. "The most common reason people over sixty-five give for not being active isn't heart disease or diabetes or poor vision, it's arthritis," says Marian Minor. That's why people with arthritis need both *specific therapeutic exercises*—to maintain flexibility and strength in affected joints and muscles—and *general exercise* to maintain their overall health. Exercise boosts both physical and mental fitness, says physician Doyt Conn, senior vice president of medical affairs for the Arthritis Foundation. "After two to three months of exercising, most people report less pain, anxiety, and depression," he notes. "Exercise helps people take charge of their condition."

EXERCISE ℞

To achieve the best results, a person with arthritis should get a physician's referral to a physical therapist who can design an individualized exercise program that takes into account the kind of arthritis, the affected joints, and the person's overall conditioning. Most insurance companies will pay for at least three visits to a physical therapist for assessment and exercise instruction. It's also important to consult a physician for a specific diagnosis of the type of arthritis, since some forms can be treated with medication that may halt the progression of the disease.

In general, people with arthritis need a balanced fitness program consisting of three kinds of exercises: range of motion, endurance, and strength:

A. *Range of motion (flexibility) exercises.* These exercises help reduce stiffness and keep joints flexible by taking them through a full range of motion, which is the normal distance your joints can move in certain directions. Daily activities, such as housework or climbing stairs, do not move your joints through their full range of motion. So it's important to do these exercises once or twice *every day.* If your joints are painful and swollen, move them gently through their range of motion. But be sure to move them daily. If you don't, they are likely to become stiff.

B. *Endurance exercise.* Sometimes called aerobic exercise, because it demands large quantities of oxygen for a prolonged period of time, endurance exercise strengthens the heart and lungs. Like anyone interested in good health, people with arthritis need to accumulate 30 minutes of aerobic activity each day to reduce their risk of chronic diseases such as diabetes, heart disease, and certain cancers. In addition, regular endurance exercise boosts mood, improves sleep, reduces

stress, and helps manage weight—all critical for people with arthritis.

People with arthritis should choose endurance activities that do not jar their affected joints. Typically, this means selecting low-impact activities such as walking or line dancing, and picking environments or equipment that reduces the load on affected joints, such as water exercise in a warm pool or stationary bicycling. Avoid high-impact activities that involve abrupt stopping and starting and any sudden changes of direction that cause pain.

If you've been inactive, be sure to start slowly, with as little as 3 to 5 minutes of your chosen activity, preferably several times a day. Add a few more minutes to your exercise bouts each week, with the goal of being able to exercise continually for 30 minutes per day. When you can continue moving for 30 minutes, you can gradually increase the intensity if you wish. Strive to exercise at a moderate intensity, where your heart rate and breathing accelerates some but you can still comfortably carry on a conversation.

Be sure to start out exercising slowly, with a good warm-up of at least 10 minutes, since studies show that as body temperature rises, so does the range of motion of your joints. One of the best ways to warm up is to do your chosen activity at a low level. So if you're planning on taking a brisk walk, start with an easy stroll. If you're going for a swim, bob around gently in the water first and gradually ease yourself into your laps.

Here are guidelines for some of the

most popular activities for people with arthritis.

Walking: Find a flat, even surface such as a school track, sidewalk, or mall. Avoid gravel roads or unplowed fields since uneven surfaces can be stressful on the leg joints. Be sure to wear good supportive athletic shoes.

Water exercise: Swimming and aqua-aerobics are excellent choices for people with arthritis, since water helps support your body, so there is less stress on your hips, knees, and spine. Be sure to exercise in warm water, with a temperature between 83 and 90 degrees, in a depth that's at least midchest, so that your weight is supported by the water. If you want to exercise in a shallow pool, do your movements while sitting. In a deep pool, use an inflatable tube or vest.

Some people with arthritis in their hands and wrists find that disposable surgical gloves offer added warmth and comfort. Wearing a T-shirt, wet suit, or spandex leggings may also help. Swimmers with neck pain can try using a snorkel and mask, so that they don't have to turn their head from side to side to breathe. After you leave the pool, take a warm shower or sit in a hot tub.

Stationary bicycling: A good choice for people who want to avoid putting too much stress on their hips, knees, and feet, stationary bicycling should be started slowly, with beginners careful not to pedal faster than 15 to 20 miles per hour (or 50 to 60 revolutions per minute). If you have knee problems, use minimal to no resistance. Adjust the seat height so it allows your knee to straighten comfortably on the downstroke.

Group exercise classes: Check with your local YMCA, health club, or senior center for special "arthritis exercise" classes, such as the Arthritis Foundation's PACE (People with Arthritis Can Exercise) Program. (Check the resources section at the end of this chapter for the phone number of the Arthritis Foundation, which will refer you to classes in your area.) Both land and water classes are offered by certified instructors who typically incorporate flexibility, aerobic, and strengthening exercises in each session. In addition to providing a safe and effective workout under the guidance of an informed leader, they also foster camaraderie and support among participants.

Tai chi: This ancient martial art has been used in China as an exercise for older individuals for three centuries and is now undergoing an explosion of interest in the United States for its ability to help seniors become stronger and reduce their risk of falls. The practice is well suited to seniors because it is geared to generating energy through slow, carefully choreographed movements that stretch and strengthen all the muscles in the body. Be sure to study under an experienced, well-qualified teacher who understands your condition and any specific joint problems you have. Don't compare yourself with others in the class. Focus on your own body and the signals it sends you. And remember to keep breathing along with your movements—never hold your breath.

C. *Strengthening exercises:* The idea of people with arthritis "pumping iron" is very new. But several recent studies indicate that resistance exercises with weights may be helpful, with rheumatoid arthritis in particular. "High-intensity strength training is feasible and safe in patients with well-controlled RA (rheumatoid arthritis) and leads to significant improvements in strength, pain and fatigue without exacerbating disease activity or joint damage," notes an article published in the April 1996 issue of *Arthritis Care and Research,* a journal of the American College of Rheumatology.

But any exerciser—with or without arthritis—must do resistance exercises with weights properly to achieve benefits and avoid injury. For people with arthritis, expert instruction is especially critical because good technique is essential. So before you lift, be sure to:

✳ Check with your physician for individualized guidelines. Ask about referral to a physical therapist, occupation therapist, or qualified athletic trainer for expert instruction. (See the resources section at the end of this chapter for groups that can make referrals.)

✳ Use any type of resistance device that's available and comfortable for you, such as exercise machines, free weights, elastic bands, rubber tubing, or resistive water devices (such as webbed gloves).

✳ Start very easily, with no or small weights, and increase very gradually. Your goal is to work out with a weight you can lift at least ten times without being too tired (if you can't, it's too heavy).

✳ Do eight to ten exercises using the large muscle groups in the body, two to three times a week. But don't lift on consecutive days, since your muscles need a day to rebuild.

If you don't have access to weights, or if your doctor tells you not to use them, you may still be able to strengthen your muscles through isometric exercises, in which you push or pull against a fixed object. (See Healing Moves to Strengthen Muscles and Bones, page 138.)

CAUTIONS

Be sure to discuss your exercise plans with your physician or other health-care provider. Remember that even if you don't feel like moving, getting active will help you break the cycle of pain, stiffness, immobility, and joint damage.

If you experience a "flare," where your joints are red, hot, and swollen, don't try to stick to your regular strengthening and aerobic routine. Switch to easy range-of-motion exercises and daily-life activities until the flare is under control. Avoid the temptation to skip movement entirely, since immobility leads to stiff joints and weak muscles. As always, the balance between exercise and rest is critical, so respect the flare by getting adequate rest, but keep moving with gentle flexibility exercises.

Like all exercisers, people with arthritis need to listen to their bodies and heed signals that tell them when they're doing too much or not doing enough. This is an individual matter, and it's important to find personal cues that indicate when you need to push yourself a little harder and when you need to back off. When in doubt, go easy and seek advice from a qualified fitness specialist, such as an exercise instructor certified by the Arthritis Foundation (see resources section at the end of this section.)

Some soreness may be an inevitable part of starting up a new activity and using muscles that have been inactive. But one good rule of thumb for people with arthritis is this:

If exercise causes pain that lasts more than ninety minutes after you've stopped exercising, you are probably either doing an inappropriate activity for you or using improper technique. Work with your doctor or physical therapist to adjust your program.

You can try applying heat to sore joints or muscles before you exercise and icing them after exercise. But be aware that if you have swelling or pain and have to ice afterward, you may be doing too much.

Try exercising at different times of the day until you find what works best for you. Some people find that doing range-of-motion exercises first thing in the morning helps them loosen up for the day's activities, while others find they're too stiff when they get out of bed and prefer exercising later in the day or before going to sleep.

PRESCRIPTION PAD

1. Do *range-of-motion exercises* once or twice each day, particularly for your affected joints. If your joints are very painful and swollen, be sure to move them gently through their full range of motion. If you are having an active "flare"—where joints are red, hot, and swollen—do only range-of-motion exercises.

2. Gradually build up to doing an *endurance activity*—such as walking or water aerobics—30 minutes, most days of the week. Be sure to warm up and cool down adequately and finish off with gentle stretching.

3. Do eight to ten *strengthening exercises* for the body's major muscle groups two to three times a week—but no more frequently than every other day. Pay special attention to working the muscles that support your affected joints.

4. Be sure to warm up adequately by doing your activity at a low, easy level and performing some easy range-of-motion exercises.

5. After exercising, cool down for 5 to 10 minutes so that your heart rate can slow down and your muscles can relax. Finish with some gentle stretching.

6. Find an activity you enjoy that's comfortable. Remember, doing something is better than doing nothing.

7. Ask your health-care provider to refer you to a physical therapist who can give you an individualized exercise program that takes into account the type of arthritis, the affected joints, and your level of conditioning.

✳ The Arthritis Foundation offers numerous publications about arthritis, many of them free, and gives referrals to exercise classes in your community. Call 800-283-7800 or visit the Web site: www.arthritis.org. To purchase exercise videotapes created for people with arthritis and related conditions, such as fibromyalgia, call 800-207-8633.

✳ The National Arthritis and Musculoskeletal and Skin Diseases Information Clearinghouse, a public service of the National Institute of Arthritis and Musculoskeletal and Skin Diseases, provides information and public education materials. Call 301-495-4484 or visit the Web site: www.nih.gov/niams/.

BACK PAIN

"You are as young as your spine," say the yoga masters, who consider a strong and properly aligned backbone the key to good health. Millions of Americans who suffer from chronic back pain are likely to agree. Few ailments can make you feel older faster than a bad back.

Today, back pain is second only to the common cold as the nation's most prevalent affliction. Stress, sedentary lifestyles, poorly designed work sites, expanding waistlines, and bad posture have resulted in a back pain epidemic from which, it seems, no one is immune. Yet most back pain could be eliminated, experts say, through regular exercise and proper body mechanics. Once people learn how to sit, stand, lift, and move prop-erly—and do some simple but regular exercises to stay in shape—most can kiss their back pain good-bye.

In fact, some experts speculate that the reason back pain is so common in our society is that the vast majority of Americans are sedentary. Sedentary living typically results in excess weight and weak, inflexible muscles, which are primary contributors to back injury and pain. Muscles need to be relaxed, flexible, and strong to support your back and get you through a busy day. That's why, when back pain strikes—as it will for up to 80 percent of American adults—it's generally better to be active than to take to your bed.

This is a dramatic change from the traditional thinking on back pain, which advocated strict bed rest for one or two weeks, followed by limitations on activities. New research shows that excessive bed rest can actually *cause* back pain and makes most kinds of back pain worse. Regular exercise, however, can help cure back pain and prevent recurrence.

If you suffer from chronic back pain, it's essential to avoid long periods of inactivity. Inactivity can delay recovery by stiffening and weakening muscles, while exercise can promote healing by strengthening muscles, alleviating swelling, and improving hydration of spinal discs. These discs have no blood supply and are the largest nonvascular tissue in the body. For this reason, some experts consider spinal discs the "weak link" in the musculoskeletal system. Physical activity acts as a kind of pump to promote the exchange of fluids, improving nutrition of the cells and removing wastes and cell by-products.

In rare cases, however, bed rest may be indicated. If your back pain comes from an impact injury or a fall or is accompanied by fever or pain radiating down your arm or leg, consult a physician. He or she may prescribe medications to combat swelling and pain or direct you to a physical therapist for a variety of treatments, including heat, cold, or ultrasound. Surgery is the treatment of choice for only a very small percentage of back problems, and conservative measures should be tried first unless there's some imminent risk of neurological damage.

The best advice for people with acute back pain is: *Return as quickly as you can to your normal activities, without either limiting yourself or increasing what you normally do.* Rest briefly, then resume your normal activities. Don't start a new exercise program right away. Wait two to four weeks after an acute episode of back pain, then begin the back-strengthening exercise program outlined in Healing Moves to Strengthen Muscles and Bones (page 152.)

BACK BASICS

To banish back pain forever, you must exercise regularly and re-educate yourself about posture and movement. Proper body mechanics can help you avoid the mistakes that caused you to hurt your back. Remember these back basics:

Sitting. Sit up straight on your two "sit bones," not on your tailbone. Use an armchair with a high, firm back, and put your spine up against it. If you like, place a firmly rolled towel behind your waist to support your lumbar curve. Try to keep one or both knees higher than your hips. Putting your feet up on a small stool may be helpful. Be sure your chair is the proper height, so you don't have to bend over. And take a break to get up and stretch at least once every hour.

Standing. Place your weight evenly on both feet and don't slump into one hip. If you must stand for a long period of time, put one foot up on a phone book or low stool to keep your lower back flat. Don't let your shoulders roll forward or hunch over. To get a feel for how erect your shoulders should be, try standing with your arms crossed behind your back, with each hand holding the opposite elbow.

Sleeping. Pick a firm mattress and set it directly on a wooden frame. Try sleeping on your side with your legs bent at the knees and hips. Back sleepers can put a pillow under their knees. If you must sleep on your stomach, use a pillow under your hips. Avoid foam-rubber pillows, which can lift the head too high. Pick feathers, down, or manufactured fiber.

Lifting. Keep objects as close to the middle of your body as possible. The farther away from your body the object you're holding is, the more force it puts on your back. If you're reaching for something on or near the floor, bend your knees to lower your body to the object. This puts less stress on your back muscles and more on your stronger leg muscles. If you're reaching for something high up, stand on a stool to raise your body to the object.

Pushing and pulling. Always push rather than pull. Pushing, especially with your knees bent, uses your stomach and leg muscles more and your back muscles less. It also puts less pressure on your back.

At your computer. Adjust the height of your chair or computer so the top of the computer screen is slightly below eye level. Position the computer so it's directly in front of you. Use an adjustable copy holder that lets you place material either just beneath your screen or slightly off to the side, to avoid having to twist your neck. Consider using a footrest that allows you to keep your knees slightly higher than your hips.

At your desk. Sit up straight in a chair that provides good lumbar support, turns easily, and has casters. Keep your body close to the desk and rest your forearms on your desk or chair arms. To avoid slumping over your desk, consider using a slantboard to hold any copy placed on the desk. Use a headset if you're on the phone for extended periods of time.

Grooming. Stand erect when brushing your teeth or shaving; don't lean over the sink. It may help to place another mirror on the wall away from the sink so you can get close to it without leaning over. If you must get closer to the mirror to see, support yourself with one arm. Wash your face with a washcloth, rather than leaning over to splash water from the sink.

Driving. Position the seat back so you can sit as erect as possible, and as close to the steering wheel as is comfortable. For extra support, roll a towel into a firm, tight tube that you secure with rubber bands. Place it behind your waist to provide a lumbar support. (Similar props can be fashioned for airplane trips.) Stop frequently to get out and move around.

Sex. Try intercourse positions that allow the partner with back pain to be less active and more supported by the firm mattress and pillows. Pick appropriate music to encourage slow, controlled movements, not frantic thrusting. Remember that keeping your knees bent can help protect your lower back.

Posture. As often as practical throughout the day, take a minute for a posture check, scanning your body to see if you are standing or sitting with good alignment. Check to make sure that your shoulders and jaw are relaxed and you are not stooped or hunched over. If you find yourself standing around at a cocktail party or waiting in line, try this posture pointer taught to West Point cadets: Stand firmly on both feet and try to raise up the top of your head to touch an imaginary hand held a quarter-inch above you. Let your spine extend, shoulders relax, and arms fall to your sides.

RISK FACTORS

In addition to poor body mechanics, certain habits and conditions also make people more prone to back pain. These include:

Overweight. If your extra weight is in your belly, it can pull your spine out of alignment and place stress on your lower back. Plus, if you're overweight, chances are you aren't physically fit, which also puts you at risk of back injury.

Inactivity. When you're sedentary, the muscles that support your back—the paraspinal muscles, abdominals, and buttocks—become weak and tight. Also, inactive people typically have little endurance, which boosts the risk of injury.

Risky movements. Certain movements

increase the stress on your spine. Repetitive motions, such as working on an assembly line or pitching a softball for nine innings, can tire muscles and cause pain. Lifting, particularly if you lift and twist, can also lead to back pain.

Smoking. Numerous studies have shown a relationship between smoking and back pain, although the specific mechanisms are unclear. Some experts speculate that smoking causes coughing, which stresses back muscles. Others say smoking reduces blood flow around the discs, depriving them of nutrients and leading to pain. One study showed that smoking for twenty to thirty minutes decreased disc nutrition by as much as 30 to 40 percent. It can take as long as two hours for disc circulation to return to normal after smoking.

Bad posture. Slouching or slumping can lead to back pain. Sitting with the all-too-common round-shouldered posture places severe pressure on the lower back.

Stress. Stress causes muscles to become tense and tight, which makes them more prone to injury.

Age. Back pain is not necessarily a part of growing older. However, older adults tend to be less fit and more sedentary, both of which are risk factors for back pain. In addition, older adults are at greater risk of osteoporosis, the bone-weakening disease that affects more than 25 million Americans (80 percent of them women) and leads to more than 1.5 million fractures each year. Regular exercise and consuming adequate calcium can help prevent this potentially disabling condition. (See the section on osteoporosis, page 127.)

EXERCISE ℞

By now you probably realize that both the way you move your entire body and the way you live your entire life will affect your back. To eliminate back pain, it's essential that you pay attention to your back throughout your day and that you begin a program of regular exercise that boosts all aspects of your fitness—endurance, strength, body composition, and flexibility. That's why experts advise a combination of aerobics, strengthening and stretching exercises, and relaxation practices.

A. *Aerobic exercise: 20 to 60 minutes of continuous activity, at a pace you consider moderate to somewhat hard, three to six days a week.* Regular aerobic activity will help improve cardiovascular fitness and muscular endurance, which lessens the risk of fatigue that can lead to back injury. Fit people are less likely to "throw" their backs out than unfit people, in part because regular exercise increases blood flow to the back muscles. Plus, aerobic exercise helps overweight people lose the excess pounds that can force the spine into an exaggerated curve, increasing the risk of injury. For many overweight people, losing as few as five to ten pounds can significantly reduce stress on the back and decrease the chance of injury.

Swimming, walking, jogging, and bicycling are all appropriate aerobic exercises for people who suffer from back pain. However, aerobic activities that put major twisting or bending forces on the spine—such as rowing or certain types of aerobic dance—and those that involve falling—such as skiing and karate—should be individually evaluated by your physician.

If, in addition to chronic back pain, you have other health problems or conditions—such as arthritis or obesity—consider getting your aerobic workout in the water. Water aerobics has several advantages. First, since water is buoyant, there is less stress on your joints and movement is more comfortable. Second, the water provides mild resistance that helps you work your muscles with little risk of injury. Also, frail people concerned with falling may find water a much more inviting place to exercise than land. The simplest exercise is to walk in chest-deep water for 5 minutes. For variety, walk forward heel-toe, heel-toe, then walk backward toe-heel, toe-heel. Or consider enrolling in an aqua-aerobics class led by a qualified instructor.

B. *Strengthening and stretching exercises: 10 to 15 minutes daily.* These exercises target the muscles that support the back, which are the paraspinal muscles alongside the spine, the abdominals, the quadriceps, and hamstrings. The common advice to just do sit-ups to avoid back pain ignores these other important muscles, which can lead to back problems if they are weak and inflexible. Strengthening these core muscles minimizes stress on the lower back, especially when bending and lifting, and also helps you maintain proper posture and healthy body mechanics. Stretching them helps reduce the risk of back pain, since tight back muscles can easily tear when you twist, turn, or lift.

Surprisingly, increasing the flexibility of your shoulders and hips also will decrease the demands on your back. If you can't stretch your arms fully overhead or you can't fully straighten your legs at the hips, you place excessive demands on your lumbar spine. Flexibility also allows your spine to rotate properly. The muscle groups that must be stretched to provide this improved flexibility include the hip flexors (the muscles that bend the leg up toward the chest), the hamstrings (the muscles in the back of the thigh), and the paraspinals (the muscles on either side of the spine.) (For specific exercises, see Healing Moves to Strengthen Muscles and Bones, page 141.)

C. *Relaxation exercises, as needed.* Relaxation exercises can help prevent "back attacks" because, in susceptible people, stress can lead to back pain. Many back-pain sufferers note that their back "goes out" at exactly the wrong time—when they are stressed with excess responsibilities. Of course, there is no "right time" to experience back pain, but incorporating mini–relaxation practices into your day—such as shoulder shrugs while driving or neck stretches at your desk—can help ease tension before it builds to the critical point of injury. In addition, doing a simple restorative yoga pose for five minutes when you get home from work or during a break in the middle of the day can be a powerful tool for relieving stress and avoiding back problems.

CAUTIONS

Almost any exercise you enjoy will reduce your risk of back pain. But if you have chronic back pain, check with your physician before doing activities that involve forceful contact or falling, such as martial arts or downhill skiing, or that result in major twisting or bending forces on the spine, such as rowing or certain types of aerobic dance.

Consult a doctor if your back pain:

✳ follows an impact injury or fall

✳ is accompanied by tingling, numbness, or weakness in your legs or lower trunk

✳ runs down your leg or arm

✳ is associated with loss of bowel or bladder control

✳ is accompanied by a fever or chills

If an exercise hurts you, stop doing it and consult a physical therapist or other medical professional for advice. The exercise may not be appropriate for your condition, or you may be performing it incorrectly. However, it's vital to understand that even if an exercise causes some discomfort, it's important to continue working through mild pain—unless the pain radiates down the leg, which may indicate a pinched nerve. Continuing to exercise through discomfort can help break the vicious cycle of back pain where pain prompts inactivity, which leads to more pain.

Set a realistic exercise goal, such as working toward a certain number of repetitions of an exercise, then keep progressing slowly until you achieve it.

PRESCRIPTION PAD

1. *Aerobic activity*. Walk, bicycle, swim, or do any other aerobic activity for 20 to 60 minutes, at a pace you consider moderate to somewhat hard, three to six days a week. If you don't have the time to exercise continuously, you may accumulate the activity in 10-minute bouts.
2. *Strengthening and stretching exercises*. Perform the "back series" of exercises in Healing Moves to Strengthen Muscles and Bones three to six days a week.
3. *Relaxation practices*. Do "spontaneous stretches"—such as those described in Healing Moves to Strengthen Muscles and Bones—throughout the day. Perform relaxation practices, such as relaxation breathing (page 155), as needed. If possible, schedule a brief relaxation practice into your day, such as doing a 5-minute legs-up-the-wall pose (page 223) or 3 minutes of relaxation breathing.
4. *Posture pointers and body mechanics*. Remember to stand and sit with good posture and to use proper body mechanics at all times.

ADDITIONAL RESOURCES

Many YMCAs offer an excellent exercise program for people with back pain. It is outlined in the *YMCA Healthy Back Book* (Human Kinetics Publishers, 1994, $11.95), and the *YMCA Healthy Back Video* ($19.95; 800-747-4457).

Other good books and videotapes include:

✳ *Back Care Basics*, by Mary Pullig Schatz, M.D. (Rodmell Press, 1992), $19.95.

✳ *Priscilla's Lower Back Repair Kit*, an

exercise video hosted by Priscilla Patrick of the PBS yoga program *Stretching for Life* (44 minutes, $27.45; 800-383-8811).

✳ *Freedom from Back Pain* (90 minutes, $24.95; 828-254-7756). This video by yoga teacher Lillah Schwartz includes 30 minutes of back-care education, 30 minutes of instruction, and a 30-minute yoga program designed to stretch and strengthen the back.

REPETITIVE STRESS INJURY

Repetitive Stress Injury (RSI) has been called the workplace epidemic of the modern age. A disabling ailment whose symptoms range from minor pain to loss of function in the affected body part, RSI affects millions of people who spend long hours at computers, switchboards, and other work sites where they perform a repetitive motion—such as clicking a mouse—over and over and over again.

While a single mouse click isn't strenuous, performing thousands of clicks for hours on end can be extremely irritating to overused body parts, causing microscopic tears in tendons, nerves, muscles, and other soft tissues. These tears become inflamed, and without adequate time to rest and repair, this gradual, continued accumulation of small—sometimes unnoticeable—micro-traumas can lead to the overuse injury known as RSI.

Also called repetitive strain injury, repetitive motion injury, or cumulative trauma disorder, RSI is an umbrella term for a broad array of ailments that cause pain, numbness, and loss of strength, usually in the hands, wrists, arms, shoulders, or

neck. Carpal tunnel syndrome is the most frequently diagnosed form of RSI, accounting for nearly half of all reported cases. Other common forms include, "mouse elbow," trigger finger (a popping or catching sensation when you bend your finger), and tendinitis—often in the shoulder or wrist.

Telltale symptoms of RSI include:

✳ Stiffness, tingling, burning, or numbness in the hands, wrists, fingers, forearms, or elbows

✳ Recurring pain in the neck or shoulders

✳ Clumsiness or loss of strength and coordination in the hands

✳ Waking at night with a disturbing numbness and tingling in the hands

RSIs aren't new. For decades, workers in jobs requiring repetitive motions—from seamstresses and musicians to assembly-line operators and meat packers—have experienced RSIs. But in the last decade, as more and more people spend their days glued to computers, complaints of RSIs have exploded. In years past, most jobs involved at least some varied, manual tasks, such as reaching to return the typewriter carriage, fixing a mistake with correction fluid, or getting up to file a document or give a message to a colleague. Such brief pauses give our hands and wrists a rest.

But today's sophisticated, multifunction technology often chains a worker to one position, since new computers let workers do everything—from communicate with co-workers to correct errors—right at their desks with a keystroke or mouse click.

About half of the workforce now uses computers, typically with pointing devices (such as a mouse or trackball) and light-touch keyboards for high-speed typing, so that they can make more than 100,000 keystrokes a day. As a result, reports of RSIs have increased nearly eightfold in the last decade, according to the National Institute for Occupational Safety and Health (NIOSH). In 1993, the most recent year statistics are available, 2.73 million U.S. workers collected workers' compensation for RSI, costing employers more than $20 billion and making RSI the largest category of workers' compensation costs.

CONDITION BASICS

RSI includes a broad array of overuse injuries linked to performing repetitive physical movements—typically hand-intensive activities such as keyboarding or cutting. Two of the most common RSIs are carpal tunnel syndrome and "mouse elbow."

More than five million Americans suffer from **carpal tunnel syndrome,** one of the most common conditions affecting the hand and wrist. The ailment occurs when the major nerve that carries impulses from the brain to the hand becomes compressed. Called the median nerve, it begins in the neck and runs underneath the collarbone, across the armpit, and down the full length of the arm before it passes through a narrow passageway in the wrist called the carpal tunnel. The tendons that enable the hand to close also pass through the carpal tunnel. When these tendons are stressed—as can occur when they perform repetitive

motions—they swell inside the tunnel and compress the median nerve. This results in numbness, tingling, pain, and burning sensations in the hand, often accompanied by clumsiness or pain. Symptoms often begin in the wrist and move down into the thumb and the index and middle fingers or back toward the elbow. Sometimes there is associated pain in the arm and shoulder. Frequently, sufferers awaken suddenly in the middle of the night with discomfort or a "pins and needles" feeling in the hand.

One of the most common reasons why the membrane linings (or sheaths) surrounding these tendons swell is in response to an overuse injury caused by repetitive hand movements, such as keyboarding. Other conditions also are associated with swelling and compression of the median nerve, including pregnancy, diabetes, kidney problems, hypothyroidism, rheumatoid arthritis, and obesity. Women are more likely than men to get carpal tunnel syndrome; they may be more vulnerable because they have smaller wrists than men but tendons that are the same size. Also, hormonal fluctuations of the menstrual cycle can result in fluid retention, which can cause wrists to swell and compress the median nerve.

Mild cases of carpal tunnel syndrome may be treated by applying a brace or splint at night to allow the wrist to rest so that swollen membranes will shrink and relieve pressure on the nerve. Wearing splints by day is controversial, however, since some physicians believe this can cause the muscles to atrophy and lead to further problems. Medications may also be prescribed to help reduce swelling. Exercises can be essential in preventing and treating carpal tunnel syndrome, since specific motions can help relieve pressure on the median nerve.

Severe cases of carpal tunnel syndrome may require surgery to release the pressure on the median nerve by cutting the ligament that forms the roof of the carpal tunnel. An estimated 240,000 such surgical procedures are done each year. This surgery is controversial and is considered by many to be a last-resort procedure, since many people who have the surgery continue to have some symptoms, such as pain or loss of grip strength.

Mouse elbow is an increasingly common RSI in which people experience elbow pain after long hours of clicking the computer mouse. Like its sports counterpart tennis elbow, mouse elbow is an inflammation of tendons in the elbow—specifically the lateral epicondyle of the humerus, which forms the origin of several muscles of the forearm and hand. Typically caused by low-grade, repetitive overuse, mouse elbow can also result when a single trauma initiates a small tear to the tendons. The ailment is associated with motions that combine rotating the wrist with applying force, such as in using a screwdriver, golf club, or tennis racquet.

Mouse elbow can take a long time to heal since tendons don't get much time off to rest and have a modest blood supply. Treatment includes medication and ice massage to reduce inflammation, wearing a tennis-elbow band for support, and doing exercises to stretch and strengthen the muscles of the forearm.

Indeed, for all RSIs—including carpal tunnel syndrome and mouse elbow—health-

care providers are increasingly recognizing the importance of exercises to stretch and strengthen the muscles of the entire upper body, including the hands, arms, shoulders, neck, abdomen, and back. Exercise is one of the "three Es" many experts now consider essential to relieving RSIs:

1. **Education,** to understand the many factors contributing to the problem and learn strategies—such as frequent stretching—to prevent overuse injuries.
2. **Ergonomics,** to fit the workstation to each individual with the proper size and height of chair, keyboard, and monitor.
3. **Exercise,** to ensure that the individual is strong and supple enough to perform the deceptively difficult task of working at a computer all day.

RISK FACTORS

Jobs that require repetitive motions put people at risk of RSI. In particular, people who perform hand-intensive activities—such as keyboarding, cutting, or using vibrating tools—have a higher-than-normal incidence of carpal tunnel syndrome.

Weak or tight muscles, poor posture, and improper technique also increase your risk of RSI. Certain conditions can make people more prone to these injuries, including pregnancy, diabetes, kidney problems, hypothyroidism, rheumatoid arthritis, and obesity. And, as explained above, women are more likely than men to suffer from carpal tunnel syndrome.

Badly designed computer workstations heighten the risk of RSI. Since prevention is the best cure, be sure that you:

* Keep the video screen straight ahead of you, about an arm's length away, with the center of the screen where your gaze falls naturally (typically a few inches below eye level).

* Set the keyboard at a height so that the forearms, wrists, and hands are aligned, parallel to the floor or bent slightly down from elbow to hand. Don't let the hands bend back.

* Position your mouse pad within easy reach, directly next to your keyboard on the same level as your keyboard.

* Don't rest your wrists on anything while you're typing and don't bend them up, down, or to the side.

* Set your chair's height properly, so that your thighs are parallel to the floor. If your feet don't reach the floor, place them on a footstool. An ergonomically designed chair with good back support may also be helpful.

* Sit with good posture, keeping your spine against the back of your chair and your neck and upper body in a relaxed, comfortable position—but not slouched over.

* Vary your tasks. Avoid long stretches of a single activity by breaking up typing with filing, phone calls, or visits to the copy machine.

* Don't use excess force in typing or clicking the mouse.

* Keep your fingernails short and your fingers curved so that you don't see the nails.

HOW EXERCISE HELPS

One of the toughest physical challenges the human body can face is sitting all day. Standing is our natural posture, and sitting increases the pressure on the lower back. Plus, the common habit of rounding the shoulders and leaning forward while sitting worsens the problem, because it puts even more pressure on the back.

It's no wonder that people in sedentary jobs often experience neck and back pain. But sitting isn't the hardest part. Sitting *still* is. Keeping a body part in a fixed position can be just as hard on the muscles as lifting a twenty-five-pound load. Even a movement as innocuous as reaching repeatedly for your computer mouse can create a "static load," which means that continuing to hold your arm up to reach puts a subtle strain on your shoulder muscles.

In recent years, the tendency to spend our days sitting in a fixed position—coupled with improper posture, low fitness, stress, and poorly designed workstations—has led to the current epidemic of RSIs. While many people focus on changing the workplace to improve ergonomics, that approach addresses only one component of the problem. It's also critical to change bad physical habits—such as being out of shape and having poor posture—to completely resolve these injuries.

That's why more and more companies and health-care practitioners are encouraging employees to think of themselves as "computer athletes" who must be in shape to tackle the physically demanding job of sitting at a desk all day.

Like any athlete, computer athletes must train for their event: the eight-hour desk marathon. Their training should include frequent "microbreaks" to stretch their arms, wrists, shoulders, and neck, which can be done throughout the workday at the desk. Workers should avoid sitting in a fixed position for too long and try to stand up and move around briefly as often as possible. In addition, "desk jockeys" need to stay fit with aerobic activity and weight training to maintain a healthy weight, improve their posture, boost their circulation, and enhance the oxygenation of their tissues.

Being fit can help reduce the risk of RSIs for several reasons. People with strong and supple muscles can better maintain good body mechanics and proper posture, which can minimize stress on tendons and nerves. Fit people are more likely to have improved circulation and a healthy weight. Improved circulation enhances the body's ability to repair itself. Lower levels of body fat may lessen the impingement of nerves, which may alleviate symptoms of carpal tunnel syndrome. And people at a healthy weight are more likely to be able to "fit" into conventional workstations.

Since stress is also a major contributor to RSIs, exercises that promote relaxation also can help people avoid overuse injuries. For example, people under stress tend to hike up their shoulders, which can cause pressure on the nerves in the neck. Neck and shoulder stretches can relax these muscles and relieve this pressure. Frequent stretching and walk breaks also give muscles, tendons, and ligaments a chance to relax and change position, relieving the stress of repeated use and enhancing oxygenation, which encourages repair of overused muscles, tendons, and ligaments.

Yoga classes are an excellent way to help people learn good posture, relaxation breathing, and stretching and strengthening

techniques that can help reduce the risks of RSIs. Movement therapies that help people improve postural habits—such as the Alexander technique and the Feldenkrais method—can also help. (See Additional Resources at the end of this chapter.)

If injuries do occur, therapeutic exercises can help tendons heal properly so that they don't become shortened and weakened. *It's important that people who have RSI consult a health-care practitioner about specifics of exercise, since the first stage in treatment is typically rest for the injured part.* People with painful injuries who exercise too soon or do too much may cause further damage. However, once the healing process has begun, exercises under the guidance of a health professional can play an essential role in recovery.

EXERCISE ℞

Several different kinds of exercises can help prevent and treat RSIs:

✳ *Stretching.* Just as athletes stretch before their event, people in hand-intensive occupations—such as computer operators or grocery clerks—should do a few minutes of warm-up stretches for the hands, wrists, neck, shoulders, and arms before starting their shift and another few minutes of cooldown stretches at the end of work. A study of patients who performed a simple four-minute series of stretches developed by surgeons at the Hand Institute of the Orthopaedic and Reconstructive Center in Oklahoma City showed that the exercises substantially reduced the incidence of RSIs. Some patients scheduled for carpal tunnel surgery experienced so much relief from the exercises that they were able to cancel their operations.

Stretches should also be done frequently throughout the day, particularly for any body parts that experience tension. Shoulder shrugs, neck rolls, wrist curls, and other simple stretches can be performed at regular intervals, such as while waiting for the computer to boot up, download files, or print out documents. Try spontaneous stretches of any body parts that tend to tighten up. For example, people who keyboard all day might grasp the fingers of one hand with the other hand and gently pull backward until they feel an easy stretch in their wrist. And if you tend to hunch over while sitting, raise your arms up and stretch back over your chair, looking up at the ceiling, every half hour or so that you're at your desk.

If you find it difficult to remember to stretch during long hours at your computer, install one of the new stretching software programs that regularly remind you to stretch. For example, one program, called Stretch-ercise, has a pop-up screen that appears at regular intervals (set by time, keystrokes, or mouse clicks) to lead the user through stretches. It was designed by Robert Gamburd, a physical medicine and rehabilitation specialist in California's computer-intensive Silicon Valley and a team physician for the San Francisco 49ers and the Stanford University athletic department. Another program, Cyber-Stretch, is marketed by the international exercise fitness program Jazzercise. Cyber-Stretch works in a screen-saver format, bringing up stretches on the screen whenever the keyboard isn't used; it also lets users call up stretches at will. Flexibility guru Bob Anderson, whose classic guide to stretching has been translated into 17 languages, also offers excellent stretching software called Stretch-ware. (See the Additional Resources list at the end of this section for more information.)

✳ *Walking breaks.* Getting up and moving around boosts circulation and gives overused muscles a chance to rejuvenate. Shorter, more frequent breaks (such as two or three minutes each hour) are more effective than longer, less frequent ones (such as fifteen minutes every two to three hours). In jobs that don't permit frequent walk breaks, standing up and stretching at the desk can be helpful. A good time to stand and stretch is while talking on the telephone.

✳ *Strengthening exercises.* Computer operators need to recognize that they're upper-body athletes, and they need to do exercises that will strengthen the entire upper body, including the back and abdominals. A strong torso is essential to correct posture, so exercises such as crunches for the abdominals and extensions for the back muscles can be extremely helpful. (See Healing Moves to Strengthen Muscles and Bones, page 138.) To strengthen muscles, it's important to work the body against resistance. This resistance can come from the water, in aqua-aerobics; from weights, such as dumbbells or exercise machines; from your own body in calisthenics, such as push-ups; or from elastic tubing. Do six to eight exercises that strengthen all the muscles of the upper body, including the arms and shoulders (both front and back), neck, wrists, chest, abdominals, and back.

* **_Aerobic activity._** Walking, running, group fitness classes, and other aerobic exercises are essential to improving circulation, boosting oxygenation of tissues, enhancing "stress hardiness," and maintaining a healthy weight. Do an aerobic activity, such as walking, cycling, or swimming, three to six days a week, at a pace you consider moderate to somewhat hard, for 20 to 60 minutes. If you don't have time to exercise continuously, you can still get benefits by accumulating exercise in 10-minute bouts.

CAUTIONS

While exercise is essential to helping prevent and treat RSI, _people who have painful symptoms should do exercises only under the guidance of a health-care professional._ If you experience painful symptoms, it's important that you consult a physician immediately. Early diagnosis is essential to limiting damage, and trying to ignore pain could result in further injury and possibly permanent impairment. There are no quick fixes for RSIs, and healing typically takes months. Gentle stretching is usually helpful, although some strengthening exercises should be done only after an injury has healed—usually marked by the absence of sharp pain or numbness.

Follow commonsense wisdom: If an exercise hurts, don't do it. If you have a diagnosed RSI, consult your physician about specific exercises and consider working with a physical therapist to learn stretching, strengthening, and range-of-motion activities.

PRESCRIPTION PAD

* **_Stretch._** Before beginning any hand-intensive activity, such as keyboarding or knitting, do several minutes of warm-up stretches for your hands, wrists, arms, shoulders, and neck. Stretch spontaneously throughout the workday, especially when a body part feels achy or tired, even for just five or ten seconds. After finishing a hand-intensive activity, be sure to do several minutes of cooldown stretches for the upper body.

* **_Take walk breaks._** Get up and walk around briefly at least once an hour if you work at a desk for long periods of time. Shorter, more frequent breaks are better than longer, less frequent ones. If you can't walk around, at least stand up and stretch.

* **_Do strengthening exercises._** Two to three times a week, do six to eight exercises to strengthen the muscles of the upper body, including the hands, arms, wrists, shoulders, neck, chest, back, and abdomen.

* **_Aerobic activity._** Do some form of aerobic activity—such as walking, swimming, or cycling—three to six days a week, at a pace you consider moderate to somewhat hard, for 20 to 60 minutes.

ADDITIONAL RESOURCES

* Dr. Gamburd's Stretch-ercise software is available from Ergonomic Sciences Corporation: Call 650-964-3134 or visit www.ergosci.com.

* Cyber-Stretch software. Call 760-434-2101 or visit www.cyberstretch.com.

* _Stretching at Your Computer or Desk,_ by Bob Anderson (Shelter Publications,

1997), and Bob Anderson's Stretchware software. Call Stretching at 800-333-1307 or visit www.stretching.com.

✳ The American Academy of Orthopaedic Surgeons offers materials about a variety of musculoskeletal concerns, including carpal tunnel syndrome. Call 800-824-BONES or visit www.aaos.org.

✳ The Feldenkrais Guild can refer you to a practitioner certified in the Feldenkrais Method of techniques to improve posture and breathing and reduce stress. Contact them at P.O. Box 489, Albany, Ore. 97321. Call 800-775-2118 or visit www.feldenkrais.com.

✳ The Alexander Technique teaches people proper posture and movement habits to reduce strain on the body. For referral to a certified practitioner contact the North American Society of Teachers of the Alexander Technique, 800-473-0620 or visit www.alexandertech.org.

OSTEOPOROSIS

The word *osteoporosis* means "porous bones," and the condition affects more than 28 million Americans, 80 percent of them women. Yet despite the widespread incidence of this bone-weakening disease, most people with osteoporosis don't know they have it. In fact, many people discover they have osteoporosis only when they fall and, instead of merely getting a bruise, they wind up breaking a bone. Sadly, at this point the condition is far advanced.

Bone loss usually occurs slowly over the years without any symptoms, which is why osteoporosis is called a silent disease. Most people who suffer osteoporotic fractures are older adults, but the disease often gets its start in childhood. Poor diet and inactivity during important growing years can result in a weakened skeleton that isn't as strong or dense as it could be. Then, in midlife, when humans begin to incur a small loss of bone mass each year, this silent disease can progress—particularly in people who have insufficient nutrients and/or physical activity to help keep their bones healthy. In women, bone loss can be dramatic after menopause, since females lose bone at an accelerated rate when estrogen levels decline.

The amount of bone people lose depends on some factors they can't control, such as genetics and gender, and other factors that they can directly influence, including nutrition, exercise, and cigarette smoking. Because osteoporosis can progress silently, awareness and attention to these healthy habits is essential to prevent bones from becoming so porous and fragile that they fracture from a minor trauma. Besides breaking a bone, there are some other signs of osteoporosis, but many people don't recognize them. One clue is the forward curvature of the spine called *kyphosis*, the classic dowager's hump. Another is diminished height. Older people often seem to "shrink" because weakened, osteoporotic vertebrae—the bones in their spine—are slowly crushed by gravity.

One-third of American women over age fifty will eventually have a spinal fracture, as will some younger people, according to the National Osteoporosis Foundation (NOF). Usually painful, these fractures may also occur without any symptoms. They frequently happen when someone with low bone density in the spine does a routine activity they've performed countless times before—like bending over to get the newspaper or feed the cat. But in a spine weakened by osteoporosis, this simple forward bend can literally be the straw that breaks their back.

Each year, about 300,000 people wind up in hospitals with hip fractures associated with osteoporosis. Half of these people never go home again, and one in five dies from complications within a year. *In fact, a woman has a greater likelihood of dying as a result of a hip fracture than from breast cancer, uterine cancer, and ovarian cancer combined.* Those who survive frequently wind up in nursing homes, and even those lucky enough to retain their independence often live in fear of future falls.

This sad picture illustrates the unhealthy cycle of inactivity: Lack of exercise leads to weak bones, which leads to fracture, which leads to hospitalization, which leads to inactivity, which leads to further medical complications. In 1995, the estimated medical, nursing home, and social costs of osteoporotic fractures exceeded $13.8 billion in the United States alone, estimates NOF. Experts expect this figure to exceed $60 billion by the year 2030. As the population ages, the number of people with osteoporosis will continue to increase dramatically in the United States and throughout the world.

BONE BASICS

Many people think of their skeleton as solid and lifeless, when in fact bone is porous and very much alive. Although the bone's outer shell is hard, the tissue inside is a soft, honeycomblike structure with blood vessels running through it. At the center is the bone marrow, where blood cells are formed. The bones provide structural support for your body, protect your vital organs, and store the calcium you need to function. About 99 percent of your body's calcium is contained in the bones and teeth. The amount of bone tissue you have is called **bone mass.** How much calcium there is and how tightly it's packed is called **bone density.**

Like many other tissues in the body, bone tissue constantly repairs and renews itself. This process is called bone remodeling and consists of two stages: bone breakdown, or **resorption,** followed by bone formation. Complex chemical signals prompt bone cells called **osteoclasts** to break down and remove old bone, releasing calcium into the blood. Then bone-building cells called **osteoblasts** draw calcium from the blood to create new bone and deposit it in the skeleton. If the bone removed by resorption is completely replaced, bone strength is maintained. *But in osteoporosis, too much bone is removed, too little bone is formed, or a combination of both occurs.* This imbalance leads to a loss in the mass and density of bones.

The bone remodeling rate is affected by the basic building block, calcium, and three catalysts that affect how that calcium is used: *vitamin D, hormones, and exercise.*

Calcium

The body needs calcium for many functions, such as muscle contraction, blood-pressure regulation, blood clotting, and new bone formation. Adequate calcium in the diet is critical to bone health because the body not only can't make calcium but loses calcium daily through shed skin, nails, hair, sweat, urine, and feces. When people don't consume enough calcium, the body robs bones of this mineral to meet its needs, accelerating the loss of bone density. Most Americans don't consume enough calcium to protect themselves from osteoporosis. In fact, studies show that *many adults and children get less than half the calcium their bodies need for strong bones*. To encourage Americans to consume more of this important mineral, the National Academy of Sciences in 1997 increased the recommended intake of calcium to between 1,000 and 1,300 milligrams per day.

Vitamin D

Vitamin D stimulates the intestines to absorb calcium. Children with vitamin D deficiency can develop rickets, a condition characterized by growing bones being "soft" or poorly mineralized. Adults with vitamin D deficiency also can develop soft bones or *osteomalacia*. The body makes enough vitamin D naturally, when the skin of the face and arms is exposed to just fifteen minutes of sunlight daily. But the skin can't manufacture vitamin D in people wearing sunscreen or during the winter months in latitudes above 42 degrees north, such as Boston or Milwaukee. That's why people in northern climates can lose up to 4 percent of their bone density during winter months. Younger, more active people can gain this amount back during the summer months, but older or more sedentary people may not

be able to totally regain this loss. Seniors in particular may benefit from food sources of vitamin D, such as fortified milk or dietary supplements.

Hormones

Estrogen has a powerful stimulating effect on the bone-making cells (osteoblasts). When a woman's estrogen levels drop after menopause (either natural or surgical), bone formation slows down. If a young woman stops menstruating—sometimes as the result of an eating disorder—the associated lack of estrogen can prevent her bones from growing properly.

Exercise

Physical impact and weight-bearing exercise stimulates bone formation. Just as a muscle gets stronger and bigger the more you use it, a bone becomes stronger and denser when you regularly place demands upon it. The best bone builders are exercises that put force on the bone, such as weight-bearing activities like running and resistance exercises like strength training. In general, the greater the impact involved in an activity, the more it strengthens the bones. That's why the bones in the racket arms of tennis players are denser than the bones in their nondominant arms. When muscles and gravity aren't pulling on the bone, humans can lose bone mass rapidly. This is dramatically illustrated when people are forced by injury or ill health to undergo complete bed rest and, as a result, lose about 1 percent of their bone mass per week. This is similar to the devastating effects on bone mass seen in young, healthy male astronauts in outer space, due to the loss of gravity.

PEDIATRIC DISEASE WITH A GERIATRIC OUTCOME

Some experts describe the human skeleton as a kind of bank account where you "deposit" and "withdraw" bone tissue. Childhood, adolescence, and early adulthood are major deposit years, where new bone is added to the skeleton faster than old bone is removed. The skeleton grows and bones get larger, denser, and stronger. About 90 percent of an adult's bone mineral content is deposited by the end of adolescence, with peak bone mass achieved between the ages of twenty and thirty. Proper nutrition and regular exercise are essential during this time to build optimal bone mass and density, which helps protect against the inevitable losses that occur with aging. More and more experts are recognizing that osteoporosis prevention begins with good health habits in childhood.

The bone bank's withdrawal period typically begins after age thirty, in men and women alike. But until about age fifty, this bone loss occurs at the relatively slow rate of about half a percent per year in most people. However, if people become sedentary and eat poorly, they may lose bone more rapidly and begin a transformation toward *osteopenia*, which means "bone loss." Osteopenia, which is a negative bone-calcium balance, is often a precursor to the clinical diagnosis of osteoporosis. In females, menopause (which usually occurs between the ages of forty-five and fifty-five) is accompanied by a drop in estrogen production that results in more rapid loss of bone. Some women lose up to 20 percent of their bone mass in the five to eight years after their monthly cycles stop. After age sixty-five, women and men tend to lose bone mass at the same rate.

While losing some bone is a natural part of the aging process, osteoporosis isn't. The disease represents an extreme imbalance between the natural processes of bone formation and bone breakdown. Restoring a sound bone balance through healthy lifestyle habits can help prevent this common disease. Proper diet and exercise in youth can help you build a strong skeleton, and in the middle and later years they can help you maintain bone health.

RISK FACTORS

Certain characteristics put people at greater risk of osteoporosis. Those over which people have no control include:

✳ *Gender.* Women are four times more likely than men to develop osteoporosis, for several reasons. First, their bones are usually lighter and thinner than men's bones. Second, they lose bone rapidly after menopause in response to declining levels of estrogen. Third, they usually live longer than men and have more years at risk.

✳ *Age.* The longer you live, the greater your likelihood of getting osteoporosis. While not every older person gets the disease, the number increases from about 15 percent of women in their fifties to half of all women in their eighties.

✳ *Race.* Caucasian and Asians of Japanese and Chinese descent are at greatest risk.

✳ *Body type.* The smaller and thinner your frame, the greater your risk.

* **Early menopause.** Reaching menopause before age forty-five—whether naturally or surgically—increases your osteoporosis risk.

* **Family history.** If your grandmother or mother had low bone density and osteoporotic fractures, you're at greater risk.

If you have some or all or these risk factors, it's particularly important that you pay attention to the following risk factors that you *can* influence:

* **Sedentary lifestyle.** Inactivity puts people at greater risk of having weak, fragile bones. Sedentary kids don't build strong bones, and sedentary adults can lose bone at an accelerated rate. In contrast, people who are active and fit have stronger muscles and bones, as well as better balance, so they are less likely to suffer an injurious fall.

* **Calcium consumption.** Inadequate calcium intake is harmful to bone health. An expert panel convened by the National Institutes of Health recommended a calcium intake of 800 to 1,200 mg per day for older children, 1,200 to 1,500 mg per day for adolescents and young adults ages eleven to twenty-four, 1,000 mg per day for adult men and women, and 1,500 mg per day for elderly people and for women over age fifty who are not taking estrogen. The NIH said the preferred source of calcium was "calcium-rich foods, such as dairy products." Be aware, too, that *a high intake of certain foods—including excess caffeine, protein, and salt—can hasten the loss of calcium in the urine, increasing the risk of bone fracture.*

* **Vitamin D.** Called the "sunshine vitamin" because the skin can manufacture it when the face and arms are exposed to sunlight for just fifteen minutes, vitamin D aids the absorption of dietary calcium. Most people can get what they need through brief exposure to sunlight in the summer months or by consuming fortified dairy products. The combination of calcium and vitamin D is particularly effective for preventing bone loss in older individuals, which is one reason why *the National Academy of Sciences in 1997 tripled the recommended intake of vitamin D for people over seventy to 600 I.U. per day.*

* **Hormones.** While hormone-replacement therapy (HRT) remains controversial, many experts feel strongly that women at risk for osteoporosis should start taking hormones or other "antiresorptive" medications at the time of menopause, when bone loss can be rapid and severe. A bone-density test can help women make the decision about medication by detecting osteoporosis before a fracture occurs and predicting the chance of fracture. Hormones will enhance the action of calcium and exercise, notes the NOF, which states that "in the absence of adequate estrogen, bone loss will occur even in vigorous exercisers with high calcium intakes."

* **Smoking.** Women who smoke have lower levels of estrogen compared with non-smokers and go through menopause earlier. Postmenopausal women who smoke may require higher doses of hormone-replacement therapy and may have more side effects.

* **Excess alcohol consumption.** Regularly drinking two to three ounces of alcohol a

day may be damaging to the skeleton, even in young women and men. Drinking heavily puts people at greater risk of bone loss and fracture, because it interferes with calcium metabolism and increases the risk of falling.

✳ *Amenorrhea.* Women who have irregular menstrual periods, often because of conditions such as anorexia or bulimia, may lose bone tissue and develop osteoporosis early in life. Female athletes in sports with a "thin aesthetic"—such as ice skating and gymnastics—are at heightened risk, since many engage in overtraining and unhealthy weight-control practices that can lead to a condition known as athletic amenorrhea. The alarming prevalence of female athletes in their twenties who have the thin, fragile bones of women in their seventies has prompted the American College of Sports Medicine to identify this condition in a statement entitled "The Female Athlete Triad: Disordered Eating, Amenorrhea and Osteoporosis." The college advises parents and coaches to be aware of the serious health hazard posed by unhealthy weight-loss practices and to encourage female athletes concerned with weight issues to seek assistance from a qualified sports nutritionist or other health professional. Adolescence is a critical time for building bone, but with poor diet and inadequate estrogen, many young female athletes are losing this peak opportunity to develop a strong skeleton.

Certain health conditions also can put people at increased risk of osteoporosis. These include hyperthyroidism, multiple myeloma, and kidney, lung, and gastrointestinal disorders. People with genetic defects that affect the production of sex hormones, such as Turner's or Klinefelter's syndrome, may develop osteoporosis early in life. Cancer treatment can also put people at risk of osteoporosis, especially if it reduces estrogen levels in women or testosterone levels in men. Plus, the inactivity and inability to eat well that accompanies cancer treatment may harm bone health. Long-term use of certain medications also can increase osteoporosis risk: aluminum-containing antacids, GnRH (used to treat endometriosis), steroids, barbiturates, and anticonvulsants. If you are under treatment for a chronic disease—such as asthma or lupus, which are commonly treated with steroids—ask your doctor how long-term use of the medications you take can affect your bone health.

THE EXERCISE-CALCIUM CONNECTION

Calcium's critical importance to bone health has received a lot of attention. But calcium consumption is just part of the picture, since exercise is essential for stimulating the calcium to build bone in youth and prevent bone loss with age.

In fact, some research suggests that calcium and exercise "may not act on bone independent of each other," reported South Dakota State University epidemiologist Bonny L. Specker in the *Journal of Bone and Mineral Research*. Specker performed a meta-analysis of seventeen studies examining the effects of physical activity and calcium on bone and found that "a positive effect of physical activity appears to exist only at calcium intakes greater than 1,000 mg/day. And the beneficial effect of a high calcium intake only appears to be present when there is physical activity."

This study shows that "you need both calcium and exercise," she says, "for optimum bone health."

Just as you can eat lots of protein and not gain any muscle unless you strength-train, you can consume lots of calcium and not build bones unless you exercise. Through a complex system of chemical reactions, the physical demands of activity "kick-starts" the calcium to make bones stronger and denser. "Physical activity, through its load-bearing effect on the skeleton, is likely the single most important influence on bone density and architecture," concludes the *U.S. Surgeon General's Report on Physical Activity and Health*. "Bone cells respond to mechanical loading by improving the balance between bone formation and bone resorption, which in turn builds greater bone mass. The higher the load, the greater the bone mass; conversely, when the skeleton is unloaded (as with inactivity), bone mass declines."

The two kinds of exercise most important for bone health are those that put the greatest forces on the skeleton: weight-bearing activities and resistance exercise.

Weight-bearing activities are those that work bones and muscles against gravity. Walking, stair climbing, dancing, running, and racquet sports are all weight-bearing activities with differing degrees of impact. In general, the higher the impact, the more the activity strengthens the bones. Exercises in which the body weight is supported by the feet and legs during vigorous movements are more effective in maintaining the density of the leg and spinal bones than non-weight-bearing activities, such as bicycling and swimming. Although a few studies have shown some positive effect on bone from swimming, possibly from working muscles against the resistance of water, it typically isn't recommended as a bone builder since the water reduces both the strengthening effect of gravity and the impact. Upside-down weight-bearing activities—such as inverted postures in yoga and handstands in gymnastics—can boost bones in the arms and upper body.

Resistance exercise, such as working out with free weights or weight machines, is particularly effective at strengthening both muscles and bones. A study by Tufts University physiologist Miriam Nelson, published in the *Journal of the American Medical Association*, showed that postmenopausal women who performed just two 40-minute strength-training sessions a week for one year gained 1 percent in bone density—comparable to the bone benefit in hormone-replacement therapy. Women in the sedentary control group lost 2 to 2.5 percent.

"People who do weight-bearing activities have bone density that is up to 10 percent higher than people who don't exercise," notes Gail Dalsky, an assistant professor of medicine at the University of Connecticut Health Center. "People who do resistance exercise have bone density up to 30 percent higher."

In addition to boosting bone health, exercise is also a critical strategy for preventing and treating osteoporosis because it improves strength, flexibility, and coordination, which may all indirectly, but effectively, decrease the likelihood of falling. Since most fractures are sustained in falls, fewer falls means fewer broken bones. In Nelson's study at Tufts, the women who did strength training improved their balance by 14 percent, compared with a 9 percent decline in balance in the control group. And spontaneous physical activity increased by almost 27 percent among weight trainers, while sedentary women decreased their activity by about that same amount.

"After one year of strength training, these women emerged physiologically younger by fifteen to twenty years," Nelson says. "They started walking, gardening, canoeing, and carrying two large grocery bags at a time instead of one small one."

EXERCISE ℞ FOR BONING UP

Three kinds of activity are important to prevent and treat osteoporosis: weight-bearing workouts, resistance training, and postural exercises.

A. *Weight-bearing activity: 30 minutes, most days of the week.* Jogging, walking, dancing, stair climbing, aerobics, and hiking are all good weight-bearing activities that will boost bone health, improve overall fitness, and reduce the risk of falling. Pick any activity that suits your bone status, fitness level, and personal interest. For example, if you are strong and healthy, try a high-impact activity such as jogging. If you don't like jogging, try brisk walking or stair climbing. However, if you have osteoporosis or

have lost a significant amount of bone in the spine and hip, you should avoid activities with too much impact or a high risk of falling. Older, frail adults can minimize their risk of falling by engaging in weight-supported exercises such as deep-water walking, chair exercises, or cycling on a stationary bike. While this won't be as beneficial for bones as weight-bearing exercise, it can help strengthen muscles, improve coordination, boost overall fitness, and reduce the risk of falling. Remember, when it comes to being physically active: *Doing something is better than doing nothing.*

For most adults, particularly those who have been sedentary, walking will be the weight-bearing activity of choice. If you've been inactive, be sure to start slowly and progress gradually. Begin by walking as little as 5 minutes per day, increasing the duration over time until you're walking for at least 30 minutes most days of the week. If necessary, you can break your walking sessions up into several shorter bouts, such as three 10-minute sessions.

Children and adults in good health should pick an activity that involves running and jumping—such as jogging, basketball, rope skipping, soccer, or racquet sports—to maximize bone health. To gain the benefits of high-impact activity while minimizing the risks of injury, adults may want to alternate high-impact workouts with low-impact activities. For example, jog on Monday, Wednesday, and Friday and walk on Tuesday, Thursday, and Saturday.

For the extra bone-building boost of

vitamin D, exercise outdoors in the sunshine. Wait fifteen minutes before putting on sunscreen, so your skin can manufacture vitamin D.

B. *Resistance training: two to three 20- to 40-minute sessions per week.* A good strength-training program includes eight to ten exercises that will work all the major muscle groups of the body: chest, shoulders, front and back of arms, back, abdominals, buttocks, and front and back of legs. This is particularly important if your weight-bearing exercise involves mainly the legs, such as walking, since a well-rounded resistance routine will also strengthen the bones and muscles of your upper body.

Use a heavy weight that you can lift between eight to twelve times. *Doing lots of repetitions with a very light weight won't do much for your bones.* To find the right weight, start by using an obviously light weight—or no weight at all—to perform a specific exercise. If you can do that exercise twelve times easily, add a little more weight and try again. Keep going until you find a weight that challenges you enough so you can do at least eight but no more than twelve repetitions of the same exercise. (Older and more frail people may find it more appropriate to choose a lighter weight they can lift at least ten, but no more than fifteen, times.) Once you build up enough muscle so that twelve repetitions become easy, increase the amount of weight gradually—by no more than 10 percent per week. Once you've achieved the strength you want, you don't need to keep increasing the weight. Just keep going with the resistance you have mastered to maintain your strength.

Be sure with each exercise that you use good technique, and always warm up first and cool down afterward. Be sure to stretch your muscles, too, since strength building without stretching can actually shorten and tighten the muscles. Stretch gently after you've warmed up, before starting your strength-training workout, and stretch again as part of your cooldown.

Consider taking several sessions with a personal trainer or physical therapist to learn proper technique. This is particularly important with resistance training, since poor technique can lead to injury. Many people will find it easiest to join a gym, where they can get expert help and choose from a wide variety of resistance machines and free weights. But most people can also do a good strength-training workout with minimal equipment at home. (For specific exercises, see Healing Moves to Strengthen Muscles and Bones, page 140.)

C. *Postural exercises: several minutes daily, plus practicing good postural habits throughout the day.* Stress, excessive sitting, and weak, out-of-shape muscles result in postural disasters that leave people slouching toward their doctors. Poor posture is linked to a host of problems, ranging from back pain to digestive disorders and heart palpitations caused by decades of crunching the internal organs by slumping over when sitting and standing. Maintaining proper posture throughout the day not only helps prevent injury, but it also can enhance appearance and boost mood. People whose posture reflects a physical "slump" often appear to be in a mental slump as well. Similarly, people who carry themselves with good alignment seem confident and at ease. Posture mirrors emotional state: The way you hold your body affects the way you feel, and vice versa.

When standing, try to distribute your weight evenly between both legs. If you must stand on one leg, use good body alignment and alternate the weight-bearing leg. Imagine a hand floating slightly above your head and gently extend the top of your head up to touch that imaginary hand. When sitting, distribute your weight evenly on both "sit bones," or ischial tuberosities, which feel like knobby bumps on your rear. Keep your feet firmly on the floor or on a footrest, with your thighs about parallel to the floor, the knees slightly higher than the hips.

In addition to practicing good posture throughout the day, it's a good idea to add a few postural exercises to your resistance-training workout. (Specific exercises are described in Healing Moves to Strengthen Muscles and Bones, page 149.)

CAUTIONS

If you already have low bone density of the spine or osteoporosis—particularly if you've suffered a fracture—consult a physician or physical therapist for an individualized program.

It may be important that you avoid:

✳ High-impact or sudden, jerking movements.

✳ Exercises that call for the spine to directly support your body weight, such as a yoga shoulder stand.

✳ Activities that round the back, such as sit-ups or rowing.

✳ Sports that involve bending forward and twisting, such as bowling or golf.

These activities can put undue stress on the vertebrae, increasing your risk of spinal fracture.

Always use these good body mechanics during activities of daily living:

Bending and lifting. Never bend all the way over with straight knees. Instead, bend at the knees and keep your back up straight. Keep the object you are carrying close to your body and lift with your legs.

Pushing and pulling. When you sweep, rake, or mop, stand with your feet apart, one slightly in front of the other and pointing forward. Do not bend forward from the waist; instead, bend your knees and move forward and back or side to side rhythmically.

Coughing and sneezing. Place one hand on your back or knee to support your back whenever you cough or sneeze.

PRESCRIPTION PAD: EXERCISE ℞ THROUGH THE LIFE CYCLE

Osteoporosis results from three factors that occur in different life stages, concludes the surgeon general's report: "a deficient level of peak bone mass at physical maturity, failure to maintain this peak bone mass during the third and fourth decades of life, and the bone loss that begins during the fourth or fifth decade of life. Physical activity may positively affect all three of these factors."

But since bone growth and loss differs during different life stages, the exercise prescription for preventing and treating osteoporosis depends on a person's age. Here are some basic guidelines:

✳ *Youth through age thirty:* Bone is built during this period, with peak bone mass achieved between the ages of twenty and thirty. To help youngsters reach their full growth potential, they should get 30 to 60 minutes of physical activity most days of the week. For optimum bone health choose sports that involve jumping and running, such as basketball, volleyball, and soccer. Activities like gymnastics and dance can also be beneficial, unless a girl's menstrual periods become irregular, since amenorrhea puts girls at increased risk of osteoporosis early in life.

✳ *Thirties and forties:* Bone loss may begin to occur in some parts of the skeleton at a rate of up to 1 percent per year. To help maintain bone, do at least 30 minutes of weight-bearing exercise three to five days a week and 30 minutes of resistance exercise two or three days a week.

✳ *Menopause (around ages forty-five to fifty-five) and up to eight years beyond:* Bone loss is most rapid at this time, with women losing up to 20 percent of their bone mass. Many experts recommend hormone-replacement therapy or other antiresorptive medications at this time to help prevent osteoporosis. To help make the decision about medication, women with osteoporosis risk factors (such as family history) should get a bone-density test at menopause. "Exercise

cannot be recommended as a substitute for hormone replacement therapy at the time of menopause," notes the American College of Sports Medicine in its position stand on osteoporosis and exercise. However, weight-bearing and resistance exercises can be an essential adjunct therapy for women taking hormones or other medications. The surgeon general's report notes that "there is evidence [that] this effect [of estrogen-replacement therapy] is enhanced with physical activity." And for those women who can't—or won't—tolerate medications, exercise and calcium can be essential interventions.

✳ *Age sixty and above:* Men and women tend to lose bone mass at a similar rate during this period. People who've been sedentary should start exercising gradually with a walking program, working up to walking 30 minutes or more most days of the week. Twice-weekly sessions of resistance exercise may also be beneficial.

ADDITIONAL RESOURCES

✳ The Osteoporosis and Related Bone Diseases National Resource Center is funded by the National Institutes of Health and offers free materials for consumers and health-care providers. Call 800-624-BONE.

✳ The National Osteoporosis Foundation has numerous fact sheets and brochures, some free and some at minimal cost. One of the best is *Boning Up on Osteoporosis,* a comprehensive 70-page booklet about prevention, diagnosis, and treatment that is available for $4 by writing to NOF, 1150 Seventeenth Street, N.W., Suite 500, Washington, D.C. 20036-4603.

* *Strong Women Stay Young*, by Miriam Nelson, Ph.D., with Sarah Wernick, Ph.D., (Bantam Books, 1997), $23.95.

* *Strength Training for Women*, by James A. Peterson, Cedric Bryant, and Susan Peterson (Human Kinetics, 1995), $15.95.

* *The American College of Sports Medicine's* statement "The Female Athlete Triad: Eating Disorders, Amenhorrea and Osteoporosis" is available to persons who send a self-addressed, stamped envelope to ACSM, P.O. Box 1440, Indianapolis, Ind. 46206.

* * *

HEALING MOVES TO STRENGTHEN MUSCLES AND BONES

*

Back in the aerobic 1980s, legions of Americans laced up their athletic shoes to exercise that most important of muscles—the heart. Today we continue to appreciate the importance of cardiovascular fitness, but it's clear that the body's other muscles deserve equal time. Without resistance exercises to strengthen muscles and bones, most people face a midlife slide into flabbiness and its associated ills. *And as we age, strength training becomes even more important* to offset age-related declines in muscle and bone mass that can lead to frailty and fracture—the primary reason older adults wind up in nursing homes.

Many people don't realize that even the most dedicated aerobic exercisers will lose muscle mass with age, starting at about age thirty, if they don't do strengthening exercises. Sedentary adults lose about a half pound of muscle a year, which means they'll drop 15 percent of their muscle mass between the third and eighth decades of life. So if you're an inactive fifty-year-old who weighs the same as you did in college, you've simply replaced ten pounds of muscle with ten pounds of fat. Although your body weight may remain the same, your body composition will change markedly with age if you don't exercise.

This is much more than just a cosmetic issue. Muscle is one of the body's most metabolically active tissues, which means that the more muscle tissue you have, the higher your metabolic rate. The metabolic rate is a measure of how many calories your body needs to function, and a variety of factors affect it, including age, gender, height, weight, activity level, and food consumption. But the biggest component is the amount of lean tissue (muscle, bone, and organs) that you have.

When you lose muscle mass, your metabolic rate declines. This metabolic slowdown can have wide-ranging consequences, including obesity, impaired glucose tolerance, and changes in the body's ability to regulate temperature. Since muscular contractions help keep bones strong, muscle loss can also mean weaker bones.

Although some age-related muscle loss is inevitable, much of the decline attributed to age actually comes from inactivity. Extensive research has shown *that muscles and bones will get stronger in response to strength training regardless of your age.* And when you build muscles through strength training, you get the added bonus of revving up your metabolic rate—which means that your body will burn more calories, even at rest. This is why some health experts call strength training "the closest we've come to a fountain of youth."

To keep your bones and muscles in maximum working order, this workout includes four components:

Part One: Weight-Bearing Activity

An activity (20 to 30 minutes, three to six days a week) to boost bone health, improve balance, and increase overall fitness.

Part Two: Resistance Exercises

Exercises (20 to 30 minutes, two or three days a week) to strengthen muscles and bones.

Part Three: Stretches

Stretches (5 to 10 minutes at least three days a week) to boost flexibility and decrease chance of injury.

Part Four: Posture Exercises

Posture exercises (5 to 10 minutes, two or more days a week) to counter the tendency to become stooped and round-shouldered with age.

In addition, we've included a special series of exercises to help prevent and treat each of these muscle- and bone-related health conditions: **back pain, carpal tunnel syndrome,** and **arthritis.** *If you have any of these conditions, or if you suffer from another chronic health problem, bring this workout to your doctor and ask if there are any precautions or individualized guidelines you should follow before proceeding.* (See Pre-Participation Checklist, page 29.)

Mix and match the components of this workout over the course of a week to suit your individual needs and time constraints. For example, if you can devote 30 to 60 minutes to your exercise, five days a week, here's a possible schedule:

Monday: 30-minute walk, 5-minute posture workout, 5-minute stretch
Tuesday: 20-minute strengthening session, 10-minute stretch
Wednesday: 60-minute step-aerobics class
Thursday: Rest (perhaps do some gardening or other easy activity)
Friday: 20-minute strengthening session, 10-minute stretch
Saturday: 30-minute walk, 10-minute posture workout, 5-minute stretch
Sunday: Rest (perhaps take a stroll or hike with family and/or friends)

PART ONE:
WEIGHT-BEARING ACTIVITY

Any exercise in which your feet and legs are bearing your weight (so that your bones and muscles work against gravity) is considered a weight-bearing activity. Walking, running, rope skipping, racquet sports, stair climbing, martial arts, hiking, and dancing are all weight-bearing activities with differing degrees of impact. In general, the higher the impact, the more the activity strengthens bones. That's why, if your goal is optimum bone health, high-impact activities like running or jogging may be a good choice. (For a guide to starting a running program, see page 238.)

But not every body is suited to high-impact activity. For example, people with advanced arthritis or osteoporosis may need to avoid high-impact activities that may jar affected joints or increase the risk of falling. So it's important to choose a weight-bearing aerobic activity that suits your bone status, fitness level, and personal interest. If you are strong and healthy, you might try a high-impact activity that involves running and/or jumping, such as rope skipping or step aerobics. If you are healthy but have a previous injury or other reason to be cautious about your joints, you might be able to gain the benefits of high-impact activity while minimizing the risks by cross-training—that is, do high- and low-impact activities on alternate days. This means you might jog on Monday, Wednesday, and Friday, then walk on Tuesday, Thursday, and Saturday. Or do step aerobics Mondays and Thursdays, walk Tuesdays and Fridays, and bike Wednesdays and Saturdays.

If you cannot tolerate high-impact activities or don't enjoy them, pick a low-impact weight-bearing activity, such as walking. For most people, walking is the activity of choice, offering the maximum muscle and bone benefit at the minimum risk. (For a step-by-step guide to starting a walking program, consult Healing Moves for Heart Health, page 214.) If you can't tolerate walking, try weight-supported exercises, such as water aerobics, chair exercise, or cycling on a stationary bike. These activities won't strengthen bones as much as weight-bearing activities, but they will help strengthen muscles, improve coordination, boost overall fitness, and promote leanness, which can reduce the risk of back and knee pain and repetitive stress injury.

No matter what exercise—or exercises—you choose, it's essential that you start slowly and progress gradually. If you've been inactive and want to take a group fitness class, don't jump right into a "boot camp" workout. Look for a class geared to beginners and discuss any special health concerns you have with the instructor. If you're working out on your own, start with as little as 5 minutes per day, increasing the duration over time, gradually, until you're moving for 20 to 60 minutes at a pace you consider moderate to somewhat hard, three to six days per week. Or think of it this way—do 30 minutes of weight-bearing activity most days of the week.

PART TWO:
RESISTANCE EXERCISES

A good strength-training program doesn't have to be time consuming. Twenty minutes two or three times a week is all you need. In that time, you can easily perform one set each of eight to ten exercises that work the body's major muscle groups (chest, shoulders, front and back of arms, back, abdominals, buttocks, and front and back of legs) against resistance—such as lifting weights or using a strength-training machine or elastic tubing.

When it comes to strength training, more is not necessarily better, because it's essential to give muscles time to repair. That's why it's important to wait forty-eight hours between each strength-training session. Bodybuilders who strength-train every day follow this principle by doing what's called split sets—they work certain muscle groups one day (such as those in the lower body) and other muscle groups the next day (such as those in the upper body). This way, each muscle group still has forty-eight hours to rest before being challenged again.

One set (eight to twelve repetitions) of each exercise is sufficient to boost strength and prevent loss of muscle mass in most adults, according to the latest guidelines from the American College of Sports Medicine. If you have extra time, the guidelines note, a three-set regimen may provide slightly greater benefits.

It's not necessary to join a gym or buy expensive home equipment to do resistance workouts. These strengthening moves can be done at home, using the resistance of your own body weight, dumbbells, and ankle weights. Dumbbells and ankle weights are inexpensive and available at most sporting goods stores. An acceptable substitute for dumbbells (if you prefer not to buy them) is an old sock filled with coins or sand.

To find the right weight, start by using an obviously light weight—or no weight at all—to perform a specific exercise. (For people who've been sedentary, this may be challenging enough for the first few weeks.) If you can do the exercise 12 times easily, add a little more weight and try again. Keep going until you find a weight that challenges you enough so you can do at least 8 but no more than 12 repetitions of the same exercise. (Older and more frail people may find it more appropriate to choose a lighter weight they can lift at least 10, but no more than 15, times.) Once you build up enough muscle so that 12 repetitions become easy, increase the amount of weight gradually— by no more than 10 percent per week. When you've "maxed out," keep going with the resistance you have mastered to maintain your strength.

Before you start these exercises, be sure to warm up first with five minutes of easy walking or other light movements, such as slowly pedaling a stationary bicycle. As you perform them, be sure to:

＊ *Move slowly, with good form.* A good basic tempo is to count to two as you move the weight (counting one one thousand, two one thousand), pause slightly, then count to four as you return to your starting position. Remember that rushing can lead to injury and won't provide as good results.

＊ *Exhale on exertion, inhale on release.* Let your breathing help you lift, and never hold your breath while lifting a heavy weight, since this can cause a sharp rise in blood pressure.

1. Dumbbell Lunge (Works the Buttocks, Quadriceps, and Hamstrings)

Stand erect, holding a dumbbell in each hand. If you've been sedentary, do this exercise without a weight at first.

Keeping your back upright and straight, step forward with the right foot, being sure

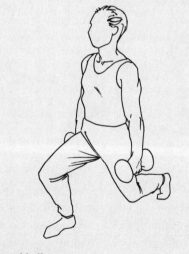

Dumbbell Lunge

to keep your front knee directly over your ankle. (The bigger the step you take, the more difficult the exercise.) Step back with the right foot to the original standing position. Repeat with the left foot.

Perform 8 to 12 on each side.

2. Knee Extension (Works the Quadriceps)

Sit tall in a chair and strap on an ankle weight. (Beginners may want to try this without a weight at first.) Keep your knees slightly apart. Extend your right leg so it is as straight out in front of you as possible, then lower it slowly. Repeat 8 to 12 times, then switch legs.

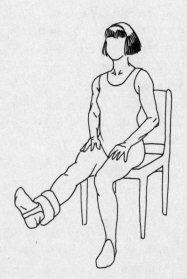

Knee Extension

3. Toe Raise (Works the Calves)

Basic: Face a wall and stand close enough to it to rest your fingertips lightly on the wall at about shoulder height. Keeping your back straight, head erect, and feet shoulder width apart, rise up on your toes as high as possible. Hold the position momentarily, then return to the starting position. Repeat 8 to 12 times.

Intermediate 1: Perform the exercise above on one foot, raising the other foot slightly behind you. Repeat 8 to 12 times, then switch legs.

Intermediate 2: Place a small, secure raised object, such as an aerobic step, next to a wall. Stand with the balls of both feet on the step, balancing yourself by placing your palms or fingertips on the wall. Rise up on your toes as high as possible, then lower your heels down as far as possible. Repeat 8 to 12 times. (See illustration page 144.)

Advanced: Perform the preceding Intermediate 2 exercise on one foot, securing the opposite foot against the heel of the working foot. (See illustration page 144.)

4. Seated Arm Curl (Works the Biceps)

Sit on a chair with your legs open and your feet flat on the floor. Hold a dumbbell in your right hand, palm up. Rest your left

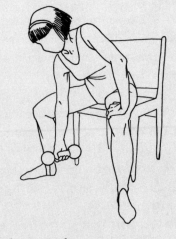

Seated Arm Curl

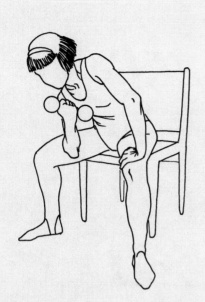

Seated Arm Curl

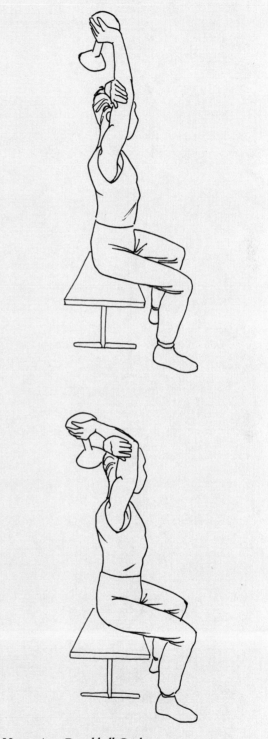

hand on your left thigh and let your right arm drop forward, so that your right upper arm touches the inside of your right thigh. Curl the dumbbell up to shoulder height, then lower it back to the starting position. Repeat 8 to 12 times, then switch arms.

5. Upper-Arm Dumbbell Curl (Works the Triceps)

Sit tall on a chair or bench. Hold a dumbbell in your right hand and raise that arm straight overhead, keeping your upper arm in close to your head. Reach over with your left hand and hold on to your right arm near the elbow for support. Slowly bend your right elbow, keeping it close to your head, and lower the dumbbell behind you. Then lift the dumbbell back up to the starting position. Repeat 8 to 12 times, then switch arms.

Upper-Arm Dumbbell Curl

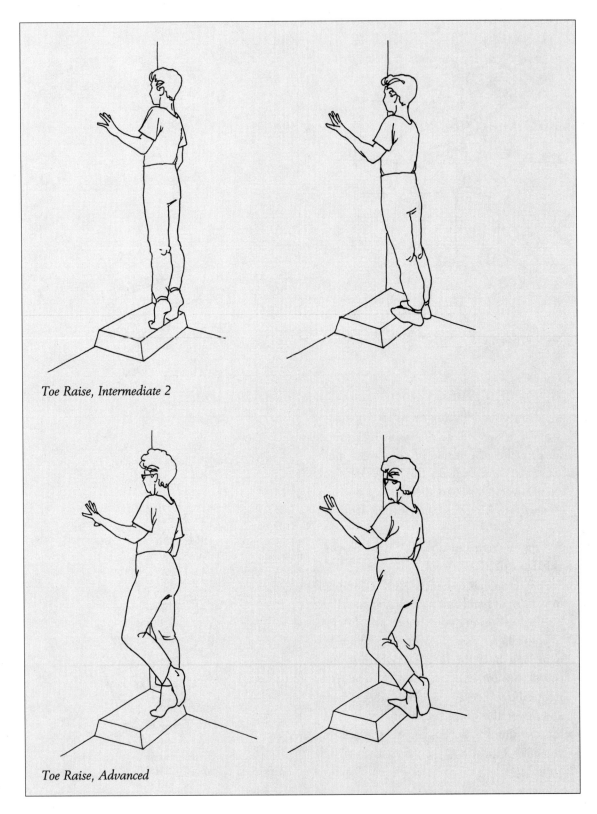

Toe Raise, Intermediate 2

Toe Raise, Advanced

6. Push-up (Works the Shoulders, Chest, and Arms)

Advanced: Position yourself on the floor with your weight on your palms and toes. Keep your feet together, your palms a little wider than your shoulders, and your back straight. Bend your elbows and lower yourself down until your chest is about a fist's distance away from the ground, then push yourself back up. Repeat 8 to 12 times.

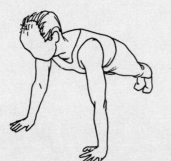

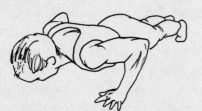

Push-up, Advanced

   Modified: Position yourself on the floor with your weight on your hands and knees. Be sure that your palms are flat on the floor, directly under your shoulders, and that your body is straight. Bend your elbows and lower your chest toward the floor, then push back up to the starting position. Repeat 8 to 12 times.

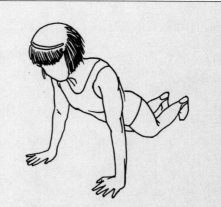

Push-up, Modified Starting Position

7. Curl-up (Works the Abdominal Muscles)

Lie on your back with your knees bent and your feet flat on the floor. Leave your arms at your sides, if you're a beginner. (The farther away your arms are from your belly, the harder the exercise will be. As you get stronger, you may want to cross your arms over your chest or place your fingertips behind your ears.) Contract your abdominal muscles, squeeze your buttocks together, and tilt your pelvis up so that your lower back is pressed into the floor. Slowly curl your head up, just until your shoulder blades lift off the floor. Ease back down. Repeat 8 to 12 times, being sure to exhale as you curl up and inhale as you release.

   To work different parts of the abdominals, try these variations:

   Alternating angles: To work the obliques, the muscles on the sides of the stomach, perform the curl-up at alternating angles, reaching with the shoulder (not the elbow) across the body to the opposite knee. Repeat on the other side.

   Reverse curls: To work the lower abdominals, raise your legs in the air with ankles

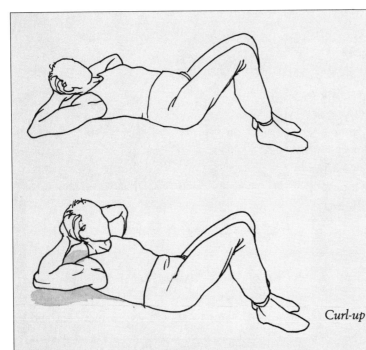

Curl-up

crossed and knees slightly bent. Place both hands under your tailbone, palms toward the floor and keep your head on the floor. Press your abdominals toward the floor, then raise your hips, buttocks, and tailbone slightly off the floor. This is a very small movement, so be sure to use your lower abdominal muscles to lift your hips, not the momentum of swinging legs.

Once these strengthening exercises become easy, or if you start craving variety, try the strength-training exercises featured in Healing Moves for Health and Fitness, page 38.

PART THREE: STRETCHES

Forget the bouncing, ballistic stretches you learned in gym class. Proper stretching should be as relaxed and natural as a yawn. For expert instruction, watch a dog or cat: These animals instinctively stretch, slowly and deliberately, whenever they get up from sitting or lying down. *The key is to stretch by a feeling, not by how far you can go.* Don't have a predetermined notion that you must touch your toes or wrap your foot around your neck. Instead, just stretch until you feel a point of slight tension. *You should feel this tension, but it shouldn't hurt.* If it hurts, you've gone too far and need to back off, just until you feel that point of slight tension. Inhale deeply, then exhale, while you imagine that you're sending your exhaled breath right through this point of tension to relax it. If the tense feeling diminishes and you feel like stretching a bit farther, go for it. Be sure not to stretch to the point of pain. Take a few more breaths, then back off.

Many people have difficulty learning this simple stretching technique because they find it hard to do something so easy. In America, we don't equate something that feels good with physical improvement. Too many of us were indoctrinated by coaches who told us to "give 110 percent" and "do it till it hurts." Also, we tend to be so competitive that if the next guy is touching his toes, we figure that's what we've got to do, too. But it's important to recognize that everyone is unique, with his or her own muscular structure, flexibility, and tension levels.

Remember, in stretching a little bit less is better than a little bit more, since overstretching can lead to injury. When you stretch too far, it activates a nerve reflex that contracts the muscles in a manner similar to what happens if you accidentally touch something hot. By overstretching, you tighten the very muscles you're trying to elongate.

Stretching to the point of mild tension helps the muscles relax, increases your range of motion, helps prevent injuries, promotes circulation, improves sports performance, and helps loosen the mind's control of the body. Think of it this way: Stretching is the bridge from the sedentary to the active life.

This is why the American College of Sports Medicine (ACSM) recently added stretching exercises to its guidelines for adult fitness. ACSM recommends doing stretches for the body's major muscle groups a minimum of two to three days a week. Our workout recommends adding five minutes of stretching to the end of any workout, whether aerobic or strength training. *Contrary to what many people practice, stretching should never be done first thing, when the muscles are cold.* Stretching a cold muscle is like trying to bend a dry sponge—it may break. Instead, start with a few minutes of light activity to get your blood circulating, then stretch gently. But the best, most effective

time to stretch is *after* your workout, when your muscles are warm and receptive. If you don't stretch after exercise—particularly after strength training—your muscles may actually lose flexibility, because strengthening alone can shorten and tighten the muscles. Stretch gently after you've warmed up, before starting your strength-training workout, and stretch again as part of your cooldown. It's also a good idea to stretch spontaneously throughout the day—just as the "stretch master" animals do. Try stretching while you talk on the phone, watch TV, or wait in line. If you sit a lot, stretch throughout the day with exercises from the Carpal Tunnel Syndrome and RSI Series that appears later in this section (page 156).

1. Stretch for the Shoulders, Back, Arms, and Hands

Sit or stand with good posture, interlace your fingers, and raise your arms above your head, turning your palms upward toward the ceiling. Straighten your arms and try to get your upper arms as close to your ears as possible. Take several slow, deep breaths, focusing on the stretch going up the sides of your rib cage, through your arms and hands. Relax and repeat. (Illustration on page 44, Upper-Body Stretch.)

2. Stretch for the Quadriceps

Stand near a wall or a countertop that you can hold on to lightly for balance. Bend your right knee and raise your right heel toward your buttocks. Grab your heel with your right hand, using the left for balance. Breathe in, then exhale as you gently pull your heel toward your buttocks, being sure not to arch your back or strain your knee.

Hold for a few cycles of breath, then relax and repeat with the left leg. (Illustration on page 46, Front of Thigh Stretch.)

3. Stretch for the Hamstrings

Lie on your back with your knees bent and your feet flat on the floor, your heels as close to your buttocks as possible. Extend your right leg upward. With your head, back, and shoulders on the floor, reach for your right leg and grab it wherever you can—at the ankle, calf, or thigh. (But be sure not to grab and pull on your knee.) Inhale, then exhale as you gently pull your right leg toward your face. Hold the leg through several cycles of breathing, then release it and repeat with the left leg. You may also place a belt or strap around your foot to perform this stretch.

4. Stretch for the Back, Hips, and Buttocks

Lie on your back with your arms out to your sides so that your body forms the letter T. Lift your buttocks and shift your hips slightly to the left. Raise your left leg into the air above you and slowly lower your left leg toward your right hand, being sure to keep your elbows, head, and both shoulders flat on the floor. Turn your head so that you look to the left. Hold the position for several cycles of breathing, then relax and repeat on the other side.

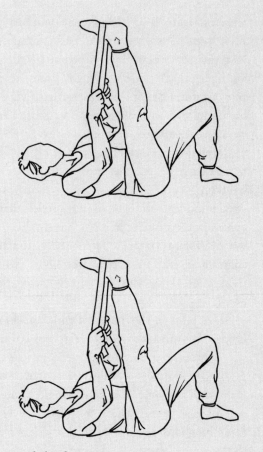

Stretch for the Hamstrings

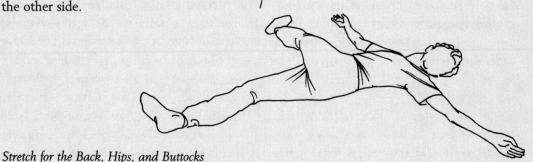

Stretch for the Back, Hips, and Buttocks

5. Stretch for the Torso, Arms, Legs, and Feet

Sit on the floor with your legs extended in front of you. If you like, you can sit on one or two folded blankets. Reach forward without bending your knees until you can hold the sides of your feet. If you can't reach your feet without bending your knees, place a belt or strap around the balls of your feet and hold on to the strap. Keeping your spine elongated, pull yourself forward, reaching your rib cage toward your thighs and bending as far forward as you can go. Try to maintain an even stretch down both legs and both sides of the body. Hold the stretch through a few cycles of breathing, then release.

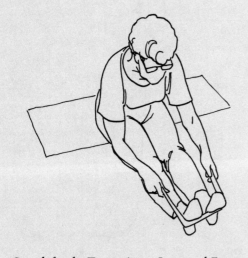

Stretch for the Torso, Arms, Legs, and Feet

Once the province of nagging mothers and finishing schools, posture has become a hot topic in today's health and fitness industry as gravity and years of lazy habits take their toll on an aging society. Stress, excessive sitting, and inactivity are all resulting in postural disasters that leave people slouching toward health-care professionals.

Many people have bad posture habits for years, but their problems don't surface until middle age. Then, one day, they reach for a toothbrush and their back goes out and they have no idea why. Back pain is the most common result of poor posture, but a host of other ailments—from digestive disorders to heart palpitations—can result from decades of crunching the internal organs by slouching. The typical American male tends to have a potbelly and a swayback. This posture leads to excessive wear on the discs, which can cause serious problems. Many older American women have a round-shouldered posture linked to osteoporosis.

Posture can also mirror a person's emotional state, which is why people with poor alignment may literally appear to be in a physical and mental "slump." When people are depressed, their body often reflects collapse. When you're tense, your body is often in a constant state of contraction. The way you hold your body affects the way you feel, and vice versa.

But don't try to *force* your body into a good posture, because that can actually create additional stress. Proper body alignment should reflect a natural state of being centered and relaxed. To practice good posture be sure that you:

✳ Stand firmly on both feet, with your shoulders and arms relaxed.

✳ Center your body, with your weight evenly distributed on both legs.

✳ Slightly tuck your pelvis, extend your spine, and let your head float gently upward on your neck.

The following exercises can help prevent common postural problems, such as swayback and rounded shoulders:

1. Posture Perfect (Works the Upper Back and Shoulders)

Stand tall with your back against a wall, your heels about six inches from the baseboard, and your feet hip width apart. Your shoulders, buttocks, and head should be touching the wall, but your back should not be overarched. Raise your arms and bend your elbows so that each elbow makes a ninety-degree angle and your upper arm rests against the wall in line with your shoulders. Keeping your elbows and wrists touching the wall for as long as possible, raise your hands up the wall, reaching for the ceiling, until your arms are straight. Don't lift your shoulders; keep them pressed down, away from your ears. And don't hyperextend your back. Slowly lower your arms back to the bent-arm position. Repeat five times.

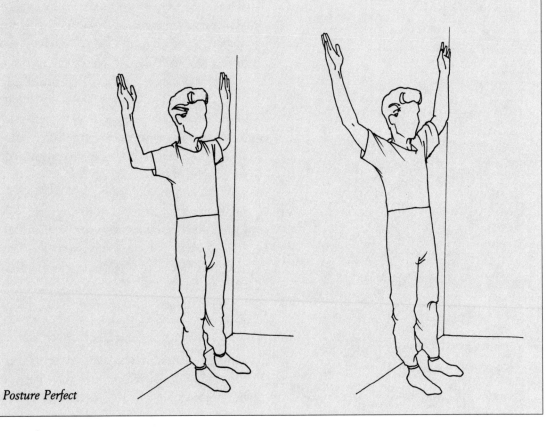

Posture Perfect

2. Wall Reach (Works the Arms, Back and Shoulders)

Face a wall with your feet hip width apart and your toes about six inches from the baseboard. Stretch your arms up to touch the wall, reaching your fingers up toward the ceiling and being sure to keep your pelvis tucked so your back doesn't overarch. Bring your arms down and repeat three times.

Variation: From the same position, try reaching up with one arm while stretching down with the other. Alternate arms.

3. Chin In (Works the Neck and Shoulder Muscles)

Sit up tall on a straight-backed chair or bench, with your feet flat on the floor. Be sure you're sitting on your "sit bones," not on your tailbone. Press your hands down against your thighs, let your breastbone gently lift, and pull your chin in, as if you could move it to the back of your neck. Keep your eyes looking forward and your head erect. (Try this exercise balancing a bean bag on your head if you like.) You should feel a stretch in the back of your neck and a flattening of your upper back.

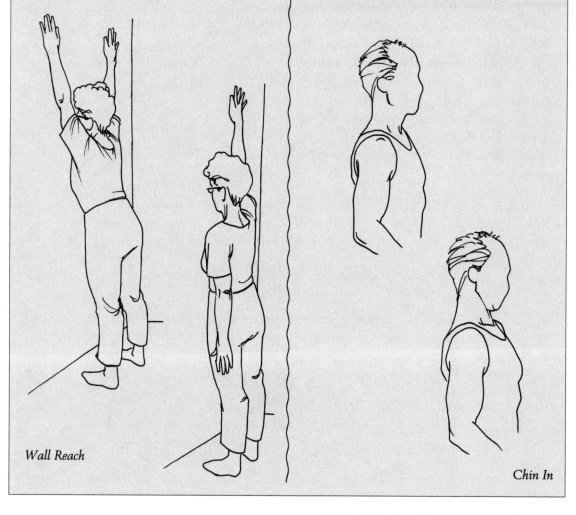

Wall Reach

Chin In

The exercises throughout this entire workout will help eliminate back pain by stretching and strengthening all the body's muscles. Here are some specific exercises, however, that can boost back health by working the muscles that support the back. If chronic back pain is a concern, do these exercises daily, with your doctor's approval.

1. Back Extension

Lie on the floor on your stomach, with a rolled towel under your forehead. Keeping your arms at your sides and feet on the floor, lift your head and shoulders a few inches off the ground, pinching the shoulder blades back. Hold for a second, then slowly lower back to the starting position. Exhale up, inhale down. Beginners should start with 3 repetitions, progressing gradually over several weeks until you can do 8 to 12 repetitions.

2. Back Flexion

Lie on your back with your arms at your sides, knees bent, and feet flat on the floor. Inhale. Then exhale and bring your knees up toward your chest. Place both hands around your knees and gently but firmly pull them as close to your chest as you comfortably can. Keep your knees together and your shoulders flat on the floor. Maintain this position for a second or two and inhale.

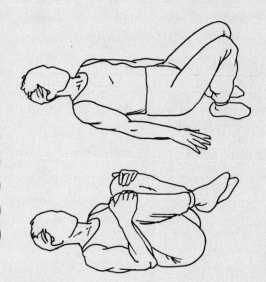

Back Flexion

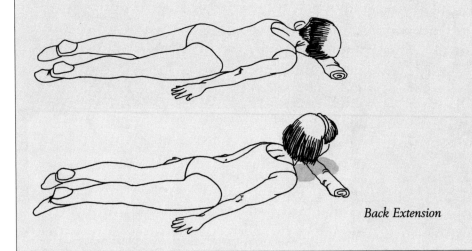

Back Extension

Then exhale while lowering your legs back to the starting position. Be sure that you *do not* raise your head as you perform this exercise or straighten your legs as you lower them. Each time you repeat this movement, try to pull your knees in a little closer to your chest. Start with just 3 to 5 repetitions per session, working up to 10 repetitions.

Here's an alternative version that you can do at your desk:

Seated flexion: Sit on a hard chair with your arms folded loosely in front of you. Exhale and let your body drop until your head is down between your knees. Inhale. Then exhale while raising your body back up into a sitting position and tightening your abdominal muscles. Relax, inhale, and repeat the exercise 3 to 10 times.

3. Pelvic Tilt

Lie on your back with both knees bent, feet flat on the floor, and arms at your sides. Place a small pillow under your head or neck, if you like. Inhale. Then exhale and rotate your pelvis so that your lower back comes in contact with the floor. Tighten your lower abdominal muscles and hold this "pelvic brace" position for two to five seconds. Repeat 15 to 20 times.

4. Basic Spinal Twist

Lie on your back with your neck supported by a rolled towel and your head on a folded blanket or pad. Keeping your left leg straight, bend your right knee and place your right foot on top of your left knee. Roll over onto your left side, so that your right knee touches the floor or comes as close to the floor as possible. Use your left hand to stabilize your right knee on or near the floor. Keep your right shoulder on the floor, turn your head toward your right, and

Pelvic Tilt

Basic Spinal Twist

stretch out your right arm. Try to keep both shoulder blades in contact with the floor. Keep your left leg active by stretching out through the heel and pulling the toes back toward you. Stay here for several breaths, imagining your spine lengthening and the muscles along the spine softening. Breathe out tension from any tight spots you feel.

To come out of this twist pose, roll your right arm up along the floor and over your head until your entire body folds toward the left. Then roll over onto your back and repeat on the other side. Do 2 or 3 times.

When you can do the previous four exercises with ease, try this advanced exercise to help strengthen the legs, abdominals, and buttocks.

5. Wall Slide

Stand with your back against a wall, feet shoulder width apart, heels twelve to eighteen inches from the wall, knees slightly bent. Inhale. Exhale and rotate your pelvis so that your lower back comes into contact with the wall. Tighten your lower abdominal muscles and hold. Inhale, then exhale as you bend your knees while sliding your back down the wall. At first, just bend your knees slightly. When you are comfortable with that, bend your knees more and more, going farther down the wall. But don't ever bend your knees to more than a ninety-degree angle. Hold the bottom position for ten to twenty seconds, breathing comfortably. Exhale as you slide back up the wall. Repeat 5 to 10 times. Try to build up to holding the bottom position for two minutes. If your knees hurt, bend them only slightly.

Since stress can exacerbate or trigger back pain, we've added two basic relaxation techniques to the back series: relaxation breathing and relaxation pose. You can practice relaxation breathing while standing up or lying down. In fact, you can practice it virtually anywhere you encounter stress—like in traffic jams, while waiting in line, when-

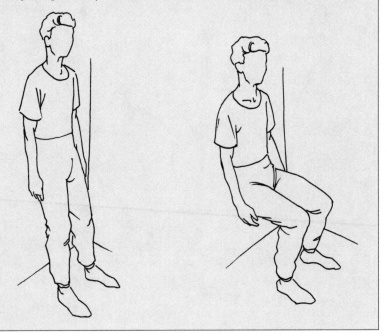

Wall Slide

ever you look at your watch, or just before you pick up the telephone.

1. Relaxation Breathing

Inhale slowly and deeply through your nose; exhale slowly and deeply through your mouth. Try to make the cycles of inhalation and exhalation slow, even, and regular. Think about inhaling energy and exhaling tension. If you like, recite this phrase taught by Vietnamese Zen Master Thich Nhat Hahn: *Breathing in I calm myself, breathing out I smile.* (This is relaxation breathing in its simplest form. For more detailed instruction, see the "paced respiration" exercise in Healing Moves for Women, page 282 and Relaxation Breathing in Healing Moves for Health Fitness, page 48. For other stress-reduction practices, see Healing Moves for Mind-Body-Spirit, page 98.)

2. Relaxation Pose

Support your body in a position of good alignment, in which tired, overworked muscles can completely relax. One of the best ways to do this is to lie on your back on the floor, with a rolled towel or blanket beneath your knees and another beneath your head and neck. If you like, place a scented eyebag over your eyes and a light blanket over your body. Let your arms rest comfortably out by your sides, palms up. If you aren't comfortable lying on your back, lie on your side, with a rolled towel or blanket under your head and neck, another under the top leg, and a third under the top arm.

Relax your jaw and let your tongue drop gently off the roof of your mouth. Let your muscles relax and sink into the floor, allowing the floor and blankets to receive their weight. Inhale slowly and deeply, filling your lungs and abdomen with healing breath. Exhale softly, letting the muscles of your diaphragm, lungs, and ribs contract to

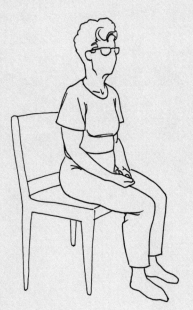

Relaxation Breathing

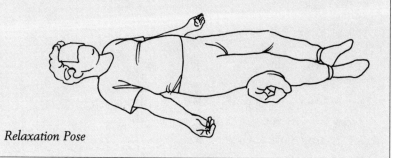

Relaxation Pose

press the breath out in a steady stream. Repeat the focused breathing several times, then return to normal breathing. Concentrate on your breath and try to keep your awareness in the present moment. If you begin to think about the past or future, simply recognize that thought and set it aside, returning to your focus on the breath, in the present moment. Stay in this position for at least ten minutes. When you're ready to rise, be sure to roll over onto your side and push yourself up with your hands to avoid straining your back.

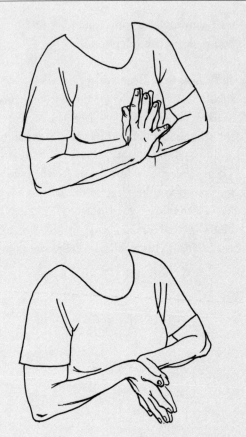

SPECIAL CONDITIONS: CARPAL TUNNEL SYNDROME AND RSI SERIES

Just as athletes warm up before their event, "computer athletes" need to warm up before their keyboard marathon. Do these stretches before and after performing any hand-intensive activity, such as working at a computer. Also, do some or all of these stretches spontaneously at least every hour during a long period of sitting.

1. Prayer Hands

Place your palms together, fingers pointing upward as if in prayer, with your thumbs lightly touching your breastbone. Gently rotate your fingers out, so they point away from your body, as far as you comfortably can, then return to the prayer position.

Prayer Hands

2. Rise and Shine

Interlace your fingers, then turn your palms outward and extend your arms out in front of you as far as you can. Inhale, exhale, and feel the stretch through your arms. Release.

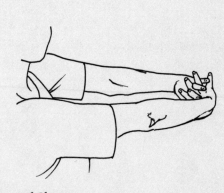

Rise and Shine

3. Fist Fling

Make a loose fist with your right hand. Release your fingers and let them fan out as far as they comfortably can. Repeat five times with each hand. (You may exercise both hands together if you like.)

4. Bye-bye

Stand or sit and extend both arms out in front of you, fingers pointing straight ahead. Inhale and flex your fingers upward, so your palms face out as if you were pushing against a wall. Then exhale as you gently move your hands so that the fingers point downward. Inhale as you raise the fingers up, then exhale as you move them down again—as if you were waving "bye-bye." Repeat five times.

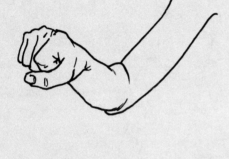

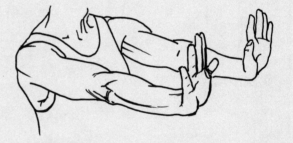

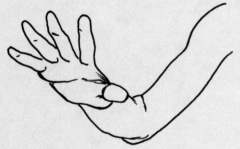

Fist Fling

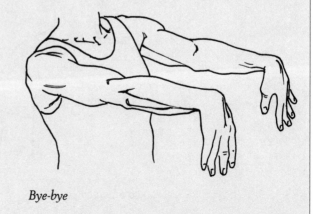

Bye-bye

5. Shoulder Shrug

Stand or sit and raise your shoulders up toward your ears. Hold them there for a count of five, then relax and let your arms hang loose by your sides. Repeat two or three times.

6. Ear to Shoulder

Sit or stand with your shoulders relaxed and your hands hanging loosely at your sides. Gently bring your right ear down toward your right shoulder, keeping both shoulders still and relaxed. Repeat on the other side.

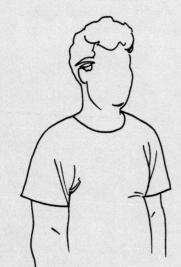
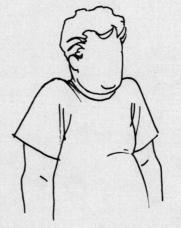

Shoulder Shrug

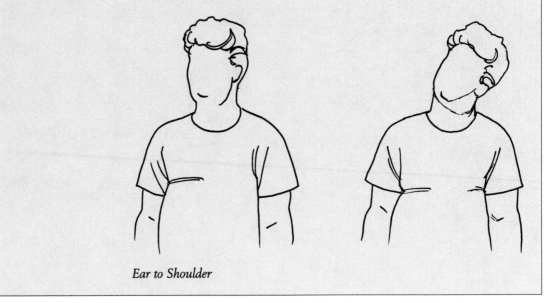

Ear to Shoulder

SPECIAL CONDITIONS: ARTHRITIS SERIES

Here are some simple range-of-motion exercises recommended by the Arthritis Foundation, for frequently affected joints. Be sure to:

* Do each exercise 3 to 10 times.
* Move slowly; don't bounce.
* Breathe while you exercise. Counting out loud will help ensure that you don't hold your breath.

* Don't overdo it. *Stop* exercising if you have pain.

1. Knee and Hip

Lie on your back with one knee bent and the other as straight as possible. Bend the knee of the straight leg, and use your hands to pull your knee to your chest. Lift the leg into the air and then lower it to the floor. (If you feel pain in your knee, do not kick it into the air, just lower it to the floor.) Repeat using the other leg.

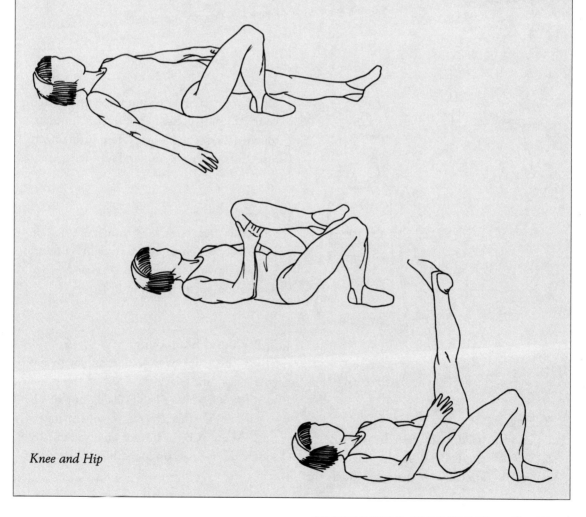

Knee and Hip

2. Shoulder

Lie on your back (or stand) and raise one arm over your head, keeping your elbow straight and your arm as close to your ear as possible. Return your arm slowly to your side. Repeat with your other arm.

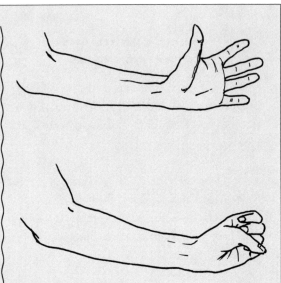

Fingers

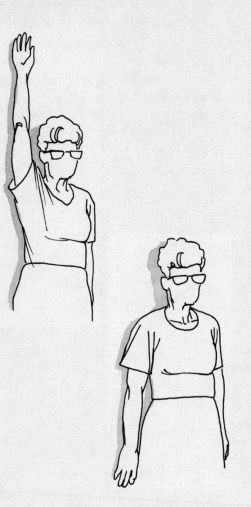

Shoulder

3. Fingers

Open your hand, with your fingers straight and spread apart. Bend all the finger joints except the knuckles so that you touch the top of your palm with your fingertips. Reach your thumb across your palm until it touches the second joint of your little finger. Stretch your thumb out and repeat.

4. Neck

Pull your chin back as if to make a double chin, keeping your head straight without looking down. Hold for three seconds. (See illustration page 151, Chin In.)

5. Back and Shoulders

Reach one palm over your shoulder to pat your back, and place the back of the other hand on your lower back. Slide your hands toward each other, trying to touch fingertips. (Many people are not able to actually touch their fingertips together.) Alternate arms.

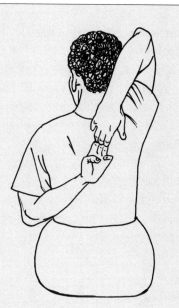

Back and Shoulders

6. Ankle

While sitting, lift your toes as high as possible, still keeping your heels on the floor. Return your toes to the floor, then lift your heels as high as possible, keeping your toes on the floor.

Ankle

Here are some exercises to strengthen the knee, the joint most often affected by osteoarthritis.

1. Knee Isometric

Sit in a straight-backed chair and cross your ankles. Push forward with your back leg and press backward with your front leg; exert pressure evenly so that your legs do not move. Hold and count out loud for ten seconds. Relax and repeat with the legs crossed in the opposite direction.

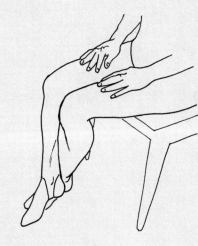

Knee Isometric

2. Quadriceps (Front of Thigh) Strengthener

Lie on your back on a firm, flat surface with one leg straight and the other leg bent. Tighten the muscles at the front of the thigh of the straight leg and slowly lift it about six inches off the floor. Hold for five seconds, then release. Repeat 12 times, then work the other leg. When this becomes easy, add a one-pound ankle weight. When that's easy, try a two-pound ankle weight.

3. Hamstring (Back of Thigh) Strengthener

Lie on your stomach. Lift one leg slowly until it's about three inches off the floor. Hold it in the air for five seconds, then release. Build up to three sets of 12 repetitions with each leg.

4. Calf Strengthener

Stand, leaning lightly against a countertop. Slowly rise up on your toes. Build up to two sets of 12 repetitions.

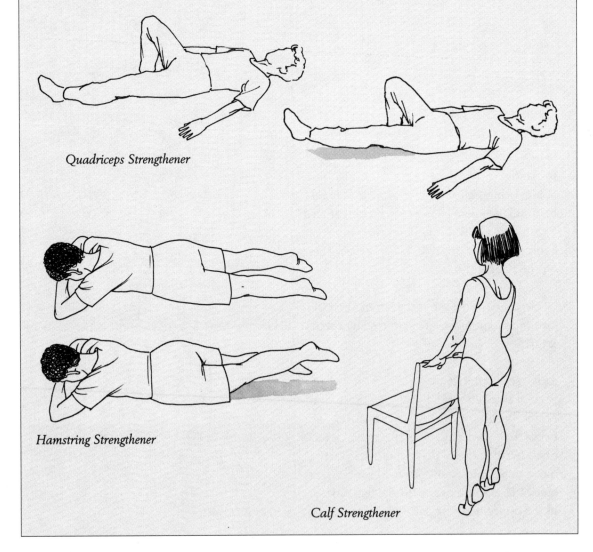

Quadriceps Strengthener

Hamstring Strengthener

Calf Strengthener

5

Immunological Conditions

COLDS, CANCER, AND HIV/AIDS

The immune system is the body's police force, patrolling the bloodstream to battle a constant bombardment of viruses, bacteria, and other harmful invaders. Scientists still do not completely understand many of the complexities of this intricate molecular defense system. Yet it has become increasingly clear that our actions and emotions have a powerful effect on our immune system's ability to protect us from disease. One of the most potent immunological enhancers is moderate exercise.

More than six hundred scientific papers have been published on the relationship between physical activity and immune function. Current research suggests that moderate exercise strengthens the immune system through a variety of mechanisms, including increasing the number and activity of certain kinds of immune cells (such as natural killer cells and macrophages), and slowing the release of stress hormones, which can hamper immunity. Regular exercise also appears to help counter the decline in immune function that typically comes with age.

"When you compare the immune systems of old and young people, the most striking finding is the decline in T-cells, which are an important type of white blood cell," notes David C. Nieman, one of the world's foremost authorities on exercise and immunology and a professor of health and exercise science at Appalachian State University in Boone, North Carolina. Nieman's study of highly conditioned elderly women showed that their T-cell activity was nearly equal to that of a control group of college-age women and 60 percent greater than another control group of elderly, sedentary women. This indicates that some of the decline in immune function associated with age may actually occur not from growing older but from becoming more sedentary.

Although moderate exercise boosts immunity, it is possible to get too much of a good thing. Prolonged or excessive exercise appears to impair immune function and leave people more vulnerable to infection. Research on marathon runners indicates that they are particularly at risk in the six to nine hours following a race, with one study showing that runners who completed a marathon were six times more likely to get sick afterward than equally experienced runners who didn't compete.

These reports point again to the essential truth about health: *A person is healthy when his or her body is in balance or harmony.* It's clear that too much or too little exercise can disrupt this healthy harmony and depress immune function. It's also clear that a more balanced program of regular, moderate exercise helps establish and maintain physical and mental equilibrium and boost immunity.

In addition to *how much* you exercise, physical activity's effect on the body's defensive capability depends on the state of the immune system itself. In that light, it's important to consider the three states of immune system activity:

1. *Normal immune functioning.* In a healthy person, the immune system is constantly active, patrolling for foreign "invaders," capturing and eliminating waste products, and protecting against infection. Moderate exercise stimulates cells of the immune system to do their job more effectively. Normal immune function can be depressed, however, by too little physical activity—the "sedentary" immune system—or by excessive activity—the "exhausted" immune system—both of which compromise host protection.

2. *Immune suppression.* In people with diseases that compromise immunity (such as cancer, HIV or AIDS, diabetes, and conditions requiring chronic use of steroid medications) the cells of the immune system function poorly or not at all due to the underlying illness itself. "Invaders" such as common bacteria, viruses, and fungi that exist in synergistic "peace" with a normal immune system may not be "recognized" or responded to in an immunosuppressed individual, leading to unusual, difficult-to-treat, and even life-threatening infections. Appropriate activity (usually moderate exercise, balanced with rest) can effectively enhance immune function in this setting.

3. *Immune reactivity.* When invaded by a foreign object, from a splinter to a cold virus, the immune system revs into an "angry" state of combat, the so-called inflammatory reaction, deploying erosive enzymes and other internally created proteins that act like cellular bombs. These immune system weapons not only take a toll on the local landscape (the site of the invasion itself) but also produce fallout elsewhere in the body. Local inflammation is characterized by areas of warmth, tenderness, and itching. Fallout may include a variety of symptoms, from fever and generalized achiness to kidney failure. Thus the runny nose and sore throat

of a cold are actually "friendly fire," casualties of the immune system's battle against a cold-virus infection in the throat and nose—the site of invasion. The general achiness, fatigue, and loss of appetite represent some of the secondary fallout associated with this war.

Exercising when you have an "angry" immune system is generally not advisable. Further stimulating the immune system when it is already hyperactive may worsen symptoms. Furthermore, what is "moderate" exercise under normal circumstances may be exhausting to a system that is fighting a war, producing immune suppression and opening the door to spread or worsening of the infection itself.

In this chapter, we'll explore how exercise affects several diseases related to immune function:

* **Colds and flu.** A walk a day keeps colds away. Even if you're fighting a cold, it's helpful to do moderate activity—as long as your symptoms are all above the neck.
* **Cancer.** Physically fit people have a lower incidence of cancer, and studies show a correlation between regular exercise and decreased risk of certain cancers, including colon, breast, endometrium, and prostate. Exercise's affect on the immune system is just one reason why it appears to provide protection. Physical activity's influence on hormones and on reducing body fat also are thought to be mechanisms by which exercise may decrease cancer risk.
* **HIV and AIDS.** At this time, there is no evidence that exercise can help prevent AIDS infection. But there is significant data showing that physical activity has many benefits for individuals who are HIV positive, such as helping maintain lean body mass, avoid excessive muscle wasting, improve appetite, and enhance mood.

THE COLD FACTS

The ailment we call a cold is actually an infection of the lining of the nose, sinuses, and throat. Caused by a virus, the cold is indeed very common. The most frequently occurring illness in humans worldwide, colds strike the average American adult two or three times per year and the average American child from six to seven times annually. The flu is also a viral infection of the upper respiratory tract, but it makes a person much sicker. In addition to the symptoms typical of a cold (such as sneezing, coughing, and congestion), the flu frequently causes a fever, headache, and chills. More than 425 million colds and flus occur annually in the United States, according to the Centers for Disease Control and Prevention, resulting in $2.5 billion in lost school and work days and medical costs.

Over two hundred different viruses cause these upper-respiratory infections, and they are very easily transmitted. For example, if you shake hands with an infected person, then touch your eye, mouth, or nose, you could become infected. Whether or not you get sick with a cold after the virus has entered your body depends on many factors, one of which is the strength of your immune system. Certain behaviors and experiences are known to impair immune functioning and increase your risk of infection. These include cigarette smoking, aging, stress, poor nutrition, quick weight loss, fatigue, and heavy, prolonged physical exertion. Healthy behaviors that can enhance immune function include eating a nutritious diet, getting adequate sleep, minimizing stress, and getting regular, moderate exercise.

Fit people report getting fewer colds than their inactive peers. For example, one survey showed that 61 percent of recreational runners said they'd experienced fewer colds since they'd started to run, compared to only 4 percent who felt they experienced more, according to the American College of Sports Medicine (ACSM). In another survey of 170 experienced runners, 90 percent said they "definitely" or "mostly" agreed with the statement that they "rarely get sick."

Research backs up this perception. Several studies by David C. Nieman of Appalachian State University show that people who walked for forty-five minutes five days a week for twelve weeks suffered half as many days of cold and flu symptoms as people in a nonexercising control group.

When people exercise, the increased circulation encourages the spread of beneficial immune cells throughout the body, boosting protection against viruses and other pathogens. Exercise can increase the number, activity, and delivery of immune cells during physical activity and for about ninety minutes afterward. When people exercise daily, or almost every day, "it's like a house cleaner coming in for a few hours every day," Nieman says. "So the house stays clean."

Exercise also may enhance immunity through its stress-relieving effects. Stress is known to impair immune function, and numerous studies show that exercise helps reduce stress and enhance mood (see chapter 3, Mental Health Conditions, page 89). By helping people balance their emotions and relieve tensions, regular exercise may offer another kind of immunological boost.

But there's a flip side to this relationship between exercise and stress. As noted earlier, excessive exercise—such as running a marathon or training for the Olympics—can itself be a physiological and psychological stress. This may explain why prolonged, heavy exertion appears to suppress the immune system and leave athletes more vulnerable to infection. During the Winter and Summer Olympic Games, for example, team physicians report that upper-respiratory infections abound.

Nieman suggests thinking about it this way: Moderate exercise, like taking a brisk walk, gives an immunological boost similar to feeding the immune system "police force" some coffee. The molecular "cops" get a caffeinelike "buzz" and start circulating around at a greater rate than normal, which increases their chance of running into bad guys. But doing excessive exercise is like giving the police force a keg of beer. The immune system "cops" become confused by the barrage of demands for fuel and repair from the body's exhausted muscles, so they are too befuddled to do their job well.

EXERCISE ℞ FOR COLD PREVENTION

The obvious question is this: How much exercise is enough to enhance resistance to colds, but not too much to impair it? Your particular exercise prescription will depend on many factors, such as your health status, previous exercise levels, and general fitness. If you've been sedentary or if you're an irregular exerciser, try moving just a little bit more than you currently move. Gradually, but regularly, move just a little bit longer and a little bit faster. A good goal is the surgeon general's recommendation for health: Perform 30 minutes of moderate activity on most days of the week. Of course, "moderate" is a relative term, since a moderate workout for a competitive athlete may be a killer workout for someone who's been sedentary.

That's why it's critical to tune in to your body and listen to the signals it gives you. For example, you know you're exercising in the moderate range when:

✳ Your breathing rate is up, but you can still carry on a conversation.

✳ Your heart rate is elevated, but your heart isn't racing.

✳ You are working, but not straining.

✳ You can recover within ten minutes of exercise. If you do not feel normal again within ten minutes of stopping exercise, you're probably pushing yourself too much.

A good indicator that your activity is benefiting your immune system is that you're having fun. When exercise crosses the line from being physical play you enjoy to being backbreaking work that hurts, your body is probably signaling you that something's wrong. Perhaps you're using poor technique or faulty equipment or simply doing too much. If you find yourself checking your watch every few minutes and wishing it was time to quit exercising, it's time to reassess your fitness program.

"Grinding your teeth and racing through your workout can defeat the whole purpose," says Ruth Stricker, founder of the Marsh: A Center for Balance and Fitness, in suburban Minnesota. Diagnosed with the auto-immune disorder lupus in 1975 and given five years to live, Stricker credits her practice of tai chi with helping her become what experts at Johns Hopkins called "the wellest lupus patient" they'd ever seen. "When you exercise with a happy mind-set, it's much more beneficial," says Stricker, who contends that the Western "perfect body" approach to fitness leaves people with "tight abs and pecs and vacant hearts and minds." When it comes to exercise and to life, Stricker says, "my number one motto is, Protect the joy."

EXERCISE ℞ FOR COLD RELIEF

Identifying the crossover line between doing enough and doing too much can be difficult for committed exercisers, since forming the exercise habit requires developing the discipline to lace up your shoes and walk out the door even on days when you'd rather pull the covers up over your head. Plus, some fitness enthusiasts become so reliant on their daily exercise "fix" that skipping exercise is itself a major stress. That's why habitual exercisers often don't let minor nuisances like a stuffy nose or scratchy throat keep them on the sidelines.

New research suggests that it's okay—and may even be beneficial—to do moderate aerobic activity when you're fighting a cold. "Exercising moderately when you have a cold doesn't appear to alter the severity or duration of the illness," according to a study published in the journal *Medicine & Science* in *Sport & Exercise*. Researchers at Ball State University in Muncie, Indiana, examined fifty people who were inoculated with a cold virus and compared the symptoms of thirty-four who exercised moderately every other day with sixteen who didn't exercise. After ten days, the two groups showed no difference in symptoms as reported by questionnaires and determined by "mucous weights" of their used facial tissues.

Exercising moderately with a head cold is "probably acceptable and, some researchers would even argue, beneficial," note experts at the ACSM. But if you have a fever or other flu symptoms, such as muscle aches, swollen lymph glands, or extreme tiredness, the ACSM experts recommend "bed rest and a gradual progression to normal training."

Pushing yourself to work out when you have a fever or other flu symptoms is not only foolhardy but could make you sicker. When your immune system is "reactive"—in the combat mode of battling an infection—activating it further through exercise may make you feel worse, not better. Also, when immune cells are overtaxed, it may take less exercise than average to depress immune function; that is, lower levels of exercise may hit your system like excessive exercise would under normal circumstances. Depressing the immune system while it is actively fighting an infection can be dangerous, as the infection may be able to increase in severity or to spread to other organ systems.

Since many competitive athletes find the stress of missing a workout worse than the stress of exercising when they feel sick, physician E. Randy Eichner, a marathon runner and professor of medicine at the University of Oklahoma Health Sciences Center, has developed this "neck check":

✳ ***Below the neck:*** Don't exercise when you have below-the-neck symptoms, such as fever, muscle aches, or a hacking cough that produces phlegm in your throat.

✳ ***Above the neck:*** You may exercise if you have only above-the-neck symptoms, such as a runny nose, sneezing, and a scratchy throat. But take a "test drive" first. Start your workout at half speed. If your head seems to clear and you feel peppy, it's okay to finish. But if you feel like you're running through sand, go back home and rest.

Before you rush out to "just do it" when you're sick, ask yourself, "What's the point?" If you're exercising for your health, because it makes you feel good, and to boost your immunity, why work out when your body is telling you to rest? If you feel bad enough to be popping cold pills, you're probably better off not exercising that day. But many regular exercisers don't know how to cut back or take a short layoff when their bodies are fighting a cold.

Our rule of thumb about exercise when you feel under the weather is to:

1. Wait until the worst is over.
2. Then start activity slowly to see if it feels good to "get moving."
3. If movement feels good, do less than you usually do until you're feeling like "yourself" again. For example, if you're a regular runner, try walking instead. Rather than take a 60-minute aerobics class, do a half hour of yoga.

While these guidelines may be fine for recreational athletes, elite athletes often don't have the option of training moderately on a regular basis because intense training is essential to their livelihoods. Also, many competitive athletes have trouble identifying the crossover line into pain, because they've learned to push past their body's caution signals in pursuit of extraordinary physical accomplishments.

Like anyone, elite athletes can reduce their risk of catching colds by practicing good health habits, such as washing their hands. But if they are doing excessive activity, they may also help ward off infection by keeping their bodies fueled during exercise. Research indicates that something as simple as drinking a liter of sports drink per hour appears to help the immune system cope with intense exercise. It's like telling the immune system, "There's enough fuel here, so don't get so excited."

Other immune-system enhancers for elite athletes (and others) are proper nutrition, keeping other life stresses to a minimum, avoiding overtraining and chronic fatigue, getting adequate sleep, and spacing vigorous workouts and race events as far apart as possible. Some experts advise athletes who are competing in the winter months to get a flu shot. And since colds are spread by contact and breathing the air near infected people, if at all possible avoid being around sick people before and after important athletic events.

CANCER ANSWERS: THE ACTIVITY CONNECTION FOR PREVENTION

Cancer is a group of more than one hundred diseases with a common characteristic—the uncontrollable growth and accumulation of abnormal cells. These abnormal cells develop through a lengthy process called carcinogenesis, which starts with damage to one or more genes that produces unregulated cell growth. The process ends, often ten to twenty years later, with the formation of a detectable tumor. Most cancers are named for the type of cell or the organ in which they begin, even if the cancer has spread. For example, a cancer that starts in the lung is called lung cancer. If a lung cancer spreads to the liver or brain or some other organ, it is called metastatic lung cancer.

Each year about 1.4 million Americans learn they have cancer, and it is the second-leading cause of death in the United States, after heart disease. While the percentage of deaths from heart disease is declining nationally, the percentage of deaths attributed to cancer is rising. Some experts predict that cancer will become America's leading cause of death. The lifetime risk for developing cancer is a startling 45 percent for men and 39 percent for women, according to the National Cancer Institute. The most frequent form of cancer is lung cancer, followed by prostate cancer for men and breast cancer for women. Colorectal cancer is the third most common form of cancer in both sexes.

Throughout the world, industrialized countries have the highest cancer death rates. Studies show that when people from Third World countries adopt Western lifestyles, certain types of cancers—especially colon, breast, and prostate—increase. This suggests that lifestyle factors play a major role in the development of these cancers, particularly habits such as cigarette smoking, a high-fat diet, and a sedentary lifestyle.

The relationship between exercise and cancer prevention is the topic of extensive scientific research. Most experts now agree that regular physical activity can help reduce the risk of colon cancer, and there is a growing consensus that exercise may lower the risk of breast cancer. Evidence also links exercise with a reduced risk of prostate cancer in men and a lower incidence of reproductive cancers (such as endometrial and uterine) in women.

In 1996, the American Cancer Society (ACS) added regular physical activity to the list of preventive measures it advocates, in part because it's now known that physically fit people tend to have a lower incidence of cancer. "According to one large study of people at various levels of fitness, the least fit men died from cancer at a rate that was more than four times higher than that of the most fit men," notes *Informed Decisions*, the ACS's guide to cancer diagnosis, treatment, and recovery. "The least fit women had fully 16 times the cancer death rate of the most fit women."

It's easy to see the connection between exercise and some ailments, such as heart disease, because when you're physically active your heart beats faster. But the relationship between physical activity and cancer is harder to grasp. Scientists still don't know the precise mechanisms by which exercise appears to exert an "anticancer" effect, but current thinking points to physical activity's effect on the immune system, the nervous system, and the endocrine system.

Theories as to why exercise may reduce cancer risk can be placed in two main categories:

1. **"Right growing."** Exercise improves physical and mental functioning and creates a healthy metabolic and physiologic environment, which is less susceptible to cancer.
2. **"Immunosurveillance."** Exercise boosts activity of the immune system, which enhances the body's ability to recognize and eliminate abnormal cells.

"Right growing" theories include:

✳ *Increased fecal transit time.* Exercise increases the speed by which food travels through the digestive tract. This shortens the time carcinogens in fecal matter would come in contact with cells that line the colon and may explain why physically active men have half the risk of colon cancer as their sedentary peers.

✳ *Leaner bodies.* People who exercise tend to be leaner, and excess body fat is a risk factor for cancer, particularly cancer of the colon, breast, uterus, and endometrium. In postmenopausal women, adipose tissue (body fat) converts adrenal hormones into estrogen. Elevated blood levels of estrogen are linked with an increased risk of breast cancer.

✳ *Hormonal effects.* Girls who exercise vigorously begin menstruating later than their less active peers, and a later onset on menarche is associated with a reduced risk of breast and reproductive cancers. Prostate cancer is associated with higher levels of the male hormone testosterone, and studies suggest that testosterone concentrations are depressed in trained athletes. This may explain why some evidence links regular physical activity with lower prostate cancer risk.

✳ **The granola effect.** When people begin to exercise, they frequently adopt a constellation of healthy behaviors, such as eating right, not smoking, and sleeping better. Dubbed the granola effect, this association between being a regular exerciser and having other healthy habits may help explain why fit people have a lower incidence of cancer.

"Immunosurveillance" theories include:

✳ **Superior mood states.** Fit people have lower rates of depression and anxiety. Since studies suggest that stress may impair immunity and that emotions may influence the course of cancer, people with positive mood states may be at reduced risk for the disease.

✳ **More and stronger cellular defenders.** Aerobic exercise is believed to enhance the production of interferon and interleukin-2, normal body proteins that also are being used to treat cancer. It is also associated with an increase in the strength and number of certain types of immune cells, including natural killer cells, macrophages, and T-cells, which all help defend against cancer.

THE ACTIVITY CONNECTION FOR CANCER SURVIVORS

Not only does regular exercise reduce the risk of developing some cancers, but for people who already have cancer a personalized exercise program can be one of the most powerful therapies in promoting recovery. Appropriate physical activity can help counter some aspects of the disease, relieve many unpleasant reactions to cancer treatments, and boost the quality of life for survivors. This is especially important to the estimated ten million Americans who are living with cancer. About seven million of these people were treated five or more years ago and are part of a new era of cancer survivorship. Allopathic cancer treatment is frequently based on destroying cancerous tissue through radiation, chemotherapy, and surgery. These treatments often affect healthy, noncancerous tissue, too, which makes the health-enhancement effect of exercise especially critical.

Success with many therapies has led to populations in which cancer is a chronic condition, like heart disease or diabetes. And just as exercise can benefit people with these other chronic ailments, regular physical activity helps people with cancer in many ways, including:

1.   *Fighting fatigue.* The biggest problem for most cancer patients is fatigue. There is no medical treatment for fatigue except rest, and many patients find that the more they rest, the worse they feel. Exercise can help counter this fatigue spiral, where tired people stay in bed, which makes them more tired. Yoga, walking, and other moderate exercise—alternated with appropriate periods of rest—can help boost energy levels and stamina. Structured activity programs can lead to an increase in stamina, with improvements in self-image, appetite,

nutritional status, drug tolerance, and immunologic defenses.

2. *Stimulating appetite.* Some cancers, many side effects of treatment, plus emotional upset can diminish appetite, with loss of both the taste and the desire for food. Exercise can help stimulate appetite and support general nutrition.

3. *Boosting mood.* Regular exercise is associated with reduced rates of depression and anxiety and increased feelings of self-esteem, mastery, and control. This can be essential in people with cancer, who often struggle with a variety of negative emotions, including depression, hopelessness, lethargy, anger, and overall poor self-image. Researchers at Ohio State University found that breast cancer patients with the most anxiety about their medical condition had the lowest levels of white blood cells, which normally attack cancer and combat infection. By relieving stress and boosting mood, exercise may help counter negative emotions and block associated decreases in immune function.

4. *Restoring immunologic resistance.* While many suspect cancers arise due to deficiencies in the immune system, it is even clearer that most cancers, once established, further depress immune resistance. Thus many cancer patients also are vulnerable to a variety of infectious diseases from bacteria, viruses, or fungi not commonly found as pathogens in human beings. The ability of regular moderate exercise to stimulate immune responsiveness and activity in this setting may provide a patient with relief from a plague of annoying minor infec-

tions, as well as resistance to some potentially life-threatening ones.

5. *Managing pain.* Movement itself may help in pain management and assist the body's own self-healing mechanisms. For pain exacerbated by movement, such as pathological fractures or metastatic involvement of bones, yoga breathing, meditation, and visualization techniques may help relieve pain symptoms.

6. *Reducing stiffness.* Surgeries and bed rest can diminish range of motion of the body's joints. Stretching exercises can restore flexibility, mobility, and activity capacities.

7. *Maintaining strength.* Many cancers involve muscle wasting through progressively poor nutrition, response to anticancer therapies, or both. Exercise, especially with resistance training, can help some cancer patients retain muscle tissue and normal strength.

8. *Maintaining a healthy weight.* Both weight gain, especially from water retention, and weight loss from body-mass wasting can be more readily modulated when a person stays active.

9. *Helping healthy tissue compensate.* Since exercise strengthens the heart, improves lung capacity, and increases circulation, regular exercise may boost healthy tissue enough to compensate for compromised cells and organs. For example, aerobic exercise may boost lung function enough to help someone with lung cancer breathe more easily. Normal cells that suffer from radiation or chemotherapy toxicities used to kill malignant cells may recover more quickly and more

completely in active individuals compared to sedentary ones.

10. *Reducing risk of other diseases.* Cancer survivors may be at heightened risk for other diseases as a result of their cancer or its treatment. For example, women with reproductive cancers are advised against taking hormone-replacement therapy, which makes exercise especially critical for preventing osteoporosis. And exercise can help reduce the risks of some diseases totally unrelated to the cancer, such as diabetes and heart disease.

There is some suggestion, from animal studies, that exercise may slow the course of the disease by reducing tumor growth and boosting the efficiency of cancer-destroying cells. But at this time, in humans with cancer, exercise is considered primarily a way to relieve unpleasant side effects of the disease and its treatments and to enhance overall quality of life.

EXERCISE ℞ FOR CANCER PREVENTION

The whole notion of reducing cancer risk through physical activity is so new that no one knows precisely how much exercise is necessary to help prevent the disease. For now, most experts say that the best guideline is the surgeon general's exercise prescription for improved overall health: *Perform a modest amount of moderate exercise (enough to burn 150 calories) on most days of the week—for example, 30 minutes of walking, 20 minutes of jogging, or 45 minutes of gardening.*

Current research into the effect of various exercise prescriptions on certain cancers also offers some insights. Among the most intriguing findings:

✻ Researchers at Harvard University found that the protective effect of exercise on colon cancer was most evident in men who exercised an average of one to two hours a day.

✻ An analysis of the exercise habits of 67,800 women in the Nurses Health Study showed that women who walked an hour every day had roughly half the colon cancer risk of sedentary women. There was a similar risk reduction for women who swam, biked, jogged, or did any other aerobic activity for 30 minutes a day.

✻ A study of more than 25,000 Norwegian women found that those who exercised at least four hours a week had a 37 percent lower risk of developing breast cancer than did sedentary women. The more the women exercised, the less likely they were to get breast cancer.

✻ A University of California study found that premenopausal women who exercised for three to four hours a week cut their breast cancer risk by as much as half. Women who exercised for one to three hours a week lowered their risk by 30 percent.

✻ A Norwegian study found that the risk of prostate cancer was reduced by more than half in men who walked during their work hours and also engaged in regular leisure-time exercise. But this protection was found only in men over age sixty.

While there is no definitive guideline for exercise to help prevent cancer, certain criteria seem important in reducing the risk:

* Consistency. Cancer is a disease that develops slowly over long periods of time, which means that adopting the regular habit of exercise is important in the long run. Daily, or near daily, physical activity maximizes the positive effects exercise has on the body's immune, nervous, and endocrine systems.

* Healthy energy balance. Since excess fat increases cancer risk, it's important to exercise enough to achieve an appropriate balance between calories consumed and calories burned. This will help you avoid obesity and maintain a healthy weight.

* Train, but don't strain. Be sure to exercise enough to activate the immune system, while minimizing heavy, prolonged physical activity that might suppress immunity.

* Enjoy. Remember that having fun along the way may be as important as achieving a specific fitness goal. Relieving tension, boosting mood, and enhancing self-confidence aren't just great side effects of exercise—they are primary effects.

EXERCISE ℞ FOR CANCER SURVIVORS

Exercise prescriptions for people with cancer need to be individualized to take into account a variety of factors, including:

* The type of cancer and its status
* The type of therapy and its effects
* The patient's exercise history
* The patient's other illnesses independent of cancer (e.g., heart disease or diabetes)

A physician's approval is essential, since cancer patients may be at increased risk for injury as a result of their disease or its treatment. (For example, chemotherapy makes people more susceptible to infection and bleeding, so low-impact activity is advised.) Be aware that some well-meaning health professionals may overemphasize the importance of taking it easy, with little appreciation for the many health benefits physical activity can offer cancer patients. Just as the idea of heart patients exercising seemed unthinkable forty years ago, the notion of cancer patients exercising surprises many people today—even some physicians. Yet appropriate exercise can stimulate or maintain the body's functional capacity, while unnecessary rest can result in progressive fatigue or weakness. The important point is to make sure that exercise is *appropriate* for your specific condition.

A qualified exercise physiologist can help you design a personalized program and set appropriate exercise goals. In some cities, you'll be able to find exercise classes designed for patients with cancer, often offered by a hospital or university-based wellness facility or a YMCA or YWCA. Similar to cardiac rehab, these emerging "oncology rehabilitation programs" tend to feature both group and individualized exercise. For example, at Living for Life, an exercise class for cancer patients at the National Institute for Fitness and Sport in Indianapolis, participants warm up together, then each person spends about 30 minutes doing an individualized cardiovascular program—ranging from pedaling a stationary bike to walking around a track to rowing. Next comes a strength-training portion on resistance machines, followed by 10 minutes of stretching done together. In addition to the physical and psychological benefits of exercise, participating in a fitness class with other cancer survivors can also offer important social support.

Exercise programs for cancer patients need to be flexible to take into account how the person feels. The nature of the disease and its treatment means that cancer patients often experience severe fatigue, which leads to inactivity. Chronic inactivity results in decreased energy, and the unhealthy cycle continues. While it's important to encourage appropriate activity to break this fatigue spiral, it's also advisable for a patient to avoid overexertion and to get appropriate rest.

Maryl L. Winningham, a Salt Lake City nurse who has pioneered exercise programs for cancer patients, asks people, "What's the most you could do without falling over?" Then she encourages them to do half that amount. She also makes sure that patients incorporate rest periods into their training. "The idea is to do something—like walk across the room—then rest, then do something, then rest," she says. "Rest, as well as exertion, is part of training because it allows the body to rebuild."

Don't try to compete with anyone else, and listen to your body. If you've exercised to the point of exhaustion, where you're unable to do your normal activities, you've done too much. "You've got to love your body back to health, cell by cell," Winningham says. "You can't do that with an Attila the Hun approach."

Like anyone starting an exercise program, people with cancer who are beginning to be active should start slowly and progress gradually. A good program should include:

✴ *Aerobic activity.* Walking is the ideal exercise for people with cancer because it improves lung function, stimulates bone and muscle growth, and is easy on the joints. Swimming is also a good option for some people, since it is virtually stress-free.

✴ *Strength training.* Resistance exercises can help restore muscle mass and improve appetite. Be sure to work with a qualified trainer to learn appropriate exercises and technique.

✴ *Mind-body practices.* Yoga, qi gong, and tai chi can help boost flexibility, restore range of motion to affected joints, and help establish emotional equilibrium and a sense of calm and control. Deep, focused breathing can help relieve stress and manage pain and may help people cope better with difficult procedures and treatments.

Be sure to:

✴ *Set personal, incremental goals.* Recognize that moving a little bit more each day can literally "keep you going." Use self-references to establish goals—for example, if you could walk to the mailbox today, consider walking to your neighbor's mailbox tomorrow.

✴ *Protect the joy.* If an exercise prescription is just another part of your cancer therapy, it will probably benefit you less. But if your physical activity is a celebration of your ability to generate and sustain wellness in the face of illness, you may have in hand the most potent path to recovery.

HIV, AIDS, AND EXERCISE

Acquired immune deficiency syndrome (AIDS) is caused by infection with the human immunodeficiency virus (HIV), which attacks the immune system and leads to a progressive deterioration in the body's ability to defend itself against disease. HIV is spread from one person to another through certain bodily fluids: blood and blood products, semen, vaginal fluid, and breast milk. Someone who is infected with HIV may have no symptoms for years. But generally, over time, the immune system can't keep up with the rapidly reproducing HIV, and serious infections develop. These infections are called opportunistic infections because they usually don't make healthy people very sick, yet they are often the cause of death for people whose immune systems are compromised by HIV or AIDS.

AIDS is diagnosed when an HIV-infected person's immune system has become severely damaged or when certain other serious infections or cancers occur. Most HIV-infected people develop AIDS within fifteen to twenty years, but modern therapies are expected to make the incubation period even longer. Without treatment, 80 to 90 percent of AIDS patients die within three to five years after diagnosis.

At this time, there is no evidence that exercise can help prevent AIDS infection. However, researchers are studying whether exercise training can be used to delay the progression from HIV infection to full-blown AIDS. One indicator that physical activity may help slow the declines usually seen in HIV-positive people is that surveys of long-term AIDS survivors show that most participate regularly in exercise programs. Another is that stress can accelerate the progression of early-stage HIV, and exercise is known to help relieve stress. Some evidence suggests that exercise may help stabilize counts of certain immune cells, and limited data indicates that exercise training in asymptomatic, HIV-positive patients may slow the disease's progression. But more research needs to be done.

What does appear clear from existing research, however, is that appropriate exercise does not harm HIV or AIDS patients. Since heavy, prolonged exertion is known to suppress immunity and increase vulnerability to infection, many health professionals have been reluctant in the past to recommend exercise programs to people with HIV or AIDS. But now that new treatments are helping people with HIV and AIDS live longer, there has been a trend toward finding strategies to help enhance the quality of life of long-term survivors. Physical activity is one of the most promising of these strategies, and researchers are trying determine an appropriate exercise prescription for people with HIV or AIDS. Emerging evidence suggests that both aerobic and strength training have many physical and psychological benefits for people with HIV or AIDS, including:

✴ *Helping maintain lean body mass.* Muscle wasting is common in people with HIV or AIDs, and a program of resistance exercises can help prevent or reverse loss of muscle mass and body weight while boosting strength and function.

✴ *Helping maintain cardiovascular function.* Moderate aerobic exercise can help offset declines in heart and lung function often seen during the course of HIV disease.

✴ *Enhancing mood and the ability to cope.* Exercise can help people with HIV or AIDS reduce their levels of depression and anxiety and improve their quality of life.

* **Countering the toxic effects of HIV therapy.** As with anticancer drugs, HIV medications may compromise normal cells. Healthy tissue may recover more quickly and more completely in active individuals than in sedentary ones

EXERCISE ℞ FOR HIV OR AIDS

Exercise prescriptions for people with HIV or AIDS need to be individualized to account for a variety of factors, including:

* The stage of the disease
* The side effects of the disease or therapies
* The patient's exercise history
* The patient's other illnesses

A physician's approval is essential, and an exercise physiologist or trainer should work with the patient's doctor to design an appropriate exercise program with realistic fitness goals. Appropriate activities may include:

* *Aerobic exercise*, particularly moderate, low-impact activities such as walking and swimming.
* *Strength training*, monitored by a qualified fitness professional.
* *Mind-body practices*, such as yoga, tai chi, and qi gong.

In the journal *Sports Medicine*, researchers J. H. Calabrese and A. LaPerriere offer these recommendations for exercise during the three stages of HIV/AIDS disease:

Stage I: Asymptomatic HIV
Unrestricted exercise activity
Competition as tolerated
Avoid overtraining

Stage 2: Symptomatic HIV
Moderate exercise training
Terminate competition
Avoid exhaustive exercise

Stage 3: AIDS
Remain physically active
Continue exercise training on a symptom-limited basis
Avoid strenuous exercise
Reduce or curtail exercise during acute illness

CAUTIONS

People with cancer, HIV, or AIDS may find that the disease and/or its treatment may alter their ability to exercise. While it's important not to automatically give in to the impulse to rest when you're feeling "low-energy," it's crucial to tune in to your body's signals. Be aware that people with compromised immune systems may be susceptible to certain conditions that affect their ability to exercise. Common concerns include:

* **Bone stress.** Some people with cancer are at risk for fractures and may be advised not to do high-impact activity or strength training.
* **Anemia.** If you have cancer in your bones or if your treatment has affected your bone marrow, you may be at risk for bruising and bleeding if you do high-impact activity.
* **Dehydration.** Some cancers can cause electrolyte imbalances and dehydration, so

it's important to drink plenty of fluids (water or a sports drink) before, during, and after activity.

PRESCRIPTION PAD

✳ *Colds and flu prevention.* Do a moderate aerobic activity, such as taking a brisk walk, for 30 to 45 minutes, five days a week.

✳ *Colds and flu recovery.* Don't exercise if you have a fever or below-the-neck symptoms. If your symptoms are above the neck, you may try a half-speed "test drive" to see if it feels good to get moving.

✳ *Cancer prevention.* Perform an aerobic activity for 30 to 60 minutes most days of the week. Do enough exercise to keep your body at a healthy weight, and be sure the activity is something you enjoy.

✳ *Exercise ℞ for cancer survivors.* Consult your physician and a qualified exercise professional to design a personalized program that you will do individually or with a reputable "oncology rehabilitation" group. If possible, incorporate aerobic activity, strength training, stretching, and mind-body practices.

✳ *Exercise ℞ for HIV and AIDS survivors.* Work with your physician and a qualified exercise professional to design an individualized program. If possible, incorporate aerobic activity, strength training, and flexibility exercises, plus mind-body practices.

ADDITIONAL RESOURCES

✳ The American Cancer Society, 1599 Clifton Road N.E., Atlanta, Ga. 30329-4251. Call 800-ACS-2345, or visit the Web site: www.cancer.org.

✳ The National Cancer Institute, National Institutes of Health, Bethesda, Md. 800-4-CANCER, www.icic.nci.gor/nci-icic.html.

✳ *The American Cancer Society's Informed Decisions: The Complete Book of Cancer Diagnosis, Treatment and Recovery,* by Gerald P. Murphy, M.D., Lois B. Morris, and Dianne Lange (Viking, 1997).

✳ ENCOREplus, a combined peer-support group and exercise program for women with breast cancer, is offered at thirty-seven YWCAs around the country. Call 800-95-EPLUS or e-mail cgould@YWCA.org.

✳ Cancer Support Services, a nonprofit organization based in Manhattan, offers exercise, nutrition, and stress-management programs for cancer patients. Call 212-628-9728 or visit the Web site: www.cancersupport.org.

✳ National AIDS Hotline, 800-342-2437.

✳ U.S. Public Health Service HIV/AIDS Treatment Information Service; Web site: www.hivatis.org/

✳ National Institute of Allergy and Infectious Disease, 301-496-2535; Web site: www.nihaid.nih.gov/.

✳ National Alliance of Breast Cancer Organizations, 800-719-9154; www.nabco.org.

HEALING MOVES TO ENHANCE IMMUNITY

Since ancient times, healers have understood that actions and emotions have a powerful impact on our health. Today scientists are probing the intricate links between body and mind through a variety of disciplines, including new areas such as psychoneuroimmunology (PNI). Emerging evidence lends scientific support to the wisdom of the ancients. Our behaviors and thoughts *can* have a dramatic effect on our immune system, in both a positive and a negative way.

Moderate exercise and positive mood states, like optimism and faith, enhance our body's ability to defend itself from disease. Negative activity patterns, like sedentariness and exhausting, prolonged exertion, and negative emotions, like hostility and depression, suppress immune function and leave us vulnerable to illness.

In this light, we've identified two keys to using exercise to enhance immunity:

1. *Make the experience as positive as possible.* Envision physical activity as something attractive—an exciting challenge or diverting play—by selecting a kind of exercise you enjoy. Enjoyable exercise relieves tension, countering the negative effect mental stress has on the immune system. The mood boost that results from a bout of physical activity is itself therapeutic, strengthening the body's resilience and defensive capability.

2. *Train, don't strain.* It's important to do enough exercise to activate the bloodstream's molecular defenders. But try not to overdo it since excessive, prolonged exertion can produce exhaustion capable of weakening the body's innate defensive system.

Exactly how much exercise will cause you to strain is a highly individual matter that depends on a variety of factors, including your exercise history, current fitness level, exercise preferences and abilities, and—to some extent—your age. Also, what makes exercise an enjoyable experience for you is another very personal matter. That's why some specifics of your exercise routine will be individual choices that you'll plug into our Immune-Enhancing workout, which includes three parts:

Part One: Body

Pick an aerobic activity—or activities—you enjoy. From dancing to kickboxing, walking to cross-country skiing, anything you like that increases your heart and breathing rates into a moderate zone, for 30 to 45 minutes, will help boost your immunity.

Part Two: Mind-Body

The Sun Salutation is a classic series of yoga poses that offers a complete system of self-care. Created centuries ago and refined through the ages by yoga masters, the Sun Salutation is designed to stretch, strengthen, and warm up the entire body. It is also geared to relieving stress, unifying body and mind, and producing a balanced state of physical and mental calm.

Part Three: Mind-Body-Spirit

Meditative activities are important to integrate the effects of aerobic, stretching, and strengthening activities into the larger self, enhancing the effectiveness of these exercises. We present several meditations from Eastern healing traditions: a qi gong "marrow-washing" exercise, the karate technique of San Shin Kai breathing, and a restorative yoga pose you can do at your desk.

Note: Our workout is designed for healthy people who want to boost their body's natural defense mechanisms and help prevent immunological disorders. However, people who have cancer or other diseases that compromise the immune system may be able to do the mind-body practices—or all three parts—with their physician's approval and guidance.

PART ONE:
BODY—AEROBIC ACTION

The old saying "One man's dish is another man's poison" is quite true when it comes to exercise. Runners wax poetic about the joys of racing across a trail at sunrise, while others think the notion sounds like torture. Martial artists spend years learning the physical and mental skills necessary to punch through concrete, which some people consider close to insanity. So the first crucial element is one of personal self-empowerment: pick an aerobic activity for yourself, for your needs—any one you like. *Do the aerobic activity you enjoy, at an intensity you consider moderate to somewhat hard, for 30 to 60 minutes, three to six days a week.* Furthermore: *Try to keep yourself cheerful throughout the entire exercise session.*

This doesn't mean that if you're getting whipped at racquetball you have to smile and laugh through the entire match. But it does mean you'll need to work on your sportsmanship, to learn to enjoy the game even if you're losing, and recognize that *a primary goal of your exercise is to have fun.* It may also mean that if you find competition stressful and filled with negative emotion, competitive sports aren't the appropriate aerobic activity for your immune-enhancing workout. Monitor yourself with this question: When you finish your activity for the day, do you feel better? Do you feel like you enjoyed yourself regardless of the score?

To help you select the aerobic activity (or activities) that you can do with good cheer and that best suit your personality, ask yourself these questions and jot down your responses:

1. *Do you like repetitive, predictable activity that lets your mind wander?*
   If yes, consider walking, swimming, in-line skating, running, cycling.
2. *Do you prefer exercise that requires concentration and skill?*
   If yes, consider aerobic dance, martial arts, jumping rope, kickboxing.
3. *Do you like purposeful activity that accomplishes a goal?*
   If yes, consider walking your dog, gardening (raking, weeding, mowing, and so on), or active chores (chopping wood, washing and waxing a car).
4. *Do you like exercising with other people?*
   If yes, choose something you can do with a buddy, like walking, or in a class, like line dancing.

5. **Do you prefer to exercise alone?**

   If yes, pick an activity you can do solo, like running, cycling, swimming, or walking.

6. **When you were a child or teenager, what were your favorite activities?**

   List some from early childhood and some from your school years.

7. **Do you have a friend who is a regular exerciser whose activity appeals to you?**

   If yes, what is it?

8. **Have you toyed with the idea of trying a specific activity, but never gotten around it?**

   If yes, what is it?

9. **Do you enjoy competition?**

   If yes, pick a sport that requires keeping score, such as racquetball or tennis, but remember that for aerobic effect you'll need to be moving continuously for 30 to 45 minutes. A doubles game or a slow-moving beginners game isn't likely to meet the requirements for aerobic conditioning. Another option is to pick an activity that holds races or tournaments, such as 5k runs, triathlons, or karate competitions.

10. **Do you like exercising to music?**

    If yes, pick an activity choreographed to music, such as dance, or pick an activity you can do while listening to music, such as in-line skating or walking with a personal stereo.

Look over your responses. Are certain activities listed repeatedly? Can you imagine yourself doing them cheerfully almost every day? It's fine to pick just one activity and do that three to six days a week if you want. But it's also fine to pick a "menu" of several activities that you can choose from, depending on your mood, the weather, and other factors. If you've been sedentary, be sure you start slowly and progress gradually. (See Pre-Participation Checklist, page 29.) Begin with as little as 5 minutes of your selected activity at a moderate pace, then add an additional 5 minutes of activity per week until you're exercising for 30 to 60 minutes three to six days a week. And remember to smile!

PART TWO: LINKING MIND AND BODY WITH BREATH—THE SUN SALUTATION

It takes only a few minutes to complete this satisfying sequence of yoga postures, which are performed as one continuous exercise. Each position counteracts the previous pose, so that doing the entire sequence stretches and strengthens opposing muscle groups in a balanced and complete fashion. It also alternately expands and contracts the chest to regulate breathing and nourish the internal organs.

Created centuries ago as a series of prostrations to the Hindu sun god—who was considered the deity for health and long life—*Surya Namaskar* (the Sanskrit name for the Sun Salutation) is traditionally performed at dawn, facing the rising run. Today, the Sun Salutation is often used as a warm-up at the beginning of a yoga class. But it can also be performed as a complete practice in itself. With several continuous repetitions of "the salute to the sun," the practice can be mildly to moderately aerobic. If you synchronize your movements with your breath—a goal of yoga—you will generate an invigorating sense of vibrant calm in which your body and mind connect, leaving you feeling warm, relaxed, and strong.

There are many variations of this classic series of yoga poses, and we offer a basic version suitable for beginners. Since mastering the basics of yoga, as of many disciplines, is a lifetime pursuit, this sequence is also appropriate for more advanced exercisers. We have included suggestions on when to inhale and exhale, but feel free to change these breathing patterns if you like. It's important, however, that you try to coordinate your breathing with your movement, in a way that feels right for you.

To prepare for practice:

* Have an empty or near-empty stomach.

* Wear comfortable clothing and go barefoot.

* Practice on a level surface. A hardwood floor is ideal, but a tightly woven carpet or a yoga "sticky mat" is fine.

* Minimize distractions. Turn off the phone and TV and, if possible, clear the room of kids, pets, and other people. If you like, turn down the lights, light a candle, and put on meditative music.

Begin in **mountain pose**: Stand tall on both feet, with heels and big toes touching each other. Lift up your toes, stretch them, and fan them out onto the floor without gripping. Be sure your weight is distributed evenly on the heels and toes of both feet. Let the top of your head extend up, as if someone were pulling you upward from a string, so that your neck stretches up, your spine

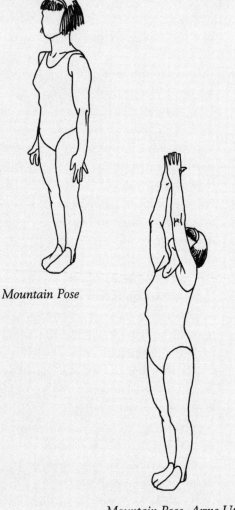

Mountain Pose

Mountain Pose, Arms Up

elongates, and your pelvis tucks slightly under. Keep your head straight, chin level, and shoulders relaxed with arms at your sides, palms facing in. Pull up your thigh muscles. Gaze straight ahead and relax the muscles of your face.

Inhale as you reach your arms out and up, until the palms touch overhead, and gaze upward. Then exhale as you bend forward from the hips and circle the arms out and down in a swan dive into **standing forward bend.** Keep the knees straight but not locked, and rest your hands on the floor, if possible, or on your shins, ankles, or toes, as your flexibility permits. (If you have a weak lower back, you may keep your knees slightly bent.) Keep your neck and head relaxed and let their weight release your upper body down toward the ground. Extend your tailbone up toward the ceiling, breathe deeply, and let the muscles in the backs of your legs lengthen. Stay here for several breaths.

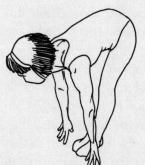

Foward Folded Arch

Exhale as you return to **standing forward bend.** Hold this pose for several breaths.

Inhale, then exhale as you step your right foot back into a **lunge** with your toes tucked under. Drop your right knee to the ground (you may rest it on a folded blanket or towel if you want) and place your palms or fingers on either side of your left foot. Inhale as you raise your arms out and up so the palms

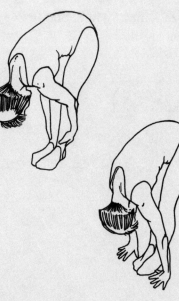

Standing Forward Bend

Inhale as you arch your back into **forward folded arch.** Lift your chest forward and up while continuing to press your fingers against the floor or your shins. Let your gaze extend upward. Hold this pose for several breaths.

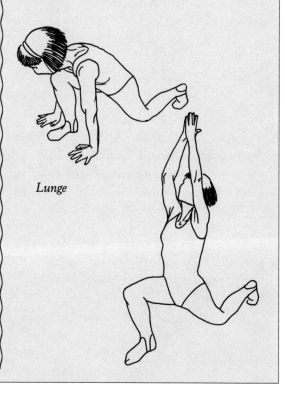

Lunge

touch overhead. Gaze forward and hold this position for a few breaths. (If you find it too difficult to lift your arms, keep your fingers on the floor, arch your back, and look up.)

Exhale as you lower your arms back to the floor, with your palms or fingers on either side of your left foot. Inhale, then exhale and step your left foot back so that your body is in the straight line of **plank pose.** Your weight should be balanced evenly on both palms and the balls and toes of both feet. Keep your arms straight but don't lock your elbows. Stay in this pose for several breaths.

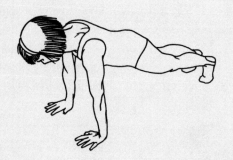

Plank Pose

Inhale, then exhale as you lower your knees to the floor and bend your elbows to lower your chest and chin to the floor in **yoga push-up.** This position is known in

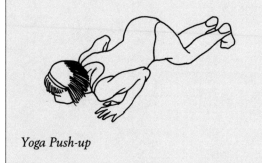

Yoga Push-up

Sanskrit as *sastanga namaskar,* or eight-curved prostration, since eight portions of the body are in contact with the floor: two feet, two knees, two hands, chest, and chin (or forehead in the traditional version). Keep your elbows close to your sides, your hips up, and your toes curled under. If you can, stay in this pose for several breaths.

Inhale as you lower your hips, push the floor away with your palms, straighten your arms, and roll over your toes into **upward-facing dog.** Lift and open the chest, looking forward or slightly up, shoulders back and down. Engage your thighs and try to bring your legs and pubic bone off the floor. Keep your buttock muscles firm. Stay in this pose for several breaths.

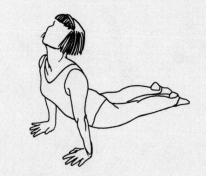

Upward-Facing Dog

Inhale, then exhale and push the floor away with your palms as you raise your hips and roll back over your toes until your body makes the inverted-V shape of **downward-facing dog.** Your feet should be parallel, about hip width apart, toes pointed ahead. Keep the legs straight, but don't lock the knees, and lift your hips toward the ceiling. Try to press your heels down toward the floor—but don't worry if they don't touch the floor. Press against the floor with your palms, fingers spread, your arms straight and your back long. Let your head relax and gaze at your navel. Stay in this pose for several breaths.

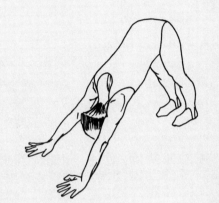

Downward-Facing Dog

Inhale, then exhale and step your right foot forward into **lunge.** Inhale as you raise your arms out and up so the palms touch overhead. Hold the pose for several breaths.

Exhale as you lower your arms back to the floor, palms or fingers on either side of your right foot. Inhale, then exhale as you bring your left foot next to your right foot for **standing forward bend.** Hold the pose for several breaths.

Inhale, then exhale as you roll your spine up, vertebrae by vertebrae, then roll your shoulders back until you're standing in **mountain pose** again. Hold this pose for several breaths.

Inhale as you raise your arms out and up, until your palms touch, then exhale as you drop both hands down to your chest into **prayer position** (also called *namaste*). Palms should press against each other, forearms

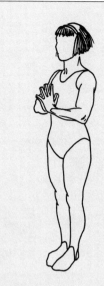

Prayer Position

parallel to the floor, fingers slightly spread, and thumbs touching your sternum.

Repeat the entire sequence, this time stepping back with the left foot.

Start by doing two or three complete rounds of the Sun Salutation (one round consists of two sequences, one leading with the right foot, then a second leading with the left foot). Work your way up until you can do twelve complete rounds. Rather than counting, some people prefer to set a timer for 10 minutes and continue flowing through the sequence until the alarm rings. Or put on some music and do the Sun Salutation until the music ends. To enhance your practice, pick a musical selection whose beat coordinates with your breath and try the sequence this way:

Stand in **mountain pose,** inhale arms up, exhale to **standing forward bend.**
Inhale to **forward folding arch,** exhale to **standing forward bend.**

Inhale in **standing forward bend,** then exhale to **lunge** (right foot back).

Inhale arms overhead, exhale hands back to the floor.

Inhale to **plank,** then exhale to **yoga push-up.**

Inhale into **upward-facing dog,** exhale into **downward-facing dog.**

Inhale in **downward-facing dog,** then exhale to **lunge** (right foot forward).

Inhale arms overhead, exhale hands back to the floor.

Inhale in **lunge,** exhale to **standing forward bend.**

Inhale and roll up into **mountain pose,** arms up, exhale to **prayer pose.**

Repeat sequence, stepping back on the left foot.

PART THREE:
MIND-BODY-SPIRIT PRACTICE

Connecting Mind and Body to Self, the Wellspring of Well-Being

Meditation, visualization, and relaxation can all help enhance your body's ability to fight disease. Eastern healing traditions consider these mind-body practices essential to strengthening the body's vital energy or life force—which is called *chi* in China, *ki* in Japan, and *prana* in India—and is the true wellspring of well-being. Traditional Chinese medicine holds that resistance to disease depends on the strength of the *chi* and its ability to flow smoothly and unimpeded throughout the body. When *chi* is blocked and becomes stagnant, the body's defensive energy is weakened, and illness results.

Here are several mind-body exercises that are designed to not only strengthen this innate life force but also enhance resistance to disease.

Marrow-Washing Breath

When performing this qi gong exercise, visualize yourself gathering healing energy—or *chi*—from nature, bringing it into your body, and storing it in the marrow of your bones.

Free your mind of all thoughts, and then try to adopt a state of cheerful indifference as you perform these movements:

1. Sit or stand with hands resting in your lap or by your sides. (If possible, do this outdoors near a tree or water.)
2. Inhale as you move your hands outward and upward, palms toward your face. Imagine that you're collecting precious healing power from nature.
3. When your hands are slightly above your head, bring them toward you and exhale as you move them slowly down the front of your body. Imagine that you're inviting the healing energy into your body, through the skin and muscle, until it settles in the marrow of your bones.
4. When your hands reach your navel area, pause momentarily. Repeat this sequence five to ten times, building up to doing twenty repetitions. Try to do the entire exercise as slowly as possible, synchronizing breath and movement in an easy, gentle flow.

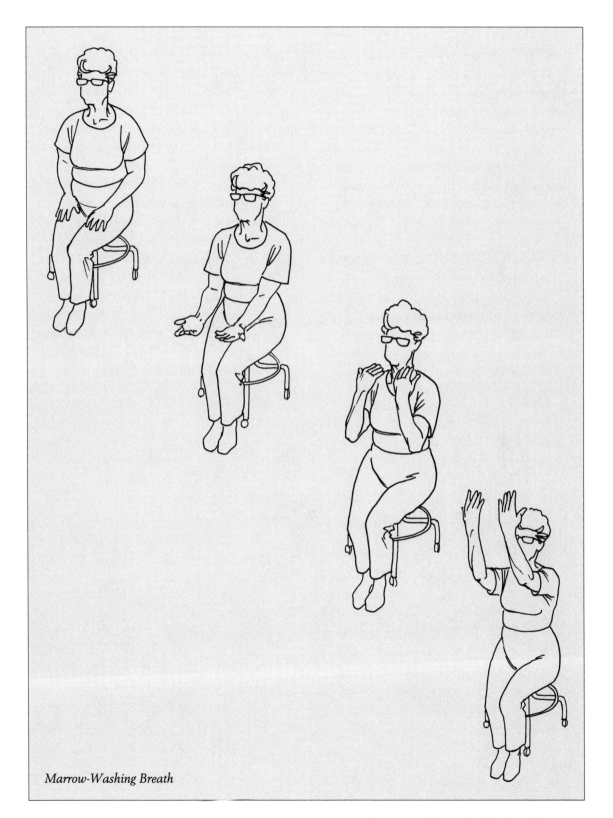

Marrow-Washing Breath

San Shin Kai Breathing

This meditative exercise is from a karate style called *San Shin Kai*, which means *mind, body, and spirit*. It is typically performed at the beginning of karate class, after warm-ups, to help unify mind, body, and spirit in preparation for intensive training. But it is also an excellent meditative practice by itself, to enhance your ability to become centered and focused.

1. Sit cross-legged on the floor, with your back straight, shoulders relaxed, and eyes gazing ahead. (If you can't sit cross-legged on the floor, you may do this exercise sitting in a chair.)
2. Extend your arms straight out in front of you, palms down. Then inhale through your nose as you turn your palms up, bend your elbows, and slide your arms back against your body while your hands close into tight fists that rest beside your ribs.
3. Exhale through your mouth as you open your fists and turn your hands forward, extending your arms out slowly and pressing both palms away from your body as if you were pushing against a force.
4. Repeat the inhaling motion, imagining yourself pulling energy into your being.
5. Repeat the exhaling motion, imagining yourself pushing an enemy away.
6. Do five rounds of inhalations and exhalations, then rest your hands on your knees, palms up, and close your eyes—do not let your spine collapse. Clear your mind and concentrate on your breathing.

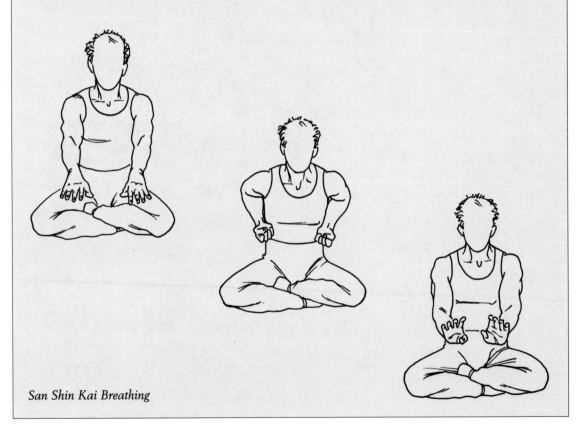

San Shin Kai Breathing

Restorative Yoga Pose: Desk Forward Bend

You can do this pose in your office, at your kitchen table, or anywhere there's a chair and a counter. This pose is not about "doing" but about "undoing" all the tension, negative thoughts, and stressed-out attitudes that can hamper immunity.

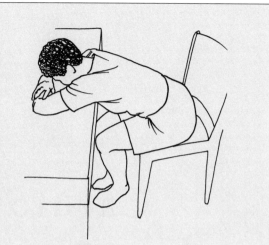

Desk Forward Bend

1. Sit on the edge of the chair with your feet flat on the floor.
2. Lean forward, place your folded arms on your desk, and rest your forehead on your arms. Tilt your chin slightly toward your chest and make any adjustments necessary so that you feel comfortably supported.
3. Close your eyes and breathe slowly and deeply for several breaths. Release the weight of your head and all its worries into the strength of the desk.
4. Breathe normally and take a few minutes to simply relax in this position.

6

Cardiovascular Disorders

CORONARY ARTERY DISEASE

Coronary artery disease (CAD) is the number one cause of death and disability in the United States for both men and women. The most common form of heart disease, CAD may lead to several different disorders—including angina, heart attack, and congestive heart failure—caused by blockages of the arteries that supply blood to the heart. An estimated seven million Americans live with some form of this ailment, and each year more than 500,000 Americans die of heart attacks resulting from CAD. Nearly half of these deaths occur in people under age sixty-five. Every year, more than 300,000 CAD patients undergo coronary artery bypass surgery, and even more have coronary angioplasty "ballooning" to restore the blood flow to their hearts.

While CAD is often viewed as a man's disease because it is more common in males at midlife, it gradually becomes an equal-opportunity killer after age fifty-five, when women reach menopause and experience a dramatic drop in production of the heart-protecting hormone estrogen. Although many women fear breast cancer as the disease most likely to cause death, heart attacks are, in fact, the leading killer of women, claiming six times the number of lives lost to breast cancer. Half of all CAD deaths are in women, and women who have a heart attack are twice as likely as men to die within the following year.

Over the last few decades remarkable new therapies have emerged to treat established CAD, yet the most profound and life-saving innovations have been in the arena of CAD prevention. Preventive strategies can be extremely effective because CAD is strongly related to the way in which people live their lives, especially surrounding behaviors such as cigarette smoking, inactivity, high-fat diets, and negative reactions to stress. As Americans have become increasingly conscious of the importance of healthy behaviors, death rates for heart disease have continued to drop; they are predicted to decline even further as those engaging in prevention in the present become the more aged of the future. New drugs, surgical procedures, and techniques such as balloon angioplasty also have contributed to the steady decline in death rates from CAD over the past twenty-five years.

But even though the number of deaths from CAD has decreased steadily, the *prevalence of CAD is increasing for both men and women*. While the United States has seen positive trends in decreased cigarette smoking and better identification and control of high blood pressure and high blood cholesterol, there have not been improvements in physical activity. Technology continues to engineer physical activity out of our lives, and most Americans are far more sedentary than previous generations, with the vast majority of adults getting little or no regular exercise. This epidemic of inactivity is a major reason why CAD remains the nation's number one killer.

Of all the lifestyle strategies geared to improving heart health, regular physical activity is one of the most powerful, affecting both the metabolic abnormalities leading to athlerosclerosis and the efficiency of the heart and circulatory system. Exercise also plays a unique role in rebuilding confidence and self-image in the context of rehabilitation programs for patients who have suf-

fered heart attacks. The positive effects of exercise on coronary artery disease is one of the most well-documented links between physical activity and health. A substantial amount of scientific literature has shown that inactivity increases CAD risk, while regular exercise reduces death and disability from the disease. In 1987, after analyzing more than three dozen of the best available studies, the U.S. Centers for Disease Control and Prevention issued a landmark report concluding that *physically inactive people are twice as likely to get CAD as those who are relatively active*. This risk level puts physical inactivity on par with the top three other risk factors for heart disease: high blood pressure, high blood cholesterol, and smoking cigarettes. In 1992, the American Heart Association added physical inactivity to this list of major CAD risk factors.

To understand the role exercise plays in protecting against CAD, it's important to distinguish between two types of prevention:

＊ *Primary prevention* is the term used for helping people who *don't have CAD* reduce their risk of ever getting blockages in their coronary arteries over their lifetime.

＊ *Secondary prevention* is the term used for helping people who *already have established CAD* to slow or reverse the buildup of fatty deposits in their arteries as well as to reduce their likelihood of death or disability from heart attack or stroke.

Regular exercise is essential to both kinds of prevention, concluded an expert panel on physical activity and cardiovascular health convened in 1995 by the

National Institutes of Health. Their consensus on exercise as *primary prevention* stated: *"Physical activity protects against the development of cardiovascular disease and also favorably modifies . . . risk factors, including high blood pressure, blood lipids, insulin resistance, and obesity."* This panel also highlighted the importance of exercise to *secondary prevention*, stating that regular exercise can help people with CAD experience a *"reduction in cardiovascular mortality, reduction of symptoms, improvement in exercise tolerance and functional capacity and improvement in psychological well-being and quality of life."*

In a foreword to the published proceedings of the NIH conference, Claude Lenfant, M.D., director of the National Heart, Lung, and Blood Institute, underscored exercise's effect on both primary and secondary prevention by noting:

✳ Sedentary people run the highest risk of coronary heart disease.

✳ About 200,000 fewer deaths a year would occur in the United States if half of those who are sedentary would engage in a low-intensity activity a few times weekly.

✳ Physical activity even helps those who already have heart disease, and regular physical activity improves chances of survival and well-being after a heart attack.

Just a generation ago, the standard treatment for heart attack survivors was up to six months of bed rest. At that time, doctors feared exercise would trigger another major "cardiac event." This thinking began to change in 1955, when Paul Dudley White— the man many consider the founder of preventive cardiology—was selected as chief

medical consultant to President Dwight Eisenhower shortly after the president suffered a heart attack. A staunch advocate of daily exercise, known for taking vigorous walks and riding his bicycle, Dr. White rejected the then-popular dogma of bed rest for heart attack survivors and promoted exercise both for prevention of heart disease and rehabilitation from its effects. Newspaper photographs of Eisenhower golfing after his heart attack helped spread the message that physical activity was important not only for primary prevention but for secondary prevention as well.

Since that time, the role of exercise in treating CAD has evolved dramatically, and today physicians recognize that exercise can be a lifesaver for people with heart disease. Cardiac rehabilitation exercise programs are now standard care for people recovering from heart attack and living with other forms of CAD. The NIH consensus statement concluded that "rehabilitation programs using both moderate and vigorous physical activity have been associated with reductions in fatal cardiac events. . . . Reductions in mortality have been particularly great—approximately 25 percent—in those who participated in cardiac rehabilitation programs that included control of other cardiovascular risk factors."

CAD BASICS

The heart is a miraculous engine that pumps blood to all the organs of the body, squeezing on average about 100,000 times per day, nonstop. Like any engine, the heart needs fuel. In human terms, fuel is blood, which carries the oxygen and nutrients that the body will convert into energy. The fuel lines feeding the heart are the coronary arteries, which carry blood to the heart muscle itself. If the fuel lines become clogged, even the best engine won't run well. In humans, the "sludge" that often clogs our arterial fuel lines is called plaque, which is made up of cholesterol, fat, calcium, blood clots, and other debris that deposits, or builds up, inside the arterial channels.

When the coronary arteries become clogged with so much plaque that the fuel supply becomes insufficient to meet the heart's demands, *ischemic heart disease* (which is sometimes referred to as coronary heart disease) results. The clinical syndromes that can result from this condition include:

* Angina, which consists of pain, pressure, or burning symptoms in the chest, neck, or arm
* Irregular heart rhythms, ranging from minor to life-threatening
* Breathlessness, easy fatigability, and loss of tolerance for exertion
* Congestive heart failure
* Heart attack
* Death

CAD refers to the disease of the fuel lines (coronary arteries) themselves. This disease begins when the arterial lining is damaged, which stimulates fatty deposits that make the damaged site more vulnerable to further injury, setting up a vicious, progressive cycle. The coronary arteries can become damaged by many sources, which are often lifestyle related. The battering force of high blood pressure can injure the arteries, as can toxic substances that enter the blood through cigarettes or an excess of fatty and fried foods. Adrenaline secreted in response to stress also can contribute to the process of artery damage.

When the arteries become damaged, a type of cell known as a macrophage travels to the injured site in an effort to repair the lining of the arterial wall. Paradoxically, this repair effort actually makes the problem worse because it generates localized inflammation and stimulates blood-clot formation, further narrowing the arterial channel.

The buildup of plaque from CAD is typically a slow process that can start in youth and worsen with age. The effects of this progressive narrowing on blood flow to the heart muscles is like what happens on an eight-lane highway if construction or an accident progressively narrows traffic flow to six, then four, then two lanes. Not only is the total flow of traffic reduced, but the likelihood of another accident increases. In human terms, the slow-forming, progressive bottleneck in a coronary artery is mostly plaque. The sudden accident that acts like a cork in the bottleneck is usually made of a blood clot. If this blood clot completely blocks the flow of blood, the heart muscle can be irreversibly damaged, which is called a heart attack, also known as a *myocardial infarction*. One and a half million Americans have heart attacks each year, and one-third of them die.

The buildup of plaque can be so gradual that it can take decades before symptoms—if any—occur. Even in the presence of severe CAD, symptoms may be highly variable. The classic symptom of ischemic heart disease is a recurring pain, pressure, or burning in the chest, under the breastbone, or into the left arm or jaw, known as *angina pectoris*. Angina typically occurs when the heart's workload increases, such as during exercise or emotional stress, and the narrowed arteries caused by CAD keep the heart from getting enough oxygen to meet its heightened need. Other angina triggers can include heavy meals, cigarette smoking, and extreme cold or heat. *Exercise during angina, or exercise that causes angina, are both potentially dangerous.* If symptoms persist or recur, call 911 and get to the nearest emergency room.

But these classic symptoms are actually very uncommon. Angina may be experienced as an amorphous feeling that "something is wrong," or it may be confused with digestive distress, or heartburn. Not everyone who has CAD gets angina or any other recognizable clues to their condition. In fact, in half of all people with CAD, the first symptom is a massive heart attack or death.

RISK FACTORS

Certain characteristics put you at greater risk of CAD. Risk factors you can't directly influence include:

✳ *Age.* Otherwise healthy men age forty-five and older and women age fifty-five and older are at greater risk.

✳ *Heredity.* Having a blood-related family member diagnosed with early heart disease increases your risk of CAD. This includes a mother or sister diagnosed with heart disease before age sixty-five or a father or brother diagnosed before age fifty-five.

✳ *Gender.* Men in midlife are at greater risk of CAD. After menopause, women's risk gradually becomes just as great.

In addition to these risk factors you can't change are equally important risk factors you can influence for both primary and secondary prevention:

✳ *Physical inactivity.* Being inactive doubles your risk of developing CAD. Regular exercise can help protect against heart disease even if you have other risk factors. Even people who've had heart attacks can reduce their likelihood of having another and can increase their chance of survival if they start to exercise regularly. People who are active regularly are also more likely to cut down or stop cigarette smoking, as well as improve other CAD risk factors such as high blood pressure or blood lipids, diabetes, and obesity.

✳ *Cigarette smoking.* Smokers are two to four times more likely to have a heart attack than nonsmokers. Following a heart attack they are 200 percent more likely to have another, and 70 percent more likely to die if they continue to smoke.

✳ *High blood pressure.* The higher your blood pressure, the greater your risk of developing heart disease or stroke. Blood pressure higher than 140/90 mm Hg (millimeters of mercury) or greater is classified as high blood pressure, or hypertension. Regular, moderate exercise can help prevent high blood pressure in people who don't have the condition and lower blood pressure in people who do have hypertension. (See High Blood Pressure, page 202.)

✳ *High blood cholesterol.* A blood cholesterol level of 240 mg/dL (milligrams per deciliter) or above is high and increases your risk of heart disease. A total blood cholesterol of less than 200 mg/dL is desirable and puts you at a lower risk of heart disease. Regular moderate to vigorous exercise is associated with decreased total cholesterol and with increased levels of HDL (high-density lipoprotein) cholesterol. HDL is the so-called good cholesterol because higher levels are linked with a lower risk of CAD. (See High Cholesterol, page 60.)

 ✳ *Stress.* A growing body of research links stress with CAD. In particular, hostility and social isolation appear to increase the risk of CAD events. Regular aerobic exercise, as well as mind-body exercises like yoga and tai chi, can help relieve stress and boost mood, which can lower CAD risk.

 ✳ *Diabetes.* The abnormalities of metabolism, tissue healing, and the immune system associated with diabetes have profound effects on blood vessel linings, including the coronary arteries. Exercise is associated with many factors that can influence this condition, including improved insulin sensitivity, cholesterol metabolism, and immune function.

 ✳ *Obesity.* In 1998, the American Heart Association elevated obesity from a "contributing risk factor" to a "major risk factor" for heart attacks. Obesity is associated with numerous conditions that put people at greater risk of CAD, including high blood pressure, diabetes, inactivity, poor diet, and an unhealthy cholesterol profile. Regular moderate exercise can play a central role in improving all of these conditions; plus, exercise is essential to maintaining a healthy weight. Even small weight losses, of just five to ten percent of body weight, can greatly reduce these risk factors and improve health.

If you have two or more risk factors, it's essential that you get regular exercise to lower your risk of CAD events. Whether or not you have suspicious symptoms, if you are in this high-risk category it is imperative that you consult a health-care professional about how to begin exercising safely. (See Healing Moves for Heart Health, page 214.)

HOW EXERCISE HELPS

Regular aerobic activity helps the heart muscle itself work more efficiently, like a well-tuned engine. It influences a wide range of physiologic factors—such as blood vessel tone and breathing patterns—that make the entire cardiovascular system more efficient. Exercise also improves many metabolic functions.

Regular, moderate physical activity **improves cardiovascular efficiency** by:

 ✳ Lowering the resting heart rate, which lowers overall oxygen demand and increases the time in each heart beat during which coronary blood can flow.

 ✳ Decreasing blood pressure, which also lowers oxygen demand.

 ✳ Improving breathing and respiratory function, which results in better oxygen exchange and in more efficient circulatory function.

 ✳ Possibly prompting the development of new blood vessels in the heart to enhance delivery of oxygenated blood.

Exercise **boosts metabolic functioning** by:

 ✳ Improving the cholesterol profile—increasing serum levels of HDL "good" cholesterol, lowering levels of LDL "bad" cholesterol, and decreasing triglycerides.

✳ Improving the digestion and metabolism of digestible fats.

✳ Increasing insulin sensitivity.

✳ Possibly decreasing the potential for clot formation.

Exercise **boosts both cardiovascular efficiency and metabolic functioning** by:

✳ Relieving stress, which relaxes blood vessels and reduces the release of chemicals such as adrenaline and cortisone.

✳ Reducing total body fat, which reduces the heart's workload and improves insulin sensitivity.

✳ Improving mood and feelings of well-being, enhancing the body's self-healing mechanisms.

✳ Helping people embrace other healthy lifestyle behaviors, such as quitting smoking and making heart-healthy food choices.

Healthy lifestyle changes are the only interventions that address the underlying causes of CAD. While medications, surgeries, and procedures can help combat the *symptoms*, only lifestyle behaviors can affect the *causes*.

For those who are able or "cleared" to exercise vigorously, boosting exercise intensity may result in even more benefits to the cardiovascular system. For example, research has shown that trained endurance athletes have more flexible arteries that expand more and become larger than those in unfit people. A 1993 Stanford University study, reported in the American Heart Association's scientific journal, *Circulation*,

showed that the coronary arteries of long-distance runners can dilate to about twice the size of similar arteries in sedentary men. When measured at rest, the runner's coronary arteries were only slightly larger than those of the inactive men. But when given nitroglycerine, which expands arteries in a manner similar to exercise, the runners demonstrated a dilating capacity about twice as great as sedentary men. This gives these athletes a tremendous capacity for increasing blood flow to their hearts.

When combined with other healthy lifestyle behaviors, regular exercise can have an even more powerful effect, which is particularly important in secondary prevention for people who already have CAD. The Lifestyle Heart Trial, conducted by Dr. Dean Ornish at the University of California at San Francisco, showed that *even severe CAD could often be reversed by making lifestyle changes alone* (low-fat, vegetarian diet, smoking cessation, stress management, moderate exercise, and emotional support) without cholesterol-lowering drugs or surgery. His research findings, published in a number of medical journals, including the *Lancet*, the *Journal of the American Medical Association*, and *Circulation*, indicate that moderate exercise—such as walking for 20 to 60 minutes—combined with a heart-healthy diet and stress-reduction techniques such as yoga can dramatically improve the health of CAD patients.

EXERCISE ℞

While experts agree that regular exercise reduces the risk of CAD, the exact intensity, frequency, and duration of exercise necessary for maximum benefit remains controversial. There is general consensus, however, that even *a modest amount of moderate exercise can confer significant benefit* and that, to some degree, a "dose response" relationship exists between physical activity and heart health. This means that, within reason, the more exercise you do, the more benefits you get.

The *U.S. Surgeon General's Report on Physical Activity and Health* advises Americans to do a moderate amount of exercise on most, if not all, days of the week. To meet this recommendation, do enough physical activity to burn approximately 150 calories, for example:

* Walk or rake leaves for 30 minutes
* Run or climb stairs for 15 minutes
* Play volleyball or wax a car for 45 minutes.

The report also suggests that activity doesn't have to be continuous to provide important benefits, and it points to several studies showing that "cardiorespiratory fitness gains are similar when physical activity occurs in several short sessions (e.g., 10 minutes each) as when the same total amount and intensity of activity occurs in one longer session (e.g., 30 minutes)."

Some experts contend that this "exercise lite" approach is not enough for those people interested in heart health. From a public health perspective, it makes sense to have activity seem as easy and appealing as possible to encourage the more than 60 percent of Americans who get little or no exercise up and moving. But it's also important to recognize that research indicates that more vigorous activity is associated with more benefits. In particular, a twenty-six-year-study of 17,321 male Harvard alumni, published in the *Journal of the American Medical Association* in 1995, found that men who expended more than 1,500 calories per week on regular, vigorous physical activity (such as swimming laps or walking briskly at four to five miles per hour) had a 25 percent lower death rate during the study period than men who expended less than 150 calories per week.

However, *intense physical activity may also have added risks compared to moderate levels of activity.* In primary prevention, for people who do not have established CAD, the risks of more intense activity are mostly orthopedic, while the increased benefits are cardiovascular. Orthopedic injury from overusing muscles and pounding joints can be moderated by good warm-up, stretching, and cross-training practices. For secondary prevention in people who have CAD, high-intensity exercise may be inadvisable. Most people who die while exercising are found to have an underlying heart condition. In people under age forty, these conditions are most frequently heart defects present at birth. In people over age forty, the heart condition is usually CAD. Often these deaths are preceded by warning signs, such as chest pain, light-headedness, fainting, and extreme breathlessness, but sometimes there are no warning signs. This is one reason why the American Heart Association recommends consultation with a health-care professional and exercise stress testing for people at high risk of cardiovascular disease (men over age forty, women over age fifty, and people of any age with two or more risk factors for heart disease, such as smoking or high cholesterol or a family history of CAD) before beginning vigorous activity.

For these reasons, exercise guidelines from the American Heart Association are divided into two main categories: primary prevention, for those without heart disease, and secondary prevention, for those with CAD. The AHA's recommendations, in a simplified form, are as follows:

Primary Prevention

Exercise should begin in the early school years, continue throughout an individual's lifetime, and include aerobic activities such as bicycling, walking, jogging, swimming, and dancing. Ideally, this activity should be done for at least 30 to 60 minutes four to six times weekly, or 30 minutes on most days of the week, at a fatigue level considered "somewhat hard" to "hard." The frequency, intensity, and duration should be individualized to personal satisfaction. As intensity decreases, frequency and duration should increase. That is, people who choose to exercise at a lower intensity need to exercise longer to achieve similar benefit.

Secondary Prevention

The emphasis of exercise in the first two weeks after myocardial infarction, angioplasty, or coronary bypass surgery should be to promote wound healing, to offset the effects of bed rest and periods of inactivity, and to enhance psychological recovery. This is one of the clearest cases where the body can lead the mind. When the individual's condition is stable and recovery is relatively complete, he or she should begin to increase the activity. Initial activities should be

supervised, and symptoms, rating of perceived exertion, heart rate, and blood pressure recorded. After safety and tolerance are documented, the activity can be performed without supervision.

Walking or riding a stationary bicycle are the recommended modes of activity unless the individual can attend supervised classes where other activities can be performed. Supervised group sessions are recommended initially to enhance psychological support and the educational process, to ensure that the participant is tolerating the program, to confirm progress, and to provide medical supervision in high-risk situations. Limited walking should begin and continue slowly with a gradual increase in duration until 5 to 10 minutes of continuous movement has been achieved. For conditioning purposes, large-muscle-group activities (such as walking or cycling) should be performed for at least 20 to 30 minutes, preceded by a warm-up and followed by cooldown, at least three to four times weekly.

An appropriate moderate initial intensity of training for secondary prevention is 60 to 75 percent of maximal heart rate (moderate) or a rating of perceived exertion of 12 to 13 on a scale of 6 to 20. Many individuals may need to begin at a lighter intensity, such as 40 to 60 percent of maximal heart rate. After safe activity levels have been established, increase duration in 5-minute increments each week. Later, intensities may also be increased.

For people not taking heart medications, a useful general formula to determine your maximal heart rate begins by subtracting your age from 220. For example, if you are forty, your maximal heart rate would be

180. To determine a "training heart rate" of 60 to 75 percent, multiply 180 by .6 for 60 percent to get 108 and by .75 for 75 percent to get 135. Your training heart rate, then, would be between 108 and 135 beats per minute. Certain heart medications—such as beta-blockers and some calcium channel blockers—can affect the heart rate, making this formula less useful. In such cases, "perceived exertion" at a light to moderate level or input from your physician may be preferred.

The American College of Sports Medicine (ACSM) offers a similar prescription in its position stand on exercise for cardiovascular fitness. For primary prevention of CAD, the ACSM recommends doing 20 to 60 minutes of continuous aerobic activity three to five days a week, at an intensity of 60 to 90 percent of maximum heart rate. (Duration is dependent on intensity, so that lower-intensity activity needs to be done for a longer period of time.) For secondary prevention, the ACSM recommends that most people with established CAD "engage in individually designed exercise programs . . . [that] include a comprehensive pre-exercise medical evaluation, including a graded exercise test and an individualized exercise prescription."

In addition to aerobic activity, careful resistance training also can be beneficial to people with CAD, since improved strength lowers feelings of exertion and decreases the heart's work during activities that involve lifting or holding objects. Strength training can be particularly helpful for people who routinely perform household or occupational activities requiring a strong upper body. The ACSM advises adults to do one set of eight to twelve repetitions of eight to ten exercises that condition the body's major muscle groups, at least two days per week. Older people (fifty and above) and more frail people should consider using lighter weights with more repetition, says the ACSM, which advises this group to do one set of ten to fifteen repetitions of each exercise.

Mind-body activities such as tai chi and yoga may be extremely helpful for people with CAD. In his book *The Healing Heart*, Norman Cousins wrote this after surviving a massive heart attack: "The human heart is not sealed off from countless processes that take place within the human body. It is a point of culmination, a collection center for all the malfunctions or deficiencies that exist in the body as a whole. It is a zone of infinite vulnerability to all the anguishes and insults and provocations of mind, soul and body."

As forms of "moving meditation," tai chi and yoga promote both physical and mental flexibility and openness and are increasingly being used in cardiac-rehabilitation programs around the world. Both integrate proper breathing with movement, which reduces tension, and can help teach people how to relax mentally and physically and to better manage stress reactions. Breathing more deeply and rhythmically gets more oxygen into the blood and so to the heart more effectively. Relaxed, rhythmic breathing also promotes more efficient general circulation, so the work of the heart itself is reduced.

While formal exercise programs (such as a regular walking routine or tai chi class) can be important to heart health, it's also essential to integrate physical activity into daily life.

For many of us who are ingrained in the habit of fighting for the closest parking space or jumping onto the escalator or elevator, this involves a whole new mind-set of actively looking for opportunities to move. Think of it this way: *One of the best ways to change your heart is to first change your mind.* Decide to park in the *farthest* space, get up and change the channel, always take the stairs.

Always remember this: Every step you take, every move you make, will benefit your heart.

CAUTIONS

While active people have a lower overall risk of heart problems than do sedentary ones, overexertion in people with uncontrolled heart conditions may cause serious cardiovascular events. That's why it's very important to consult a physician before beginning any vigorous exercise if:

✳ You do not have CAD, but you have two or more risk factors for heart disease, including being a man over forty or a woman over fifty.

✳ You have CAD. Check with your doctor, too, if you experience any suspicious symptoms (chest pain, breathlessness, dizziness) during exercise.

In addition, all exercisers should heed these commonsense precautions:

✳ *Start slowly and progress gradually.* If you've been inactive, take gentle steps toward your goal. Begin with as little as a 5-minute walk and each week add another 5 minutes until you're walking continuously for 30 to 60 minutes. Remember: Something is better than nothing.

✳ *Warm up.* Give yourself a 5- to 10-minute warm-up period of easy movement and stretching to get your blood pumping and to prepare your body for the stress of exercise. The ideal warm-up for an endurance activity is usually doing that activity at a lower intensity. For example, walking is a good warm-up for jogging.

✳ *Cooldown.* Never stop vigorous activity suddenly: Intense activity can cause the heart and lungs to pump with twice their normal effort, and if you stop moving suddenly, blood may pool in the dilated vessels of your legs. This puts a strain on the heart and can cause dizziness and increase your risk of an abnormal heart rhythm. Instead, cool down by gradually slowing your pace with 5 to 10 minutes of light activity similar to your warm-up.

✳ *Watch out for weather extremes.* Avoid exercising in excessive heat or cold. Do outdoor activities during the most comfortable parts of the day, or switch to indoor workouts, such as mall walking or using a treadmill or stationary bike. Be sure to drink plenty of fluids, and on cold days wear a hat, gloves, and layers of clothing that you can shed as your body heats up.

✳ *Avoid strenuous exercise for at least two hours after a heavy meal.* Blood you need for your heart may be otherwise occupied if your stomach is full. However, easy exercise, such as a walk, after a meal can help digestion and redistribution of blood.

✳ *Listen to your body.* Be aware of possible signs of heart problems such as:

1. *Abnormal heart rhythm.* Irregular heartbeats may feel like your heart is skipping

a beat or adding extra beats, or may cause you to feel breathless or dizzy.

2. *Chest pain, pressure, or tightness.* Discomfort in the chest during or right after exercise may be a signal that your heart isn't getting enough oxygen. In some people, these symptoms may radiate down the left arm or appear in the back, jaw, or throat.

3. *Dizziness, light-headedness, or cold sweats* during or immediately after exercise may be a symptom of a cardiovascular problem.

4. *Fatigue.* Unusual tiredness during or after exercise may be related to a heart problem.

PRESCRIPTION PAD

✳ Integrate activity into your daily life. Whenever possible, walk instead of ride, and don't push a button if you can use your muscles instead. Take the stairs instead of the elevator, rake your leaves instead of blowing them, get off the bus or train a stop early and walk the rest of the way to work.

✳ Do some form of aerobic activity for at least 30 to 60 minutes three to six times weekly or 30 minutes on most days of the week, at an intensity level you consider moderate to hard—if you don't have CAD. If you do have CAD, consult a physician for an individualized program. In general, however, people who have CAD should work toward performing large-muscle-group activities (such as walking or cycling) for at least 20 to 30 minutes (preceded by a warm-up and followed by cooldown) at least three to four times weekly at a light to moderate intensity.

✳ Try a mind-body activity such as tai chi or yoga, and incorporate into your day the practice of a moving or still meditation with emphasis on breathing.

✳ Consider doing some resistance exercises to strengthen the body and "take a load off" the heart during activities that involve lifting or holding objects. But avoid "maximal lifting" if you have high blood pressure—that is, don't lift the heaviest weight you possibly can. Stick with more repetitions of lighter weights or use your body weight in calisthenics (for example, modified push-ups).

✳ Be aware that your heart rate may be affected by medications you take for CAD, so that exercising to a perceived exertion of an intensity you find moderate may be more effective than monitoring your heart rate.

RESOURCES

✳ The American Heart Association has numerous brochures and fact sheets about CAD and stroke. Call 800-AHA-USA1 or visit the Web site: www.americanheart.org.

✳ The National Heart, Lung, and Blood Institute's Information Line offers free material about heart disease to consumers and health professionals. Call 800-575-9355, write NHLBI, P.O. Box 30105, Bethesda, Md. 20824, or check the Web site at www.nhlbi.nih.gov/nhlbi/nhlbi.htm.

✳ Healthfinder, an Internet site for health-related government agencies, such as the National Institutes of Health and the Department of Health and Human Services, can provide a wealth of information about cardiovascular disease. Access the Web site at www.healthfinder.gov, then follow the "search" cues to access material about heart disease.

✳ EHAC, or Early Heart Attack Care, is a public-education program based at St. Agnes HealthCare in Baltimore. For information write Dr. Raymond Bahr, St. Agnes Health-Care, 900 Canton Ave., Box EM, Baltimore, Md. 21229-5299. Or e-mail info@ehac.org or the Web site: www.ehac.org.

✳ *The Rockport Fitness Walking Test* is a free brochure to gauge your fitness level and start you on an individualized walking program. Call 800-ROCKPORT.

✳ The American Volkssport Association has more than five hundred clubs nationwide that run noncompetitive walking events in the outdoors. For information, call 800-830-WALK.

HIGH BLOOD PRESSURE

High blood pressure is called an "illness of civilization" because it's associated with stress, inactivity, salty junk-food diets, and other unhealthy habits endemic to modern life. This disease has become extremely common in our high-pressure culture, affecting one in four people over age six and one in two people over age sixty— or more than 50 million Americans. According to the National Heart, Lung, and Blood Institute (NHLBI) of the National Institutes of Health, more than a quarter of those who have the condition don't even know their blood pressure is abnormal. This is especially unfortunate, since the negative effects of high blood pressure occur over time. Since blood-pressure elevation itself is treatable, early recognition

and treatment can prevent most related health problems.

Like many medical problems, high blood pressure is a "silent" disease. Blood pressure usually begins to rise without any obvious symptoms and continues to climb unnoticed. Uncontrolled high blood pressure, however, can seriously damage many of the body's organs and tissues, including the heart, kidneys, brain, and eyes, by damaging the blood vessels that supply each organ. When blood pressure rises and remains elevated, it effectively turns the nourishing blood flow from the beating heart into a "jackhammer," pounding the vessels to each vital organ with every heartbeat. Since on average the human heart beats about 100,000 times a day, even seemingly small elevations in blood pressure when multiplied by 100,000 beats per day, every day, can overwhelm other protective mechanisms in the body and damage blood vessels in vital organs.

The relentless pounding of blood vessels in the brain may result in rupture of the vessel, as seen in some strokes. In the heart, this pounding may damage blood vessels' lining, an injury that accelerates cholesterol buildup and can lead to heart attack. In the kidneys, such pounding can cause a thickening of the small vessels that filter waste products out of the blood, rendering them ineffective and leading to progressive kidney failure.

In addition to this jackhammer effect, high blood pressure forces the heart to continuously work harder to sustain blood flow against higher resistance. This increased workload can cause the heart muscle itself to enlarge and thicken—becoming literally "musclebound"—so that it fails to pump effectively. These changes may contribute to the condition known as congestive heart failure.

When high blood pressure is detected early, lifestyle changes—such as regular physical activity and reduced salt intake—can be extremely effective. But if hypertension (the medical term for high blood pressure) isn't detected until later, when blood pressure is markedly elevated, physical activity is most safely introduced only after the condition is controlled by medication and with the advice of a physician.

Over the last few decades, scientists have developed an increasingly powerful arsenal of drugs to treat hypertension. These medications have helped to substantially reduce the incidence of sickness and death attributable to high blood pressure. In the United States, deaths from heart attack and stroke have decreased by 40 to 60 percent over the last twenty years, partly through more effective blood-pressure control. These new drugs are one reason why about 30 percent of people with hypertension now have their disease controlled into the normal range.

But while drugs are important, they are hardly a complete prescription and are not without risk. Their side effects may be obvious, such as dry mouth or impotence, or they can be subtle, such as blood salt imbalances that can lead to life-threatening abnormalities of heart rhythm. Some of these medications also are very expensive. But most important, *drugs that lower blood pressure do not treat the underlying causes of hypertension directly, as attention to regular exercise and diet can.* People with hypertension who think that taking a "wonder drug"

gives them license to overeat and underexercise are making a potentially deadly mistake.

Appreciation of these facts has led preventive medical specialists to view drugs as a last-resort strategy after healthy lifestyle interventions are tried. Before prescribing a pill to people with mild to moderate hypertension they urge patients to correct the dangerous imbalances in their lives that contribute to their disease: exercise regularly, lose some weight, cut back on eating salt and drinking alcohol. In 1997, the federal government endorsed this advice with new guidelines stressing the importance of healthy lifestyle habits to prevent and manage hypertension. The NHLBI's new guidelines recommend that:

✳ People whose blood pressure is mildly to moderately elevated, but who have no other disease risk factors (such as diabetes or angina), should *try regular exercise and other lifestyle strategies for at least a year before turning to medications.*

✳ Patients taking hypertensive medications also should practice healthy habits, since these *lifestyle changes may reduce or eliminate the need for drugs.*

BLOOD PRESSURE BASICS

The heart is a large, hollow muscle filled with blood. With each heartbeat, the muscle squeezes, pumping blood into the arteries with the force we measure as the **systolic** pressure—the first, higher number recorded when the blood pressure is checked. This systolic force fills and stretches the naturally elastic arteries. As the heart relaxes and refills with blood, the elastic, stretched arteries recoil, providing a second wave of pumping force. The force of this elastic recoil from the arteries themselves is measured as the **diastolic** pressure—the second, or lower, number recorded when blood pressure is checked. The systolic and diastolic force together create an almost continuous perfusion pressure, which drives blood cells throughout the circulatory system, providing oxygen and nutrients to all the body's tissues and washing out waste products. *Blood pressure is the force that pushes blood cells through blood vessels and against blood-vessel walls.*

In a healthy cardiovascular system, the heart and elastic arteries pump and recoil with sufficient force to propel the blood through the body without damaging the vessels. Hypertension literally represents the pressure levels (systolic and/or diastolic) at which the pulsing of blood also becomes the relentless pounding and damaging of blood-vessel walls. This transition from normal to abnormal is generally related to the blood vessels being either constricted or overfilled or both. That is:

1. How big is the circulatory-system "tank" (i.e., how relaxed are the blood vessels)?
2. How much fluid is in the tank (i.e., what is the combined volume of water and blood in the blood vessels)?

Your circulatory-system "tank" holds, on average, five liters of blood volume. This may vary either as the vessel tissues lose elasticity or as metabolic and autonomic stimuli cause them to dilate or constrict. The most common factor affecting elasticity is age. With advancing age, the elastic ele-

ments of the blood vessels are progressively replaced by more leathery, fibrous tissue. Progressive deposition of cholesterol plaque, known as athlerosclerosis, or hardening of the arteries, can also compromise blood-vessel elasticity. This frequently accompanies aging.

Blood-vessel size can become reduced or constricted when overstimulated by the central nervous system or by circulating substances like adrenaline. Stress, hostile emotions, and a sedentary lifestyle are all factors likely to "shrink the tank" through such mechanisms.

Exercise early in life may help preserve blood-vessel elasticity, helping prevent the effects of aging and of atherosclerosis. Exercise at any age helps condition blood vessels to "relax" and dilate. For example, watch how profusely trained athletes sweat. Even the blood vessels in their skin are conditioned to dilate effectively.

No matter what its size, the "tank" of your circulatory system can become "overfilled." This can occur when a high-salt diet causes the body to retain excess water, so that the blood volume exceeds the amount the vessels can safely hold. The resulting "too full" tank can create excess pressure on the entire circulatory system. When the "tank" becomes too full or too small or both, the blood pressure rises. If the imbalance between the size of the tank and the volume that fills it becomes too extreme, hypertension results, and the life-giving pulsation of blood pressure turns into a relentless pummeling of blood vessels everywhere in the body.

Blood pressure is routinely determined with an instrument called a *sphygmo-manometer*, which consists of a gauge and a rubber cuff that is placed around the upper arm and inflated. Blood pressure is measured in millimeters of mercury (mm Hg) and is recorded with two numbers separated by a slash. The first number, called systolic pressure, measures the maximum pressure in your arteries generated by your heart muscle squeezing. The second number, diastolic pressure, measures the pressure maintained by the recoil of the elastic arteries while your heart muscle relaxes between beats. Readings of more than 140 systolic and/or 90 diastolic are considered abnormally high blood pressure.

It's important to recognize that your blood pressure is dynamic—that is, it's more than just one set of figures determined with one measurement once a year. Your blood pressure varies throughout the day in response to physical and mental stimuli. For example, in a healthy individual it goes up during physical activity or when you're excited or stressed, and it goes down during rest, sleep, or meditation. Your blood pressure can even vary from minute to minute as a result of a wide range of factors, including caffeine, smoking, noise, a full bladder, or being cold. In some people, personal or job stress can prompt a blood pressure "spike" as high as 30 or 40 mm Hg. Just the nervousness caused by being in a doctor's office or of having their blood pressure taken by a health professional can be enough to cause an elevation in some people's blood pressure—a phenomenon known as the "white-coat" syndrome. *For this reason, the key to diagnosing hypertension is determining your average blood pressure, which means taking several readings over a period of time, such as once every two to four weeks, over a period of one to two months.*

In about 5 to 10 percent of cases, high blood pressure is only a secondary symptom of an identified primary medical condition,

CATEGORIES FOR BLOOD-PRESSURE LEVELS IN ADULTS*
(AGE 18 YEARS AND OLDER)

Blood-Pressure Level (mm Hg)

Category	Systolic	Diastolic
Normal	<130	<85
High Normal	130–139	85–89
High Blood Pressure		
Stage 1	140–159	90–99
Stage 2	160–179	100–109
Stage 3	≥180	≥110

*For those not taking medicine for high blood pressure and not having a short-term serious illness. These categories are from the National High Blood Pressure Education Program.
(< means less than; ≥ means greater than or equal to)

such as a kidney abnormality, congenital blood-vessel defect, rare tumors, endocrine abnormality, or pregnancy. High blood pressure also may primarily occur as a side effect of certain drugs, such as oral contraceptives or some cold remedies. In these cases, when the root cause can be corrected, blood pressure usually returns to normal. But in 90 to 95 percent of cases, doctors can't determine a precise cause of the high blood pressure, and the condition is classified as "essential" hypertension—a complex interaction of genetically driven and environmentally interactive processes that aren't well defined enough to be "cured." Essential hypertension involves the combined contribution of imbalanced function across various body systems, including:

* the *heart and arteries*, which generate the force that keeps blood moving through the body;
* the *kidneys*, which help regulate the amount of fluid circulating through the body;
* the *sympathetic nervous system*, which helps control the contraction and dilation of blood vessels; and
* the *endocrine system*, which produces hormones that tell the other systems what to do.

Diet and exercise may positively influence all of these components, as opposed to medications, which target just one specific element, such as the kidneys or blood-vessel tone. That's why *the foundation of blood-pressure treatment is adopting healthy lifestyle changes, such as regular exercise and good nutrition, to help all the body's systems come into a better balance.*

RISK FACTORS

Certain characteristics put you at greater risk of hypertension. Those you can't influence include:

* *Age.* In general, the older you get, the greater your chance of developing high blood pressure. Being older than sixty is considered a major risk factor.
* *Heredity.* The tendency to have high blood pressure runs in families.
* *Sex.* In general, men are more likely than women to develop high blood pressure. After menopause, however, women's risk of the disease rises significantly. In fact, more postmenopausal women have high blood pressure than do men of the same age.
* *Race.* African Americans are more likely to develop high blood pressure than Caucasian Americans. They are also more likely to get the disease earlier in life.

If you have some or all or these risk factors for high blood pressure, it's particularly important that you pay attention to the following risk factors that you *can* influence:

* *Physical inactivity.* The more sedentary you are, the greater your risk of developing high blood pressure. When compared with their more active and fit peers, sedentary individuals with normal blood pressure have a 20 to 50 percent increased risk of developing hypertension.
* *Obesity.* Being overweight can make you two to six times more likely to develop high blood pressure than if you are at your desirable weight. Many people don't realize that as they gain extra fat over the years, their blood pressure often creeps up, too.

✳ *Eating too much salt.* In people with sodium-sensitive hypertension, eating too much salt is related to an increase in blood pressure. A healthful sodium intake ranges from 500 to 2,400 milligrams, or no more than 1¼ teaspoons of table salt, daily. Yet most Americans consume five to eighteen times more sodium than they need. According to the American Heart Association, the prevalence of high blood pressure could probably be reduced if people used less salt to cook and season food and ate less fast food and processed food. Even people who don't think they eat much salt may actually consume a high-sodium diet. People are often unaware of the large quantities of sodium contained in many ready-to-eat foods and over-the-counter remedies, such as analgesics. Seventy-five percent of American's sodium intake is derived from processed food.

✳ *Alcohol.* Drinking more than one ounce of alcohol a day has been associated with increased blood pressure in some people. Whether the kind of alcohol matters— liquor versus wine, for example—and whether some alcoholic beverages, such as red wine, may have other health benefits remains controversial.

✳ *Oral contraceptives and some other medications.* Women who take birth-control pills may develop high blood pressure. Certain other drugs, including amphetamines and diet pills, also tend to raise blood pressure.

✳ *Stress.* Some health professionals consider "high stress" to be a risk factor for high blood pressure. Stress levels, however, are hard to measure and responses to stress vary. The classical physiology of the fight-or-flight stress response, with its surge of adrenaline and increase in sympthetic nervous system tone, does elevate both heart rate and blood pressure to some degree, although transiently. Whether or not this "programmed" response reaches pathological proportion may vary across individuals and across stressors.

✳ *Smoking.* Cigarette smoking may not directly cause high blood pressure, but nicotine does cause blood vessels to constrict, and smoking accelerates atherosclerosis. Thus, cigarette smoking also increases the likelihood that high blood pressure, when present, will lead to catastrophic events like heart attack and stroke.

✳ *Other disorders.* Many other chronic health conditions, including diabetes, thyroid and other glandular disease, autoimmune disorders, and many kidney abnormalities, may result in abnormally high blood pressure. In some cases, curing the underlying problem leads to normalization of blood pressure. In many cases, good control of blood pressure requires directed medical therapy. In almost all cases, regular exercise and a sound approach to diet will help make blood pressure easier to control.

HOW EXERCISE HELPS

Exercise is among the most powerful of the lifestyle strategies recommended to reduce blood pressure because it helps improve numerous regulatory functions that affect blood pressure. Regular aerobic exercise itself has been shown to decrease the resting systolic and diastolic blood pressure by approximately 10 mm Hg. (Remember: That "little" drop of 10 mm Hg is multiplied over the 100,000 heartbeats daily!)

Known positive effects of exercise include:

1. Regular aerobic exercise trains the blood vessels to dilate when the stress of exertion is applied. This conditions the vessels to dilate more readily in response to all forms of stress.
2. Exercise "processes" stress and creates a relaxation effect, which can help lower blood pressure.
3. Exercise helps develop breathing, which enhances the connections between circulatory efficiency and meditative states of mind.
4. "Exercise training has the ongoing effect of lowering blood pressure by attenuating sympathetic nervous system activity," notes the *U.S. Surgeon General's Report on Physical Activity and Health*. This means that regular exercise helps boost the efficiency of the central nervous system in regulating blood-vessel tone. One sign of this is how well-conditioned athletes have slower resting heart rates and lower blood pressure than their peers.
5. Exercise improves insulin sensitivity. This not only affects sugar levels in the blood but may also have a positive effect on sodium and water reabsorption by the kidneys, contributing to blood-pressure reduction.
6. Sedentary people who begin to exercise regularly typically lose weight, and weight loss is associated with improvement in blood pressure. (Even small weight losses of five to ten pounds can result in a significant decline in blood pressure in some overweight people.)
7. Adopting the habit of regular exercise often results in a phenomenon called the "granola effect"—that is, many people who start exercising also begin to adopt other healthy behaviors, such as quitting smoking and improving their diet. These other positive lifestyle habits can also have a positive effect on blood pressure.
8. Regular exercise affects many of the risk factors for cardiovascular disease, such as improving blood cholesterol and glucose levels. This is particularly important for hypertensives, since people don't die of high blood pressure per se, but from the cardiovascular complications that are worsened by the condition.

THE STROKE CONNECTION

High blood pressure is the main risk factor for stroke, the third leading cause of death in the United States, after heart disease and cancer, and the leading cause of adult disability. Just as regular exercise can help reduce the risk of a heart attack, physical activity may also help prevent a "brain attack"—the name some experts have given stroke to increase awareness of the urgent nature of this devastating illness. The National Stroke Association's Prevention Advisory Board recommends taking "a brisk walk for as little as 30 minutes a day" as one of ten strategies to help prevent the disease, which occurs when blood circulation to the brain fails, most often as the result of blockage to a blood vessel in the brain or neck.

One of the main mechanisms by which exercise may prevent strokes is its impact on lowering blood pressure. Regular physical activity also reduces the risk of several other conditions that put people at increased stroke risk, including heart attack, elevated cholesterol levels and diabetes. Exercise may also reduce the risk of stroke by slowing the process that leads to clogging of the arteries, keeping weight down, and helping reduce clotting of the blood. In addition, people who exercise are more health conscious and are more likely to have healthy behaviors, such as not smoking or drinking to excess and having a good diet. These habits also help prevent strokes.

Recent research has helped strengthen the link between physical activity and stroke prevention. People who exercise for one hour per day cut their risk for stroke nearly in half, according to a study of 11,130 Harvard University alumni published in *Stroke: Journal of the American Heart Association.* Researchers found that people who expended 2,000 calories each week—the equivalent of a one-hour brisk walk, five days a week—had a 46 percent lower risk of stroke than those who did little to no exercise. People who expended 1,000 calories a week—the equivalent of walking briskly 30 minutes a day, five days a week—had a 24 percent reduction in stroke risk.

"Walking, stair-climbing and participating in moderately intense activities such as dancing, bicycling and gardening were shown to reduce the risk of stroke," says the study's lead author, physician I-Min Lee of the Harvard School of Public Health. "Light activity such as bowling and general housekeeping activity did not have the same effect."

EXERCISE ℞

While exercise can ultimately be an important factor in blood-pressure control for all, when and how to get started varies depending on:

1. whether or not you have hypertension;
2. the severity of the hypertension; and
3. its association with other conditions, such as coronary artery disease or congestive heart failure, that might influence how much exercise is ideal and safe.

If you don't have high blood pressure, regular physical activity can help you avoid developing the condition. If you have mild to moderate high blood pressure, regular exercise can help lower it—possibly into the normal range. If you have very high blood pressure, it should be lowered with medication before you begin an exercise program.

Here are some general guidelines:

✳ *Normal blood pressure:* If your blood pressure is currently normal and you have a family history of hypertension or if occasional measurements of your blood pressure are abnormally high, it's advisable for you to do some form of moderate activity, such as walking, for 30 minutes, most days of the week.

✳ *Mild to moderate hypertension (up to 159/99):* Try regular exercise—and other healthy lifestyle strategies—for six months to a year before resorting to medications. Your blood pressure should be monitored about once a month during this time to make sure it stays only moderately elevated or improves. The new NHLBI guidelines advise doing *"moderately intense" aerobic activity, such as brisk walking, for 30 to 45 minutes on most days of the week.* A good indicator that your activity is in this moderate range is that it will elevate your heart rate and breathing somewhat, but you'll still be breathing without excessive effort and be able to carry on a conversation. Most people can safely exercise at this level, although some discussion with a health-care provider about your exercise program is a good idea. If you smoke or have any other health problems in addition to hypertension, a physician should definitely be involved in planning your exercise program.

❋ **Markedly elevated blood pressure (either the systolic value above 160 or the diastolic value above 100):** It's important that you have your hypertension controlled by medications before you embark on an exercise program. Once your blood pressure is under control, gradually increasing your physical activity may improve your blood pressure further. Regular activity may also decrease—or even eliminate—your need for blood pressure medications. But it's vital that people with markedly elevated blood pressure discuss their exercise plans with their health-care professional to determine what physical activity level is healthy for them and to help optimize ongoing medical therapies. Because very vigorous activity can further elevate blood pressure transiently in some people with extremely high blood pressure, strenuous athletic activity can trigger serious health complications, like stroke or congestive heart failure. However, mild to moderate activity, such as easy walking or swimming, generally lowers blood pressure and overall is likely to be beneficial.

Contrary to the "Rambo mentality," which assumes that if walking is good, running must be better, studies show that *mild*

exercises, such as walking, may reduce blood pressure just as much as or even more than strenuous activities, such as jogging. While jogging, cycling, swimming, and other more strenuous activities may be beneficial for some people with mild to moderate hypertension, adults who have been sedentary should both use common sense and consult a physician before beginning a program of vigorous exercise.

In this context, common sense can be defined as: Starting any new exercise program slowly and progressing gradually.

"You don't have to exhaust yourself to lower your blood pressure," notes the American College of Sports Medicine in its booklet *Exercise Your Way to Lower Blood Pressure*. "The physical activity required to lower blood pressure can be added without making major lifestyle changes. Park your car at the far end of the parking lot or in a different lot, so you can 'walk' to and from work. During the day, take the stairs rather than the elevator . . . walk to a restaurant with low-fat, low-cholesterol options on its menu. In the evening or on weekends, take your kids or grandkids to the park, the woods or the beach for a walk. On weekends or when it is too hot, too cold or too wet, take a 30-minute continuous window-shopping walk around the mall." In this setting, "common sense" can be defined as: Make sure to do more walking than shopping!

Remember, when it comes to physical activity, *doing something is better than doing nothing.* And, contrary to Rambo, increasing activity levels a little at a time, steadily over time, is safer and more effective than trying to do too much all at once.

Lowering your blood pressure may progress gradually, but the effect of exercise begins quickly. Changes in blood pressure may be measurable as soon as three to four weeks after you increase your physical activity levels. It is equally important that you remember that the blood-pressure-lowering effects of exercise last only as long as you continue to be active. That's why one of the most important components of exercise to improve blood pressure is frequency: Stay physically active regularly. In this context, "common sense" is:

1. Building activity into your lifestyle by always taking the stairs, parking in the farthest space, or walking to work.
2. Finding an activity you enjoy enough to make time to do it regularly.
3. Rotating activities you enjoy to avoid injury and boredom.

In addition to daily life activities and regular aerobic exercise, *meditative activity— such as tai chi and yoga—also may help lower blood pressure.* The ancient Chinese martial art of tai chi lowered blood pressure in older adults nearly as much as moderate-intensity aerobic exercise in a study by researchers at Johns Hopkins University School of Medicine in Baltimore. The slow, relaxed physical activity they performed consisted of a series of thirteen movements, each of which had ten to fifteen additional moves. After twelve weeks of practicing tai chi, a group of thirty-one previously sedentary adults ages sixty and older with mild to moderate blood-pressure elevation experienced an average blood-pressure drop of 7 mm Hg. This was nearly as great a drop as that expe-

rienced by a similar group who began a program of aerobic exercise (brisk walking and low-impact aerobics). The aerobic exercise group's systolic blood pressure fell an average of 8.4 mm Hg. The beneficial effects were seen in both groups after only six weeks.

Studies also indicate that the five-thousand-year-old Indian practice of yoga may help decrease blood pressure. This is one reason why respected institutions such as the Duke University Center for Living in Durham, North Carolina, and Dr. Dean Ornish's Preventive Medicine Research Institute in Sausalito, California, include the practice of yoga in their "healthy-heart" programs. Yoga not only boosts the health of the circulatory system but can also help people learn mental and physical relaxation techniques, so that they can better combat stress-related rises in blood pressure.

In addition to the beneficial effect of their physical movements, both of these techniques focus on breathing, which offers unique healing qualities. Breathing techniques have a quieting effect on the mind and the emotions and also improve cardiovascular efficiency, which can directly affect blood pressure. Through simultaneous stress-relaxation effects and respiratory mechanics, breathing techniques help modulate blood pressure and become an exercise that connects body and mind.

Strength training is not recommended as the only form of exercise for people with high blood pressure, says the American College of Sports Medicine (ACSM) in its position stand on physical activity, physical fitness, and hypertension. With the exception of one form of strength training—called circuit weight training—resistive exercises have not consistently been shown to lower blood pressure. Circuit weight training involves doing a series of strengthening exercises on machines or with free weights and moving quickly from machine to machine in the circuit to achieve an aerobic benefit. Some studies have associated this form of exercise with a decline in blood pressure.

In the past, people with high blood pressure were warned not to do strength training, since lifting extremely heavy weights can result in an exaggerated increase in blood pressure. But today many experts only caution against doing "maximal lifts"—that is, attempting to lift the heaviest weight you can. Instead, people with hypertension who want to do resistance exercise to increase muscle and bone strength should use lighter weights and do more repetitions, being sure to pick a weight they can lift ten to fifteen times. In addition, strength workouts should be part of an overall fitness program, with a physician's clearance.

In addition to regular exercise, the NHLBI also advises these other lifestyle modifications for blood-pressure management:

* **Lose weight if overweight.** Losing just 15 percent of body weight (thirty pounds for someone who weighs two hundred) is associated with a 10 percent reduction in systolic blood pressure, according to a report by the Institute of Medicine. Losing just 7.7 pounds resulted in a 30 percent decrease in the need for antihypertensive medications, according to a study by the Tulane University School of Public Health.

* **Limit alcohol intake** to no more than two drinks a day if you're a man or one drink a day if you're a woman.

* **Reduce sodium intake** to no more than 2.4 grams. This corresponds with approximately 6 grams of "table salt," which is actually a compound called sodium chloride that contains 40 percent sodium and 60 percent chloride.

* **Maintain adequate intake of dietary potassium** (approximately 3,500 mg), preferably from fresh fruits and vegetables, such as apricots, bananas, prunes, orange juice, spinach, dry peas, and beans. If you are taking diuretics for your blood pressure, consult your physician about taking sea salt or potassium supplements.

* **Maintain adequate intake of dietary calcium and magnesium** from foods such as low- and nonfat dairy products and whole grains, leafy green vegetables, nuts, seeds, and beans.

* **Stop smoking and reduce intake of dietary saturated fat and cholesterol** for overall cardiovascular health.

CAUTIONS

If you have high blood pressure, smoke, or have other health conditions for which you take medication, be sure to discuss your exercise program with your physician, since exercise recommendations may vary depending on the severity of your condition, the medications you take, and any related conditions you may have. If you're taking antihypertensive medications, be aware that some drugs can affect your athletic performance, which is why some sports organizations ban the use of beta-blockers and diuretics by participants in competitive events.

Follow these commonsense principles for exercise to prevent or treat high blood pressure:

* Start slowly and progress gradually. Pick a moderate exercise that you enjoy, such as walking or swimming, and begin with as little as 5 to 10 minutes a day. Each week, add a few more minutes to your exercise session until you're doing your activity for 30 to 45 minutes, most days of the week.

* Monitor your blood pressure periodically (a minimum of once every one to three months) at home, through a nurse at work, or with a machine in the drugstore or grocery store.

* Consult a doctor if you have pain or pressure in the chest or shoulder area, if you tend to feel dizzy or faint, if you get very breathless after a mild workout, or if you've been sedentary and you want to begin a vigorous exercise program. The American Heart Association advises men over age forty and woman over age fifty, as well as adults with risk factors for heart disease (such as cigarette smoking, diabetes, high cholesterol, or a family history of heart disease), to get a stress test before beginning to exercise vigorously. *But most people don't need a doctor's approval to do mild to moderate activity, such as going out for a walk.*

* Avoid lifting extremely heavy weights.

* Check with your physician before doing inverted yoga poses, such as a handstand, or performing any exercises in which your head is lower than your heart.

PRESCRIPTION PAD

* Add activity to your daily life. Climb stairs, rake leaves, park in the farthest space, go dancing.

* Take a daily 30- to 45-minute walk, most days of the week. If you prefer, you can substitute another moderate aerobic activity—such as swimming or gardening—for walking. If you want to substitute a strenuous activity, such as jogging, be sure you have your physician's approval if you have hypertension or if you've been sedentary.

* Incorporate a 10- to 30-minute relaxation session into your day. This can be a "moving meditation" session, performing a meditative activity such as tai chi or yoga, or simply the practice of breathing techniques done sitting or lying still—as a *human be-ing,* not just a *human do-ing.*

* If you are taking antihypertensive medication, be aware that your need for the drugs may be reduced or eliminated after you begin to exercise regularly. Monitor your blood pressure and never reduce dosages of your drugs without your physician's approval.

* Avoid "maximal lifting"—that is, if you have hypertension, don't try to pick up the heaviest weight you can.

ADDITIONAL RESOURCES

* *The American Heart Association* has numerous brochures and fact sheets about hypertension, heart disease, and stroke. Call 800-AHA-USA1 or visit the Web site: www.americanheart.org.

* *The National Heart, Lung, and Blood Institute's* Information Line offers free material about high blood pressure to consumers and health professionals. Call 800-575-9355, write NHLBI, P.O. Box 30105, Bethesda, Md. 20824, or check the Web site at www.nhlbi.nih.gov.

* *The National Stroke Association:* 800-STROKES; www.stroke.org.

* *Healthfinder*, an Internet site for health-related government agencies, such as the National Institutes of Health and the Department of Health and Human Services, can provide a wealth of information about hypertension. Access the Web site at www.healthfinder.gov, then follow the "search" cues to access material about high blood pressure.

---

* * *

HEALING MOVES FOR HEART HEALTH

*

Of all the body's organs, the heart is the one most associated with our emotions—love, grief, anger, sadness, fear. And increasingly, research indicates that negative emotions and stress can seriously damage the heart, while positive emotions such as faith and love may heal. That's why our program includes two parts:

Part One: Aerobic Activity

We present a walking program designed to strengthen the cardiovascular system, enhance lipid and insulin metabolism, and boost mood.

Part Two: Mind-Body Practices

We feature several exercises, adapted from yoga and qi gong, that serve as a sort of "moving meditation" to connect physical and mental energies, both relaxing and opening the heart.

This program is geared to primary prevention of heart disease, which means it's designed for people who do not have established coronary artery disease. It's also appropriate for people with normal blood pressure or mild to moderate hypertension. People seeking secondary prevention of heart disease—to reduce or reverse the buildup of fatty deposits in the arteries of those who already have CAD—and people with markedly elevated blood pressure should consult a physician for individualized exercise recommendations. (See Pre-Participation Checklist, page 29.)

Bring this workout to your health-care professional and ask him or her to advise you about specifics of your exercise program if you:

* Are a male over forty or a female over fifty who has been sedentary and plans to begin a *vigorous* exercise program

* Have two or more risk factors for CAD (smoking, family history, diabetes, obesity, high cholesterol, hypertension) or have been diagnosed with CAD

* Have had a heart attack, bypass surgery, or a procedure to open blocked arteries. (You may benefit by enrolling in a supervised program of cardiac rehabilitation.)

✳ Have markedly elevated blood pressure (systolic above 160 and/or diastolic above 100). You'll need to have your blood pressure controlled with medication before starting an exercise program.

PART ONE: AEROBIC ACTIVITY

Aerobic means "with oxygen" and is used to describe activities that boost the heart's capacity to deliver oxygen to the muscles. Any activity that uses the large-muscle groups of the legs, back, and arms in a continuous and rhythmic manner is considered an aerobic exercise. Among the most popular: walking, running, aerobic dancing, bicycling, skating, stair climbing, swimming, water exercise, and rowing.

Our program uses walking, since fitness walking is America's most popular exercise, with 17 million regular participants. Easy, enjoyable, effective, economical, and empowering, walking is an activity virtually everyone can do with very little risk of injury. Follow our gradual weekly progression and within three months you should begin to see and feel the results.

Month One: Start Your Engines

Week One: This is "contemplation and visualization week," a time to just think about and see ways to fit walking into your life. You won't be taking half-hour walks for a while yet, but it's not too early to start thinking about the time of day that will work best for you to walk: first thing in the morning, lunchtime, after work, or after dinner? Also, decide where you'll walk. If possible, try to walk outdoors, for the extra health boost of sunshine and fresh air. If bad weather or other factors make outdoor walks inadvisable, consider walking in a mall, at a gym, through hallways in an apartment building, or on a home treadmill.

In addition, make a list of three to five strategies for fitting several short "walk breaks" into your day: For example:

1. Instead of getting my coffee at the vending machine near my office, I'll take the stairs to the cafeteria and buy my coffee there.
2. When I take the kids to soccer practice, I'll walk around the field instead of sitting in my car.
3. I'll get off the elevator two flights early and climb the stairs the rest of the way.
3. I'll park my car at the far end of the lot and walk a few extra steps to my destination. (See 25 Ways to Activate Your Life, page 35.)

Week Two: This week you'll make the first small step in your program. Five or six days this week, slip into a pair of comfortable walking shoes and take an easy, 5-minute walk during the time you picked as the best for you. Consider using these walks as "contemplative" or "mindful" times, where you focus on the pleasurable feeling of moving in the fresh air.

Week Three: Continue your 5-minute walks, five or six days a week, at a comfortable pace. In addition, pick one of your "walk break" ideas and put it into action.

Week Four: Double your daily walking time to 10 minutes, five or six days a week, at a comfortable pace. Continue doing your first "walk break" strategy, and consider adopting a second.

Month Two: Experience Your Zone

Now that you've begun to establish the walking habit, it's time to pick up the pace a bit. This will help your cardiovascular system achieve the "training effect," which is a complex constellation of physiological changes that occur as your body begins to adapt to the demands of regular aerobic conditioning. There are two basic ways to determine the proper exercise intensity for you to achieve this training effect:

1. **Perceived exertion.** Find a pace you consider "moderate" to "somewhat hard," where you can feel that your heart rate has gone up some, but it's not racing. You should be able to carry on a conversation without becoming breathless. On a scale of 1 to 10 (with 1 being "very, very light" and 10 being "extremely hard"), about 4 to 7 is a desirable intensity range. One to 3 may be too light to allow you the maximum cardiovascular benefits; 8 to 10 is too hard for most people and increases the likelihood of orthopedic or cardiac problems. If your fitness level is low, you may want to begin at the lower end of this range and gradually increase your intensity over time.
2. **Target heart rate.** Exercising at 50 to 75 percent of your maximum heart rate (the fastest your heart can beat) will improve the fitness of your heart and lungs, which is why it's considered a "training zone."

(People who are already fit may be able to exercise at up to 90 percent of their maximum heart rate and may benefit from a more intense training zone. People who are recovering from a debilitating illness may, with the guidance of a health care professional, improve their fitness by exercising in a less intense training zone.) To find your maximum heart rate, subtract your age from 220. For example, if you are forty, your maximum heart rate would be 180. To determine your "training zone," multiply your maximum heart rate (180) by .5 to get 90, and by .75 to get 135. By target heart rate, then, a forty-year-old's training zone would be 90 to 135 beats per minute. A list of training zones appears on the next page.

Week Five: Walk 5 minutes at an easy pace to warm up. Then pick up your pace until you're in your "training zone"—using either perceived exertion or target heart rate to determine the right intensity. Walk for 5 minutes in your training zone, then slow your pace and cool down with 5 more minutes of walking at an easy pace for a total walk time of 15 minutes. Do this four to six days a week.

Your workouts will continue to follow this pattern, four to six days a week, increasing your training zone time slightly each week. And don't forget to keep up with your "walk break" strategies.

	Warm-up	Training Zone	Cooldown	Total Time
Week Six:	5 minutes	8 minutes	5 minutes	18 minutes
Week Seven:	5 minutes	11 minutes	5 minutes	21 minutes
Week Eight:	5 minutes	14 minutes	5 minutes	24 minutes

TRAINING HEART RATES

Age	Target HR Zone 50–75%	Average Maximum Heart Rate 100%
20 years	100–150 beats per min.	200
25 years	98–146 beats per min.	195
30 years	95–142 beats per min.	190
35 years	93–138 beats per min.	185
40 years	90–135 beats per min.	180
45 years	88–131 beats per min.	175
50 years	85–127 beats per min.	170
55 years	83–123 beats per min.	165
60 years	80–120 beats per min.	160
65 years	78–116 beats per min.	155
70 years	75–113 beats per min.	150

Month Three: A Program for Life

By the end of this month, you'll be doing a complete walking program that can help keep your heart healthy for life. To keep your muscles and joints supple and injury-free, this month we'll add some gentle stretches. The best times to stretch are after your warm-up, before you move into your target zone, or at the end of your walk, when your muscles are warm and pliable. Some people like to do both, stretching gently after their warm-up, then again at the end of their walk. Avoid stretching cold muscles.

Shins and Ankles: Stand on one foot (holding on to something for balance, if necessary), lift your other foot off the ground, and draw circles in the air with your toes. Make 5 to 10 circles in each direction, then switch legs.

Calves and Achilles Tendons: Stand an arm's length away from a wall, step forward with your right foot, and lean into the wall with your forearms, bending your right knee but keeping your left leg straight and your left heel on the ground until you feel a mild tension through the back of your left leg. Repeat with the other leg.

	Warm-up	Training Zone	Cooldown	Stretch	Total Time
Week Nine:	5 minutes	18 minutes	5 minutes	5 minutes	33 minutes
Week Ten:	5 minutes	22 minutes	5 minutes	5 minutes	37 minutes
Week Eleven:	5 minutes	26 minutes	5 minutes	5 minutes	41 minutes
Week Twelve:	5 minutes	30 minutes	5 minutes	5 minutes	45 minutes

Hips, Lower Back, and Groin: Sit in a "butterfly" position with the soles of your feet together. Hold on to your toes and feet, bend from your hips, and gently pull yourself forward. Breathe slowly and deeply for about 30 seconds, without bouncing, then release.

(For more stretches, see Healing Moves for Health and Fitness, page 44, and Healing Moves to Strengthen Muscles and Bones, page 147.)

Month Four and Beyond: Keep On Keeping On

Congratulations on working your way up to a complete, 45-minute heart-healthy walking program. To enhance your motivation and fun, and maximize your exercise's benefit, try:

✳ Walking with a friend, human or canine.

✳ Checking local newspapers for listings of walking clubs and walk with a group.

✳ Taking the scenic route. Study a map of your city and look for parks, trails, and recreation areas suitable for walking.

✳ Take quicker—not longer—steps. To pick up your pace, step more quickly and let your stride length come naturally. If you take 130 steps per minute, you'll be walking at a pace of about four miles per hour, which will give your heart a great workout.

✳ Walk tall. Avoid slouching or hunching your shoulders, and instead think about elongating your spine. Look forward, not down at the gutter.

✳ Bend your arms. For a speed boost, bend your elbows to ninety degrees and let your hands swing in an arc from your waistband to chest height.

✳ Push off with your toes. Land on your heel, roll your foot from heel to toe, then push off forcefully with your toes.

✳ Be sure to wear good walking shoes. When selecting a new pair, shop at the end of the day, when your foot is at its largest, to avoid the common mistake of buying a too small shoe. Bring along the socks you'll wear, and be sure there's a thumb's width distance between the end of your toe and the shoe. Try several brands until you find one that fits snugly at the heel but has "wiggle room" in the toes.

To keep walking for life, remember these four keys to exercising for a healthy heart:

1. Move every day. On your days "off" from your aerobic exercise, be physically active in other ways—for example, do the moving meditation practices, garden, dance, or play actively with children or grandchildren.

2. Integrate activity into your life. Embrace opportunities to move your body: Use the bathroom on another floor and take the stairs, walk a lap around the store before you start to shop, hide your remote and get up to change the channel. Every step you take counts.

3. Find an activity you enjoy, so that your workout is not another stressful chore but a welcome "play break." Just be sure to start slowly, progress gradually, and enjoy your chance to move your body and relax your mind.

4. Use exercise time for your spirit, too. If you enjoy company and scheduling permits, celebrate your exercise with the

companionship of a walking buddy or a pet. If you prefer time alone or scheduling is too complicated, use your exercise time for private contemplation, problem solving, or mindfulness.

Remember: *The most important exercise criterion for heart health is **frequency**.* It's better to do some moderate movement every day than to sit all week and do a huge workout on the weekend. Daily movement helps the body make the essential adaptations that bring all its varied systems into balance. Of course, use common sense: Sometimes rest is more healing that exercise—for example, if you've got the flu or if you ran the Boston Marathon yesterday. But on most days, your heart—and mind—needs movement.

PART TWO: MIND-BODY PRACTICE

These healing exercises are adapted from ancient Eastern arts that have been used for thousands of years to promote health: yoga from India and qi gong from China. Both of these disciplines incorporate three fundamental, interdependent parts:

1. *Posture*. Placing the body in correct alignment is essential to helping relieve stress, take unnecessary pressure off vital organs, and encourage circulation of oxygen, blood, and energy.

2. *Breathing*. Focusing on the breath helps connect the body with the mind, calming both and enhancing the flow of life-sustaining oxygen, nutrients, and energy.

3. *Mental quietness*. Encouraging calmness of mind helps adjust the nervous system, nourish the spirit, and relax the body.

Exercise 1: Fang Sung Kung (Qi Gong Relaxation Breathing)

1. Lie comfortably on your back, using a pillow to support your head and shoulders. Let your arms extend out beside your body and your legs stretch out naturally. Keep your eyes and mouth lightly closed.

2. Breathe naturally in and out through your nose. Focus on breathing soundlessly, steadily, and smoothly, so that your inhalation is as long as your exhalation, with an even speed and depth.

3. Enter into calmness by thinking of the word *quiet* as you inhale and the word *relax* as you exhale. When you think the word *relax*, consciously focus on a part of the body and relax it. For example, think *forehead relax* as you invite the muscles in your forehead to release. With each breathing cycle, move down the body, relaxing each part. After you've relaxed all your muscles down to your toes, men-

Fang Sung Kung

tally suggest to your blood vessels, nervous system, and internal organs that they also relax.

4. When you are finished, gently rub your face with your hands, massage your ears, then get up slowly.

Exercise 2: The Essential Breath (Yoga Relaxation Breathing)

1. Sit comfortably on a stool or chair with both feet firmly on the ground, about shoulder width apart. The chair height should allow your knees to form a ninety-degree angle. Keep your back and waist straight, so that your thighs and torso also form a ninety-degree angle. Place your hands gently in your lap, palms up, letting your shoulders fall naturally. Tuck your chin slightly inward.

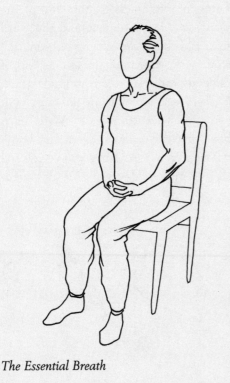

The Essential Breath

2. Breathe in slowly and gently through your nose, focusing on filling up the lower portion of your lungs first, which will make your abdomen expand. Then continue the breath so that the upper lobes of your lungs fill, which will expand your rib cage and chest.

3. When the two "balloons" of your lungs are completely inflated, exhale slowly and gently through your nose, consciously inviting yourself to relax.

4. Enjoy the momentary pause that follows the end of the exhalation, then let the next inhalation arise naturally and repeat the cycle, gently and without strain, for several minutes.

You can also practice yoga relaxation breathing lying down or standing up. Just make sure to use good posture that will allow your lungs to expand fully. Practice yoga breathing for a few minutes each morning and each evening. It's helpful to think of a cue—such as a ringing telephone—that will remind you to "belly breathe" throughout the day, whenever the phone rings. (Several variations on this basic essential breath—such as color breathing and mantra breathing—are presented in the relaxation breathing section of Healing Moves for Health and Fitness, page 49.)

Exercise 3: Frog Pose

1. Sit on your feet with your knees together (or if this is uncomfortable, sit on a bench or chair with your feet flat on the floor). Rest your palms on your knees.

2. Inhale as you lean forward, arch your back, and gaze up, stretching your throat and letting your elbows bend.

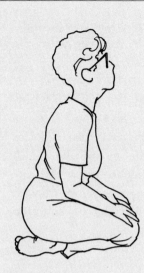

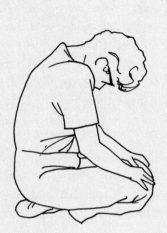

Frog Pose

3. Then exhale as you bend the opposite way, rounding your back, shifting your torso back, tucking your chin into your chest, and letting your arms straighten.

4. Repeat several times, being sure to move along with your breath—inhale and arch the back, exhale and round the back.

Exercise 4: Spinal Twist

1. Sit on the floor with both legs extended. (If you can't or don't wish to sit on the floor, see the chair variation below). Bend your left knee and lift your left leg over your right leg so that the left foot is flat on the floor. Place your left arm behind you for support.

2. Keeping your spine straight and tall, twist your torso to the left and reach your right arm past your left knee, pressing against your left knee with your right elbow and encouraging your spine to twist farther to the left. Be sure to keep your right leg straight, with energy running down the leg toward your heel.

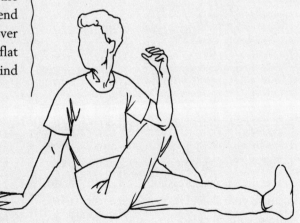

Spinal Twist

3. Inhale, then exhale and—without collapsing the spine—deepen the twist, continuing to spiral around to the left. Allow your neck to turn and your eyes to look as far around to the left as possible.
4. Hold the twist for a few gentle breaths, then slowly release and repeat on the other side.

Chair variation: Sit tall in a chair with back support, feet flat on the floor. Place your right hand on the outside of your left knee and your left arm on the back of the

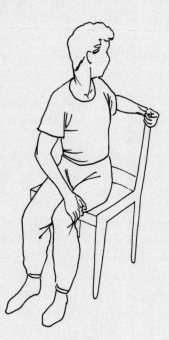

Spinal Twist, Chair Variation

chair. With your left hand, hold the seat back firmly, sit up straight, and inhale. Then exhale as you slowly turn toward the left as far as possible, pressing your right hand against your knee to encourage the twist. Allow your neck to turn and your eyes to

look as far around to the left as possible. Inhale as you release, then repeat to the other side.

Exercise 5: Bird Play (Part of Wu Chin Hsi, or Five Animal Play)
1. Stand naturally with arms relaxed, knees slightly bent, and eyes straight ahead. Take a few centering breaths.
2. Inhale as you take a full step forward with your left foot, followed by a half step

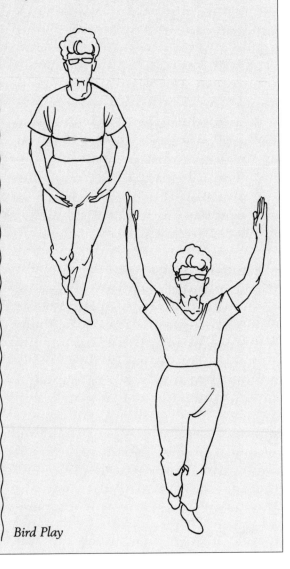

Bird Play

with your right foot, simultaneously lifting and spreading your arms wide open in a large V.

3. Exhale as you step forward with your right foot, squat down low, and lower your arms to embrace your knees. (If you can't squat down low, just bend your knees as far as comfortable as you lower your arms.)

4. Inhale and step forward with your left foot, lifting your arms into a V, repeating the sequence until you are pleasantly tired.

Exercise Six: Legs Up the Wall

1. Sit on the floor near a wall, with your thighs parallel to the wall.

2. Roll onto your back as you swing your legs up the wall. Position yourself so that your tailbone, buttocks, and lower back rest comfortably on the floor.

3. Keep your legs straight but relaxed. Allow your arms to lie comfortably out at your sides, palms up.

4. Make sure your chin is slightly lower than your forehead, but don't force it down. If your chin is lifting toward the ceiling, put

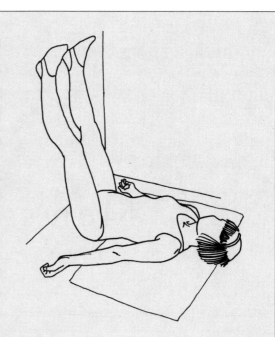

Legs Up the Wall

a blanket under your head to encourage the natural curve of your neck.

5. Breathe deeply and gently for five minutes in this position. When you're ready to come up, bend your knees toward your chest and roll to one side. Push against the floor with your arms to return to a sitting position.

7

Men's Health

SEXUAL DYSFUNCTION, PROSTATE PROBLEMS, AND "GUT" ISSUES

It's true of birds and bees, humans and chimpanzees: Males generally die younger than females. Only an estimated 2 percent of American males born in 1998 will see their eightieth birthdays, while the majority of females (52 percent) are expected to live to eighty and beyond. Forty-one percent of males will die between ages seventy and seventy-four, compared to just 14 percent of females. Thirty percent of both sexes will make it to between seventy-five and seventy-nine.

Gender-specific physiology or cultural reverse sexism?

There are many theories as to why males don't live as long as females. Physiologically, female hormones may provide greater pro-

tection against cardiovascular disease, and the procreation-designed female body is, in some ways, better equipped for endurance. But cultural factors also probably play a role: Women are less likely to go to war, participate in risky sports, abuse drugs, or be involved in violence. Traditionally, men have carried the stress of being the sole provider for the family, often in an unfriendly environment of the working world, where the prevailing "macho" ethic encourages men to suffer in silence, "tough out" problems, suppress emotion, and ignore pain. (As the gender balance equilibrates with more women wage earners, there has been an increase in women adopting "male" stress behaviors, such as smoking, and suffering from "male" ailments like heart disease and lung cancer.) Women tend to take better care of themselves, visiting physicians more frequently than men do, so that their health problems are often detected at earlier, more treatable, stages. So it's no wonder males die an average of seven years earlier than females.

To some extent, as Freud pointed out, anatomy is destiny. Some gender-specific traits lend substance to this observation. (For example, being male is a risk factor for cardiovascular disease.) But adopting positive lifestyle habits—such as regular exercise—can help modify or modulate many intrinsically male characteristics, from cholesterol metabolism to body composition to stress relief, boosting a man's chances of living a longer, healthier life. Physical activity can add more than just years to a man's life; it can add life to a man's years. From the bedroom to the boardroom, men who exercise regularly report enhanced performance and satisfaction.

The beneficial effects of exercise on the biggest threat to men's (and women's) longevity—heart disease—we examine in detail in chapter 6. In this chapter, we'll explore how exercise can prevent and treat other common men's health concerns, specifically:

✳ *Sexual dysfunction.* From erectile difficulties to loss of libido, getting fit can improve your love life.

✳ *Prostate cancer.* Among American men, prostate cancer is second only to lung cancer as the leading cause of cancer deaths (other than skin cancer) in males. Studies link exercise with reduced risk.

✳ *Gut issues.* Male-pattern obesity (a.k.a. beer belly) isn't inevitable. Physical activity can deflate the spare tire and reduce associated health risks, from heart disease to

hernia. And for the ninety-seven-pound weakling who wants to keep bullies from kicking sand in his face, exercise is essential for "bulking up."

SEXUAL DYSFUNCTION

In men, sexual dysfunction generally refers to difficulty achieving or maintaining an erection and the often-related problem of lack of interest in sex. These concerns typically surface in midlife, when a complex constellation of hormonal, physical, and psychological changes can interfere with sexual intercourse. Levels of the male hormone testosterone decline with age, and the incidence of diseases that can cause impotence rises. Men are more likely to be taking medications that can affect their ability to have an erection, specifically drugs used to treat high blood pressure or heart disease. The common "spare tire" that inflates around many midlife male middles may be accompanied by buildup of fatty plaque in the arteries, which can affect blood flow to many organs—including the penis. Emotional factors such as stress and depression also weigh in, as can cigarettes and alcohol.

The two most common forms of male sexual dysfunction are:

Inhibited sexual desire. America's number one sexual complaint, loss of libido affects up to half of all men and typically occurs after age forty. Once thought to be largely a female problem, lack of desire is now recognized as equally common in men. It is not the same as impotence; the body works, but there is little or no interest in sex. This "desire downshift" is often linked to psychological factors such as stress, fatigue, or performance anxiety, but may be tied to physical problems, such as low testosterone levels, depression, diabetes, or medications.

There is no single definition of inhibited desire, however, since there is an extremely broad spectrum of "normal" sexual activity. (A recent national survey estimates that the average American couple has intercourse seven times a month.) In general, if you've experienced a dramatic drop in sexual frequency or sexual interest, or if you or your partner are dissatisfied with your love life, you may be experiencing inhibited sexual desire.

Impotence. Sometimes called "erectile dysfunction," impotence is defined as a consistent inability to sustain an erection sufficient for sexual intercourse. While most men occasionally have difficulty getting an erection, an estimated one in ten are affected by chronic impotence. It can occur at any age, but it's more common in men over fifty. Just 5 percent of men experience impotence at age forty, according to the National Institutes of Health, while the proportion rises to between 15 and 25 percent of men at age sixty-five. Yet it is not an inevitable part of aging.

Mechanistically, the causes of impotence can be separated into physical and psychological factors. Erection difficulties linked to physical disorders are generally related to impaired blood flow to the penis or to dysfunction of the nerves that regulate penile engorgement. Psychologically, men who experience occasional impotence may lose confidence in their ability to have an erection, which can exacerbate erection problems and make the "cause" a complex combination of physical and emotional fac-

tors. NIH experts estimate that psychological factors primarily cause 10 to 20 percent of cases of impotence, but are secondarily associated with more than 80 percent of cases of impotence.

Common physical causes of sexual dysfunction include:

* **Chronic diseases.** Diseases that can lead to impotence include diabetes, kidney disease, chronic alcoholism, multiple sclerosis, atherosclerosis, and vascular disease. Damage to the arteries, smooth muscles, and fibrous tissues as a result of the specific disease process results in impotence.

* **Medications.** Many commonly prescribed drugs produce impotence as a side effect. These include some high-blood-pressure medications, heart medications, antihistamines, tranquilizers, appetite suppressants, antidepressants, and ulcer drugs. Drug effects account for about 25 percent of cases of impotence.

* **Smoking.** Excessive tobacco use can hinder blood flow in veins and arteries.

* **Hormonal problems.** In some men, low levels of testosterone can cause impotence.

* **Pelvic trauma.** "Straddle" injuries such as occur when cyclists fall against the crossbar of a bike have been linked to later problems with impotence. Some sports medicine experts contend that conventional bicycle saddles can lead to impotence by compressing nerves and blood vessels that are important for erection.

* **Pelvic surgery.** Cancer surgeries involving the prostate, bladder, colon, or rectum can result in nerve damage, causing impotence.

* **Fatigue.** Studies show that we're a sleep-deprived society in which 40 million people suffer from sleep disorders that keep them from getting a good night's rest. The average adult needs eight to nine hours of sleep each night, but most get only seven and nearly one-third get six or less during the workweek. Exhaustion may be expressed in a loss of sexual interest or in the inability to become sexually aroused.

Common psychological causes of sexual dysfunction include:

* **Stress.** Pressures and worries about job, finances, family, and health can contribute to erection difficulties, as can the stress of previous episodes of impotence.

* **Performance anxiety.** Misinformation about how men should or shouldn't be able to perform can lead to anxiety and fear of "failure," resulting in impotence.

* **Depression.** Lack of energy and reduced sex drive are common in men with depression. This can lead to difficulty producing or maintaining an erection, which can deepen depression and further exacerbate erectile dysfunction.

Since sexual problems may be transient and resolve themselves, it's not necessary to rush to the doctor the morning after a frustrating night in bed. However, men who have significant and consistent erectile problems over a period of three months are advised to consult a physician. It's more than just a matter of having satisfactory sex. Since serious illnesses can be associated with sexual dysfunction, getting to the root of sexual problems could be an important health matter.

Embarrassment often keeps men from acknowledging and discussing their concerns. The benefits of a sensitive but direct approach are clear, however, since numerous treatments exist for impotence in most age groups. Viagra, the first oral pill to treat impotence, is just one of many options available. Exercise, with its ability to positively affect underlying health conditions, circulation of blood, and emotions or mood can be uniquely effective as a medicine for impotence—a powerful therapeutic tool that serves as a kind of "sexercise."

HOW EXERCISE ENHANCES SEXUALITY

It's been touted in locker rooms for years: Getting fit improves your love life. Research supports this age-old "jock wisdom." Exercise increases sexual drive, sexual activity, and sexual satisfaction, according to numerous studies. Getting fit appears to enhance sexuality through a variety of mechanisms that affect both body and mind. Physical boosts in endurance, muscle tone, body composition, and blood flow can all improve sexual functioning. Psychological benefits, such as stress reduction, mood elevation, increased self-confidence, and heightened self-esteem can also enrich your love life.

Exercise boosts health and appearance, both of which can enhance sexuality. Healthier people may be more willing and able to have sex. People who feel more attractive may also feel more sexy. Aerobic exercise exerts a calming yet energizing effect, which many consider the ideal mindset—and body-set—for good sex. A man who looks and feels better about himself may also be better able to perform sexually.

Here's a roundup of some of the most interesting findings about exercise and sex:

* **Sexual declines with age may have more to do with poor health than years.** A Harvard University study of 160 male and female swimmers in their forties and sixties showed a positive relationship between regular exercise and sexuality in terms of both the frequency and enjoyment of intercourse. "The swimmers in their sixties reported sex lives comparable to people in the general population in their forties," reported anthropologist Phillip Whitten. "The swimmers in their forties had sex lives more like those of people in their twenties and thirties."

* **Starting an exercise program can get you in shape for sex.** A study of seventy-eight sedentary but healthy middle-aged men who started exercising vigorously three to four day a week, for 60 minutes per session, revealed that the new exercisers reported more frequent sexual activity and orgasms, more reliable function during sex, and a higher percentage of satisfying orgasms. "The degree of sexual enhancement correlated with the individual's fitness gain," reported study author James White, professor emeritus of physical education at the University of California, San Diego.

* **Running boosts sex drive.** Eighty-three percent of female runners and 75 percent of male runners responding to a poll in *Runner's World* magazine claimed that running enhanced their sex life.

* **Women also get a sexual spark from exercise.** A survey of more than eight thousand women, ages twenty to forty-five, who responded to a questionnaire published in *Shape* magazine found that 40 percent said exercising made them more easily aroused, 33 percent said exercising led to more frequent sexual activity, and 27 percent reported increased ability to climax. As a result of working out, 89 percent reported they felt heightened sexual confidence and 98 percent reported improved self-confidence.

This "sexercise" link is so strong that many sex therapists now prescribe exercise to patients with sexual dysfunction. Even low levels of exercise tend to improve mood, and moderate exercise helps maintain the condition of the equipment used for sex. Plus, sex itself is good exercise. A single act of sexual intercourse consumes about 150 calories. By comparison, eighteen holes of golf (riding a cart) uses just 118 calories. And the coach's old maxim that sex saps strength is questionable, as long as proper rest and sleep patterns are maintained. A study at Colorado State University showed that having sex within twenty-four hours of athletic activity didn't hurt performance.

The effects of exercise on the male reproductive system vary according to the intensity and duration of the activity and the fitness of the individual. Relatively short, intense exercise is linked with an increase in testosterone levels, which may enhance sexual interest and behavior. Too much exercise, however, may put a damper on both sex and fertility, since excessive and prolonged exercise is associated with a decrease in testosterone and other male hormones. Studies of female athletes have shown that intense regular exercise that leads to low body fat can affect hormone levels and result in athletic amenorrhea which, in effect turns off the menstrual cycle. Some evidence suggests that excessive exercise and overtraining may exert a similar effect in men, lowering levels of male sex hormones and possibly impairing fertility. Anecdotal reports from men involved in high levels of intense endurance training also indicate that sex drive may diminish, in part because they're just too exhausted to get aroused.

This again highlights the essential truth about balance and harmony in health. It's clear that too much or too little exercise can disrupt this healthy harmony and depress sexual function. It's also clear that a balanced program of regular exercise helps establish and maintain physical and mental equilibrium and boosts sexual desire, performance, and satisfaction.

How much exercise is ideal to boost a man's sex life, without under- or overdoing it, is an individual matter. In general, *exercising at a level you enjoy*—either moderately or vigorously—for 30 to 60 minutes three to six times a week will boost your physical, mental, and sexual health with little danger of overtraining. Aerobic exercise is important to reduce risks of diseases that can lead to sexual problems—such as cardiovascular disease and diabetes—and should be done at least three times a week for 30 minutes a session. Weight training can help build strength and rev up your metabolic rate, so you burn more calories even at rest. Two or three, 20-minute strength-training sessions can build and maintain muscle mass. Stretching after each exercise session will help boost flexibility and prevent injury.

If you've been sedentary, however, it's important that you work gradually toward this goal. (See Healing Moves for Health and Fitness, page 38.) And if you're a man over age 40 who's been inactive and wants to start a program of vigorous exercise, check with your doctor first. Even if you start slowly, however, you may quickly notice the positive effects of physical activity on sexual function.

PROSTATE CANCER

A male sex gland about the size of a walnut, the prostate secretes a thick fluid that is a vehicle for semen ejaculated during orgasm. The prostate surrounds the urethra, the tube that empties urine from the bladder, and is located just above the rectum. Of all the parts of a man's body, the prostate is the most likely to develop cancer. An estimated one out of every seven African American males and one of every eight Caucasian males develops the disease, usually after age sixty-five but sometimes as young as forty. It is the second most common cause of cancer death in American males, after lung cancer, and the most common cause of cancer death in males over fifty-five.

Prostate cancer shouldn't be confused with *benign prostatic hypertrophy*, a gradual enlargement of the prostate that occurs in more than one-third of men over forty-five. These two different conditions may have some similar symptoms—specifically difficulty urinating and the need to urinate frequently, especially at night. The most common treatments for prostate cancer are surgery, radiation therapy, and hormone therapy. Each treatment has potential side effects, including impotence and incontinence; the survival rate, however, is excellent.

General H. Norman Schwarzkopf and actors Sidney Poitier and Jerry Lewis are among the men in public life who have spoken openly about the impact prostate cancer has had on their lives; they have urged other men age fifty and older to have a digital rectal exam of the prostate as part of an annual checkup. The American Cancer Society also advises men in this age group to have a blood test, called the prostate-specific antigen test, to determine the level of a normal protein that rises abnormally in men with prostate cancer. While most men are advised to have these tests starting at age fifty, it may be prudent for black males and those with family history of the disease to start these tests at age forty. Since prostate cancer often has no early-warning signs, early diagnostic testing can be critical. Every year, thousands of men die needlessly from the disease, says the American Cancer Society, in part because they are too embarrassed to have these tests, which can spot the disease soon enough for a wide variety of lifesaving treatments.

HOW EXERCISE HELPS

The cause of prostate cancer is unknown, but research suggests it's linked to a combination of hormonal, genetic, and environmental factors. The incidence of prostate cancer has increased in recent years, in part because it's typically a disease of older men and the population is aging. Some studies also suggest that this increase reflects unhealthy lifestyle factors, such as a high-fat diet and sedentary lifestyle. Countries with low-fat diets have lower prostate cancer rates than junk-food havens like the United States, and the American Cancer Society says that men who eat high-fat diets, particularly diets high in saturated fats, are at greater risk of prostate cancer.

Inactivity also may increase a man's risk of the disease. A Harvard University study of more than seventeen thousand men found that those who burned 4,000 or more calories a week in activities such as stair climbing and walking had a prostate cancer risk that was 47 to 88 percent lower than men who burned less than 1,000 calories a week. A Norwegian study reported that the risk of prostate cancer was reduced by more than half in men who walked during their work hours and also engaged in regular leisure-time exercise. But this protection was noted only in men over age sixty.

The specific mechanisms by which exercise may exert a protective effect aren't clear. Theories point to physical activity's effect on hormones, immunity, body composition, and psychological well-being. (See Cancer Answers: The Activity Connection for Prevention, page 169.) For people with cancer, exercise can provide numerous benefits, including increases in energy, appetite, endurance, and self-esteem and reductions in weight loss, pain, depression, and fatigue. More active men may tolerate anticancer therapies better than their less fit counterparts. In addition, men who become incontinent as a result of prostate surgery may eliminate or minimize urine leakage by doing special exercises for the muscles of the pelvic floor, called Kegels. (See Healing Moves for Men, page 236.)

No one knows precisely how much exercise is necessary or optimal to help prevent the disease. For now, most experts say that the best guideline is the surgeon general's exercise prescription for improved overall health: *Perform a modest amount of moderate exercise (enough to burn 150 calories) on most days of the week—for example, 30 minutes of walking, 20 minutes of jogging, or 45 minutes of gardening.*

This amount of exercise may also help prevent the common, noncancerous condition in older men called prostate enlargement or benign prostatic hypertrophy (BPH). A survey of more than thirty thousand men, reported in the *Archives of Internal Medicine,* revealed that three hours of walking per week was sufficient to reduce the risk of BPH by about 10 percent. Couch potatoes beware: The researchers also found that the incidence of BPH increases with the number of hours of television watched per week.

GUT ISSUES

Jelly belly, spare tire, beer gut, love handles. By any name, abdominal fat carries serious health risks not associated with extra pounds stored elsewhere. Over the past decade, it's become increasingly clear that where the body stores its fat determines how risky that excess weight is. People with fat distributed in the upper body are more likely to have higher cholesterol levels, high blood pressure, and high blood sugar and are more likely to die of cardiovascular disease at an earlier age than individuals who are the same age and weight but have fat distributed in the lower body.

Humans tend to store fat in one of two patterns:

 * An apple shape with fat in the abdomen and upper body
 * A pear shape with fat in the buttocks, thighs, and lower body

Men are more likely to be apple-shaped, women are more likely to be pears. However, these fat-distribution patterns can occur in either sex. An apple shape—the typical male-pattern obesity—is associated with greater disease risk in both sexes.

No one is exactly sure why potbellies are more hazardous than thunder thighs. But scientists do know that fat isn't just an inert mass. It can affect your hormone levels, your reaction to insulin, and your cholesterol metabolism. Abdominal fat is more active, more hormonally sensitive, and more metabolically responsive than lower-body fat.

To determine if you're at risk from excess upper-body fat, take a tape measure around your waist at your belly button and divide it by your hip measurement to determine your waist-to-hip ratio (WHR). Many experts recommend that men strive for a WHR that is equal to or less than .9, while women target a WHR that is equal to or less than .80.

Where your body stores excess fat is determined largely by gender and heredity, although smoking appears to have some effect. Smokers tend to have more upper-body obesity than nonsmokers, possibly from the influence smoking has on hormones.

Not all potbellies come from excess fat. Medical problems such as tumors, bowel obstruction, liver disease, and enlarged organs can cause a belly bulge, as can poor posture and weak abdominal muscles. Sometimes just correcting posture will decrease the size of a potbelly.

Whether love handles carry the same health risk as a beer belly is the subject of some controversy. The "grab of flab" on the sides of your waist that gives your Valentine more of you to love, "love handles" are not found in any anatomy text. But they're a familiar sight around countless American middles—especially those of middle-aged men. The average American male picks up five to ten pounds between his twenty-fifth and thirty-fifth birthdays, according to the Centers for Disease Prevention and Control. Some experts feel that if these pounds are distributed on the sides of a man's waist, the problem is largely cosmetic. Fat here is "superficial," they contend, and doesn't really count from a health point of view. Genetics can play such a strong role that even men who exercise and eat right may still have little love handles and be perfectly fit.

Other experts contend that flank flab is as bad as belly bulge. Research at the University of Texas Southwest Medical Center in Dallas indicates that people who have abdominal obesity, even if it's located on the sides of the body, are still at greater health risk. The more abdominal fat there is, the greater the risk.

Most experts agree that the major health culprit is visceral, or deep body, fat. Since men tend to store fat from the inside out, fat outside may be a sign of excess fat inside. How much is too much? Unscientific tests include the "blubber fold"—if there's an obvious fold in the excess fat, it's in your best health interests to lose some weight. Another is the "pinch an inch"—if you can pinch more than an inch, your love handles are too thick.

Internist Michael Hamilton, director of the Duke University Diet and Fitness Center in Durham, North Carolina, offers this more scientific indicator: Measure your abdomen at the natural indentation of your waist, as seen from behind. In general, if the abdominal circumference is greater than forty inches in men (or thirty-five inches in women), there is a good chance you have significant visceral fat, which puts you at greater health risk.

It's not necessary (or even, for some people, possible) to totally deflate a spare tire to boost health. For people who are obese, even small weight losses of 5 to 10 percent of body fat can reduce their health risks. The best way to lose fat and keep it off is by eating healthy portions of a nutritious diet and exercising regularly. A key reason why many people gain weight in midlife is that they become less active and burn fewer calories each day, while continuing to eat the same amount. Also, after age twenty-five, people who don't exercise lose muscle mass at the rate of about one pound of muscle every two years. Since muscle tissue is one of the most metabolically active tissues in the body, as you lose muscle mass, you burn fewer calories throughout the day. (See Healing Moves to Regulate Metabolism, page 77.)

This decline can be slowed or stopped by strength-training exercises, which build muscles and rev up the metabolic rate so that your body burns a higher percentage of fat during activity and also at rest. Aerobic exercise, such as walking or running, is also essential for burning calories and reducing excess fat. When you burn more calories than you consume, your body decides where it will reduce fat stores. If you want to lose fat, be sure to:

✳ Burn about 250 to 500 calories on most days of the week through aerobic activities such as walking or jogging.

✳ Do strengthening exercises two to three times a week to build muscles and boost your metabolic rate.

✳ Eat sensible portions from a well-balanced diet with emphasis on fruits, vegetables, and grains. Be sure you eat enough to fuel your body (at least 2,100 calories per day for a man and 1,800 for a woman), since about half of the weight lost on extremely low-calorie diets isn't from fat but from muscle and bone.

✳ Reduce your intake of fats so they make up less than 30 percent of your diet.

✳ Be as active as you can throughout the day. If you expend just 10 extra calories a day, over the course of a year you'll lose a pound of fat.

✳ Remember that one pound of fat equals 3,500 calories. If you burn 150 calories a day more than you have in the past and don't eat more, over a year you'll lose 10 pounds. If you also eat 150 calories less (half a candy bar), that's an additional 10 pounds.

✳ Be aware that it's impossible to "spot-reduce." Exercise gadgets that profess to "whittle waists" or take fat from any specific spot on your body are all scams.

The healthiest and most balanced weight-loss strategy focuses on embracing appropriate behaviors while avoiding obsession—and self-loathing—about appearance. It's very common in our society to hate those love handles. They're the area most frequently targeted by men who opt for liposuction, notes the American Society of Plastic and Reconstructive Surgeons. But getting depressed and obsessed about weight can be counterproductive if your goal is optimum health, since stress and low self-esteem can contribute to ill health in a variety of ways, from suppressing immunity to actually prompting unhealthy habits like overeating and drinking. Try this reality check to determine what you can and can't control about your appearance: Look at other males in your family and see how they're shaped. Your genetic blueprint is likely to follow this pattern. If you're exercising regularly and eating well and still have half an inch you want to get rid of, you may be striving for perfection instead of reality. Keep eating right and exercising to build the healthiest body you can, and learn to love every inch of it.

The Skinny on Beefing Up

In our overweight society, skinny people are uniquely subject to ridicule. For those who are self-conscious about their "stick legs" or "scrawny arms," the struggle to gain weight can be just as frustrating as the more common battle to lose pounds.

Typically, the desire to "bulk up" is a guy thing. A large majority of those who want to gain weight are males, ranging from adolescents to men in their early forties. For most of these people, being skinny isn't a health hazard but a cosmetic issue. However, people with illnesses that can lead to weight loss—such as AIDS or cancer—may also struggle to put on pounds, which can dramatically benefit their health. People with a chronic illness, or those who have begun to lose weight without explanation, should consult a physician before embarking on a program to gain weight.

For most "underweights," the healthy way to flesh out a skinny frame is to add pounds that are mostly muscle, not fat. Athletes are notorious for trying to bulk up by devouring high-fat, high-protein diets that include huge portions of meat and up to a dozen raw eggs. For most of us, these practices can be dangerous. Eating raw eggs may lead to salmonella poisoning, and doesn't promote lean-tissue growth. Building muscle requires energy, both in calories consumed and exercise required. Most calories, about 60 percent of the diet, should come from carbohydrates, such as fruits, vegetables, breads, and grains. About 15 percent of calories should come from protein, and the rest, about 25 percent, should come from fat.

Popular high-protein diets actually deplete glycogen, the body's storage form of carbohydrate. Once available glycogen stores are emptied, the body starts burning protein from tissues (including muscle tissue) to meet its demand for energy. You lose hard-earned muscle as a result.

Seattle sports nutritionist Susan M. Kleiner offers these formulas for active, exercising people who want to build muscle:

Total calories: Men should consume 24 to 27 calories per pound of body weight, per day. This means a 150-pound man would need to consume about 4,050 calories per day. Women should consume 20 to 22 calories per pound of body weight.

Protein: Consume .6 to .8 grams of protein per pound of body weight per day. This is about twice as much as the recommended dietary allowance, but still less than the amount most Americans consume.

Carbohydrates: Consume 4 to 5 grams per pound of body weight.

Fluid: Drink a quart of fluid for every 1,000 calories of food you eat. Go into your workouts well hydrated by drinking two cups of fluid two hours before exercise, four to eight ounces every fifteen to twenty minutes during exercise, and sixteen ounces after exercise.

Nutrients are the "construction materials" for muscle building. Strength-training exercises are also essential to gain weight that is mostly lean tissue and not fat. To build muscle, you must work your body against resistance—such as lifting weights or using a strength-training machine. The American College of Sports Medicine recommends doing one set each of eight to ten exercises that strengthen the major muscle groups, two to three days a week. Most people should pick a weight that they can lift at least eight but no more than twelve times. Older and more frail people may want to choose a lighter weight that they can lift at least ten but no more than fifteen times. While one set of each exercise is sufficient to boost strength, three sets of each exercise may provide even greater benefits. (See Healing Moves to Strengthen Muscles and Bones, page 138.)

Brookline, Massachusetts, sports nutritionist Nancy Clark offers this advice for people who want to gain weight healthfully:

1. Eat consistently. Each day, have three hearty meals plus one to three snacks, such as a bedtime peanut butter sandwich with a glass of milk.
2. Eat larger-than-normal portions. Take extra helpings, choose a taller glass of milk, bigger bowl of cereal, and larger piece of fruit.

3. Select higher-calorie foods. Pick cranberry juice over orange juice (170 calories versus 110 calories), granola over Cheerios (700 versus 100 calories), corn over green beans (140 versus 40 calories).
4. Drink lots of juice and milk. Instead of "no-calorie" water, quench your thirst with calorie-laden beverages such as cranberry-apple, grape, or pineapple juice. Boost the caloric value of milk by mixing in malt powder, Ovaltine, Carnation Instant Breakfast, or other flavorings.

As for supplements, both nutritionists say: Food first.

"Your body can get almost all the nutrients it needs from a balanced diet," says Kleiner. "What's more, your body absorbs nutrients best from food." If you want "insurance," she advises a daily antioxidant multiple containing 100 percent of the daily values for vitamins and minerals.

Many supplements are expensive forms of nutrients readily available from food, say Kleiner and Clark, who offer these recipes for homemade "muscle builders":

Kleiner's muscle-building formula: 8 ounces nonfat milk, 1 packet Carnation Instant Breakfast, 1 banana, 1 tablespoon peanut butter. Blend until smooth. One serving contains 438 calories, 70 grams carbohydrate, 17 grams protein, 10 grams fat.

Clark's protein shake: ¼ cake silken tofu, ¼ cup dried milk powder, 1 cup low-fat milk, 2 tablespoons chocolate milk mix. Blend until smooth. Total calories 348; 52 grams carbohydrate, 26 grams protein, 4 grams fat.

PRESCRIPTION PAD

✳ *Exercise ℞ for better sex.* Exercise at a level you enjoy—either moderately or vigorously—for 30 to 60 minutes, three to six times a week. Be sure that at least three of these sessions include 30 minutes of aerobic exercises and at least two include resistance exercises to strengthen muscles. Stretch after each exercise session to enhance flexibility and avoid injury.

✳ *Exercise ℞ for cancer prevention:* Perform a modest amount of moderate exercise (enough to burn 150 calories) on most days of the week—for example, 30 minutes of walking, 20 minutes of jogging, or 45 minutes of gardening

✳ *Exercise ℞ to deflate a potbelly:* Burn 250 to 500 calories most days of the week, through aerobic activity such as walking or jogging. In addition, build muscles and boost metabolism by doing strengthening exercises two or three times a week.

✳ *Exercise ℞ to beef up:* Build muscles by doing strength-training exercises two or three days a week. Eat three hearty meals plus one to three snacks each day, choosing nutritious, wholesome foods.

ADDITIONAL RESOURCES

✳ *National Kidney and Urologic Diseases Information Clearinghouse,* 3 Information Way, Bethesda, Md. 20892-3580; Web site www.healthfinder.gov.

✳ *Impotence Information Center,* P.O. Box 9, Minneapolis, Minn. 55440; 800-843-4315.

✳ *Sexual Function Health Council, American Foundation for Urologic Disease,* 300

West Pratt St., Suite 401, Baltimore, Md. 21201; 800-242-2383.

✳ *Man-to-Man, the American Cancer Society*, 1599 Clifton Road, NE, Atlanta, GA 30329-4251; 800-ACS-2345; www.cancer.org.

✳ *National Cancer Institute*, National Institutes of Health, Bethesda, Md. 20892, 800-4-CANCER; www.icic.nci.gor/nci-icic.html.

✳ *Nancy Clark's Sports Nutrition Guidebook*, by Nancy Clark (Human Kinetics, 1996).

✳ *Power Eating*, by Susan M. Kleiner (Human Kinetics, 1998).

✳ ✳ ✳

HEALING MOVES FOR MEN

✳

Back in the days before spandex and aerobics, when there were no health clubs or high-tech exercise machines, men who wanted to get fit did calisthenics. Staples of the military and sports teams, these basic conditioning exercises (pull-ups, push-ups, and the like) were considered the best way to get strong and fit. In fact, the popularity of the Royal Canadian Air Forces' calisthenics program in the late 1950s helped launch the modern fitness movement.

Today these low-tech, low- (or no-) cost basic training tools are experiencing a renaissance—as evidenced by the popularity of "boot camp" workouts. In our program, you won't have a drill sergeant barking "Suck it up, maggot" in your ear. But you will have these time-tested techniques that can help you get maximum fitness in minimum time:

Part One: Aerobic Action

For cardiovascular fitness, weight maintenance, and stress reduction, it's important to do an aerobic activity you like and will commit to doing for 30 to 60 minutes three to six days a week. We suggest running, which is the most time-efficient way to achieve cardiometabolic fitness, and offer *a step-by-step plan to becoming a runner*. If running doesn't appeal to you, we also offer advice on other aerobic options, including in-line skating and jumping rope.

Part Two: Basic Training

This set of six classic calisthenics uses your own body weight to provide the resistance needed to strengthen muscles. They should be done at least twice a week. Paired with the six flexibility exercises in Part Three, they make a great "daily dozen" for musculoskeletal fitness.

Part Three: Flexibility

Strengthening without stretching can actually decrease flexibility and lead to injury. These six yoga-inspired stretches are best done after warming up at the beginning of a workout and again at the end of a workout.

Part Four: Relaxation/Moving Meditation

Designed to relieve stress and increase vitality, these restorative exercises can be integrated into your day—while you're on the telephone, for example, or when waiting in line. We also offer several "mind game" exercises to help you overcome sports performance anxiety and play your best.

Part Five: Kegels for Guys (Optional)

It's not something many guys talk about, but 20 percent of men over age sixty suffer from urinary incontinence, frequently related to prostate problems. We offer a man's version of Kegel exercises (named after the physician who developed them for women), which strengthen the muscles of the pelvic floor and help eliminate or minimize leakage.

Feel free to mix and match these elements to suit your goals, preferences, and time. Here are four options:

✳ **The Least You Can Do:** Time-crunched, but want to get fit? Run (or do another aerobic activity) Monday, Wednesday, and Friday for 30 minutes. Stretch for five minutes at the end of your run. Do the "daily dozen" of six strengthening and six stretching exercises on Tuesday and Thursday. Integrate relaxation moves and Kegels into your day. Total time: 20 to 35 minutes, five days a week.

✳ **Optimum Weight Loss.** Do an aerobic activity five to six days a week for 45 minutes to an hour, being sure to cross-train if your primary activity is high impact and your joints can't take daily pounding. (For example, run Monday, Wednesday, and Friday and swim or in-line skate Tuesday and Thursday.) Do the "daily dozen" of six strengthening and six stretching exercises two or three days a week (pick the days you do aerobics for just 45 minutes) and integrate relaxation moves and Kegels into your day. Stretch at the beginning of each workout (after warming up), and at the end of each workout. Total time: one hour, five to six days a week.

✳ **Sportsman's Weekly Workout.** If you play a sport, avoid the common mistake of trying to use your sport to get fit. Instead, you've got to *get fit to play your sport.* Otherwise, you're setting yourself up for injury. Fit your sport into your weekly workout schedule. For example, if you play basketball on Wednesday nights and volleyball on Sunday afternoons, warm up and stretch before each of those activities. Do your aerobic activity on three other days, say Tuesday, Thursday, and Saturday, and your "daily dozen" of six stretches and six strengtheners on Monday and Friday. If you want to have a rest day, combine your aerobic and daily dozen workouts so that you run for 30 minutes and do 15 to 20 minutes of stretching and strengthening on Tuesday, Thursday, and Saturday. Then you're off on Monday and Friday—good days to do light activity like walking, shooting hoops, or gardening.

✳ **Daily Dozen.** Combine the six strengthening exercises (Part Two) with the six stretching exercises (Part One) to form a "daily dozen" that you do five or six days a week. Run or do another aerobic activity of your choice for 30 minutes, three or four days a week, for a well-balanced, total fitness routine. Time: 30 minutes three days a week and 60 minutes the other three or four days a week.

PART ONE: AEROBIC ACTION

We recommend running because it's simple to do and extremely effective. But if you don't like to run, no problem. *The best aerobic exercise for you is the one you like and you'll do regularly.* So take your pick from this list of other popular options: walking, swimming, in-line skating, jumping rope, cross-country skiing, rowing, and cycling. Depending on how you do them, some racquet sports and martial arts may also be aerobic—as long as you're moving continuously.

Walking is an excellent choice and the most popular physical activity in the nation because it's easy, effective, enjoyable, economical and empowering. We present instruction on starting a walking program in Healing Moves for Heart Health (page 214).

If you're crunched for time (and who isn't?), running offers many advantages. Like walking, all you need to do is lace up a good pair of shoes and step out your door. But when you run, it takes less time to achieve similar results. For example, a 175-pound adult burns about 180 calories in a half-hour walk and 400 calories in a half-hour run. Plus, the fitness benefits of walking vary depending on whether you're strolling casually or marching briskly. *Running—even at a slow pace—is guaranteed to be a vigorous activity, with all the corresponding cardiovascular and metabolic benefits—and some risks.* If you work up to running for 30 minutes three to four times a week, you will become fit. Before you start any program of vigorous activity,

such as running, you should consult your doctor if you're a sedentary male over forty or female over fifty (or younger person with risk factors for heart disease such as smoking or obesity). People with joint problems may be advised to avoid running completely or to alternate running with a low-impact sport like swimming to give the body time to repair. (See Pre-Participation Checklist, page 29.)

While running isn't for everyone, it's the preferred activity for an estimated eight million Americans—including three of the last four presidents. The old "faster-is-better" mentality that characterized the early days of the running boom is gone. Today's runners have a kinder, gentler approach, with less emphasis on competition and more focus on health, stress reduction, and fitness. More runners are over forty, and increasing numbers are entering races, joining clubs, and getting coaching to help them reach varied goals, from starting a running program to finishing a marathon. (For referral to area running clubs and coaches, contact the Road Runners Club of America, 1150 S. Washington St., Suite 250, Alexandria, Va. 22314; 703-836-0558; Web site: www.rrca.org.)

The biggest pitfall for beginners is trying to do too much too soon. Don't expect to be a runner in one week. If you start slowly and progress gradually, you could be running in six to ten weeks. But if you push too hard, too fast, you're more likely to be set back by injury.

Here's our six-step plan to get you up and running:

1. *Be able to walk briskly for 30 minutes.* (If you're unable to do this, follow the walk-

ing program in Healing Moves for Heart Health, page 214. When you've been walking for at least 30 minutes, three to six days a week, for at least three months, you may proceed to step 2.)

2. *Get a good pair of running shoes.* Shop at a reputable athletic shoe store, in the afternoon, when your feet are largest. Wear athletic socks and be sure that when you stand up there is "wiggle room" about the width of your thumbnail between the end of the toebox and the tip of your longest toe on your longer foot. (It's not uncommon to wear an athletic shoe that is *a full size larger* than your street shoe.) Make sure the heel fits snugly and doesn't rub or slip. The shoes should feel good the day you buy them, without a "break-in" period.

3. *Commit yourself to doing 30 minutes of continuous training three to six days a week.* Schedule your run into your day—first thing in the morning, at lunch, after work—whenever's most convenient and appealing. Decide where you'll run. A track is a good place to start. If there's not a convenient track or the idea of going in circles seems dull, look for a relatively flat route with a good surface such as dirt or asphalt (avoid concrete).

4. *Start slowly.* At first, you will walk for most of your 30-minute session, and that's fine. In fact, the *best approach is to start slowly and be sure that you're never working so hard that you can't carry on a conversation.* Walk for at least the first five minutes, stretch gently, and when you feel ready, jog slowly until you feel out of breath—even if you've jogged for as little as 30 seconds. Then walk some

more until you feel ready to jog again. Continue this walk-jog cycle for the full 30 minutes, being sure to cool down with a walk during the last five minutes. Be sure you jog with a smooth, heel-to-toe motion, letting your shoulders and hands stay relaxed and your arms move freely.

5. *Progress gradually.* Each time you go out for your run, jog more and walk less. But avoid the temptation to run too hard. Labored breathing and a pounding heart are signs you're overdoing it. For the best indicator of the proper intensity, check your heart rate by taking your pulse manually or with a heart rate monitor. Your goal is to get your heart rate up to 60 to 90 percent of your maximum heart rate, which is called your "training zone." To find your training zone, first calculate your maximum heart rate by subtracting your age from 220. Then multiply that number by .6 to get your lower-limit heart rate and by .9 to get your upper-limit heart rate. (For example, if you're forty, subtract 40 from 220 to get 180. Multiply 180 by .6 to get 108 and by .9 to get 162. Your training zone is then 108 beats to 162 beats per minute.)

It's important that you exercise in your training zone to get the "training effect," a constellation of beneficial changes that occur in the lungs, heart, and vascular system in response to regular aerobic exercise. But if you find taking your pulse annoying or difficult, another way to be sure you're working in the zone is to use your personal perception of how hard you're working. Find a pace you consider "somewhat hard" to "hard," where you can feel that your heart rate has gone up some, but it's not racing. Your breathing should be accelerated, but you shouldn't be breathless or unable to talk with a running buddy. On a scale of 1 to 10 (with 1 being "very, very light" and 10 being "extremely hard"), about 4 to 7 is a desirable intensity range. If you're a beginning runner, you may want to start at the lower end of this range and gradually increase your intensity over time.

6. *Keep up the good work.* By the time you've been out there regularly for three months, you should be able to run for a full 30 minutes. Be sure you always warm up and cool down by walking for three to five minutes at the beginning and end of your run. If you like, stretch gently after your warm-up, but be sure you always stretch after your cooldown to lengthen your leg muscles, which can tighten with running. To minimize your risk of injury, avoid running hard two days in a row. Alternate hard and easy running days or cross-train by alternating running with low- or no-impact activities like swimming or in-line skating.

Alternate Aerobic Options

In-Line Skating: The hardest thing about in-line skating is the pavement you're bound to fall on, which is why protective gear is essential. While a few bruises are part of the learning curve, once you've got your "skate legs," falling is no longer inevitable. In-line skating is a terrific nonimpact aerobic activity that burns about 285 calories during a 30-minute skate, which is comparable to swimming and cycling. To skate safely, be sure you:

✳ Always wear a helmet, wrist guards, and knee and elbow pads.

✳ Take a lesson. Some health clubs feature classes, and skate shops often offer clinics for beginners. Or call the International In-Line Skating Association at 800-56-SKATE for referral to a certified instructor.

✳ Learn the basics of gliding, turning, and stopping in a traffic- and obstacle-free zone that is flat and clear of debris and cracks, such as an indoor rink, a tennis court, or empty parking lot.

✳ Be sure to keep your knees bent, so your weight is over your skates. Bend forward slightly from the waist and keep your hands in front of you. Pretend you're holding a hockey stick to get a feel for the correct posture.

✳ Head for grass, if possible, if you feel like you're going to fall. When gravity grabs, go forward onto your pads, not backward onto your unprotected tailbone.

Lapping It Up. One of the main attractions of lap swimming is its Zen of quiet meditative tranquillity—back and forth, back and forth—that lets the mind float off to peaceful levels of creativity and well-being. Released from 90 percent of your body weight, you're likely to find water activity uniquely calming and refreshing. Plus, swimming involves all the major muscle groups in the body and gives an excellent all-around conditioning effect. It's one of the few aerobic activities that cool you down while boosting your heart rate. To get the most from fitness swimming, be sure to begin with a warm-up—bobbing and moving easily in the water. Then try challenging yourself with a variety of workouts such as:

✳ **Medleys.** Swim one length of each stroke you know.

✳ **Intervals.** Swim one or two fast lengths, then one slow length.

✳ **Beat the clock.** Use a waterproof watch or pool clock to calculate how long it takes you to swim one length. Then try to swim it faster.

✳ **Pyramids.** Attempt a long swim, say thirty-six lengths, by swimming one length, then resting, then swimming two lengths, then resting, three lengths, resting, four lengths, resting, five lengths, resting, six lengths, resting, then working your way back down to one length. The decreasing numbers will give you a psychological edge for finishing.

Jump for Joy. One of the world's best exercise devices costs less than $15, fits into your briefcase, and is easy enough for a child to use. In fact, jump ropes have long been considered "kid stuff"—but that's changing. Professional athletes in a variety of sports, particularly tennis and basketball, are adding jumping rope to their training for the same reason boxers have "skipped it" for years. An unparalleled all-around workout, rope jumping strengthens the heart, muscles, and bones; promotes leanness; and improves agility, coordination, timing, rhythm, and explosive power on both sides of the body.

An extremely versatile sport that the whole family can do, jumping rope burns about 200 calories in fifteen minutes—with some variation depending on how fast you go and how much you weigh. Despite concerns that jumping rope is hard on the joints, it's easier on the knees and hips than running, since you land on the balls of your feet, so that the calves and shins absorb and control the impact. It's also a great travel workout, since a rope takes up little room in your suitcase.

Although jumping rope is child's play, active people unaccustomed to repeated jumping may find it difficult at first. But with practice, anyone can jump rope. Try these tips:

1. Be sure your rope is the right length. When you step in the center, the handles should just reach your armpits.
2. Wear a good pair of aerobic or cross-training shoes.
3. Jump to music that has 120 to 135 beats per minute.
4. Avoid concrete or hard tiles and jump on wooden floors, rubber tiles, or low-nap carpeting.
5. Keep your shoulders relaxed and your elbows in close to your body. Turn the rope with your wrists, not your arms.
6. Don't jump too high—unless you're doing tricks.
7. Warm up with 5 to 10 minutes of light activity, then stretch gently before jumping.
8. Start by alternating brief periods of jumping with resting moves, such as turning the rope alongside your body without jumping. Over time, do fewer resting moves and more jumping. Your goal is to jump continuously for at least 15 minutes.

Pedal Pushing. Bicycling offers an excellent, nonimpact cardiovascular workout. But a controversy over whether it can cause impotence has some men riding uneasy. The August 1997 issue of *Bicycling* magazine detailed the possible connection, and as a result there's been a boom in newly designed saddles that are friendlier to a man's essentials than the old-style, small, hard saddles. Since about a third of a cyclist's body weight rests on a few inches of tender flesh, many pedal pushers experience a host of "bottom-line" ailments ranging from saddle sores to genital numbness and, for some men, impotence. To minimize problems:

✳ Defend against saddle sores by wearing a clean, padded pair of bike shorts. Nothing should come between you and your shorts, since cotton or nylon underwear can act like fine sandpaper, irritating skin and trapping moisture against the body.

✳ Lubricate areas of friction with petroleum jelly.

✳ After your ride, avoid the temptation to scrub the area with alcohol, which will only dry out the skin and irritate it further. Instead, wash with tender loving care and a gentle soap. Apply talcum powder to clean dry skin after riding, but not before, since sweat can turn it into a white, sticky mess.

✳ Get immediate medical attention if you experience a "straddle injury"; any injury to the body between the legs can affect blood flow to the penis.

✳ Consider an ergonomic saddle if you experience numbness, tingling, or erectile difficulties after cycling.

PART TWO: BASIC TRAINING

You don't need fancy equipment or lots of money to get in top physical condition. These six classic calisthenics use your own body weight to provide the resistance necessary to strengthen muscles. Be sure to warm up for a few minutes first by walking in place or doing easy motions (big arm circles, light jumping jacks, easy trunk twists).

1. Push-ups (Strengthens Shoulders, Chest, and Arms)

Position yourself on the floor with your weight on your hands and knees. Be sure your palms are flat on the floor, slightly wider than shoulder width apart, fingers pointed straight ahead. With your feet together, raise your knees off the floor, so that your body is in a straight line and your weight is resting evenly on your palms and toes. Bend your elbows and bring three points on your body toward the ground at the same time: nose, nipples, and navel. Lower yourself until you're about a fist's distance from the floor, then push yourself back up to the starting position. Inhale down, exhale up. Or, to make sure you don't hold your breath, count each repetition aloud as you push back up. Repeat 10 to 20 times.

(If you are unable to do this exercise with good technique, do modified push-ups with your knees on the ground. When you build the upper-body strength to do 20 modified push-ups easily, try the regular push-ups. Illustrations of both positions are on page 145.)

Variation 1: Triangle for triceps. Place your palms on the floor so that your thumbs and index fingers touch to form a triangle. If you like, spread your feet about hip width apart. Push up 10 to 20 times.

Variation 2: One hand. Place one palm on the floor below your chest and the other hand behind your back. Spread your legs about hip width apart. Push up 10 to 20 times, then repeat with the other hand.

Variation 3: Knuckle. A favorite of martial artists, this variation helps toughen the first two knuckles of each hand, which are the striking point of punches. Make two tight fists and place them on the floor so that your weight is on the first two knuckles of each hand, palms facing in, feet together. Push up 10 to 20 times.

2. Sit-ups (Strengthens Abdominal Muscles)

Lie on your back with your knees bent and your feet flat on the floor. Cross your arms over your chest or place your fingertips behind your ears with your elbows out to the sides. Contract your abdominal muscles, press your lower back into the floor, and slowly curl up your upper back until your shoulder blades lift off the floor, then slowly lower back down. (If your fingertips are behind your ears, be sure you don't pull your head forward with your hands, since this could cause neck injury.) Repeat 10 to 20 times, exhaling as you curl up and inhaling as you release. (For an illustration, see page 146.)

To get the full definition of "washboard" abs (a.k.a. a "six-pack"), try these sit-up variations:

Side sit-ups. To work the obliques, the muscles on the sides of the abdomen, start in sit-up position and lower your knees gently to the right until the right leg touches the floor and the left leg rests on top of the right leg. Do 10 to 20 sit-ups from this position, then change sides and do 10 to 20 more.

Buns up. To work the lower abdominals, lie on your back and bring both hands under your tailbone, palms facing the floor. Lift your legs into the air, crossing them at the ankle. Use your abdominal muscles to raise your feet toward the ceiling, lifting your buttocks slightly off the ground. Repeat 10 to 20 times, being sure to use your muscles—not the momentum of the movement—to lift your legs.

Leg lowers (for advanced exercisers only). Lie on your back with your arms comfortably out to your sides, palms down. Bend your knees and bring your legs to your chest, then raise them above your head. Keeping your legs straight, slowly lower them to the ground—but don't touch the floor. Stop about one inch from the ground,

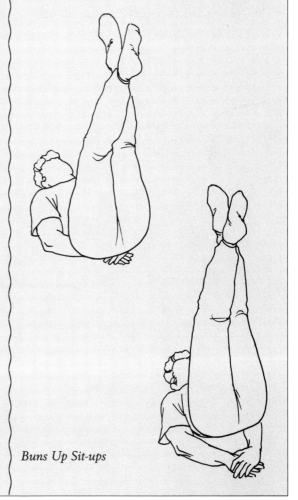

Buns Up Sit-ups

bend your knees to your chest, and repeat the whole sequence 10 times. The more slowly you lower your legs, the harder the ab workout. (If you have low-back pain, skip this exercise.)

3. Flying Bow (Strengthens Back, Legs, Abdominals and Shoulder Muscles)

Lie on the floor on your stomach, face downward, arms at your sides, palms up. Inhale, then exhale and lift your head, chest, legs, and arms off the floor as high as possible so that only your abdomen is on the floor. Be sure your buttock muscles are contracted. Breathe normally and gaze upward as you focus on stretching your legs and arms back. Stay in this position as long as you can, breathing comfortably, then rest. (If you have a weak lower back, leave your legs on the ground and lift only your head and shoulders. When you can do this, include the legs.)

Variation 1: Swan Dive. Perform the exercise with your arms out to the sides so that your body makes a T shape.

Variation 2: Superman. Perform the exercise with your arms out in front of you.

4. Dips (Works the Backs of the Arms)

Use a bench or any sturdy surface that is about two feet off the ground. Sit on the bench and place your hands at the edge of it, right beside your body with your fingers pointed forward. Stretch your legs out in front of you, knees slightly bent, and scoot forward to the edge of the bench. Pressing your palms against the bench, lift your bottom up and walk your heels forward so that your bottom is in front of the bench and your weight is resting on your palms and your heels. Bend your elbows to lower yourself down a few inches, then press back up, but don't lock the elbows. Repeat 10 to 20 times.

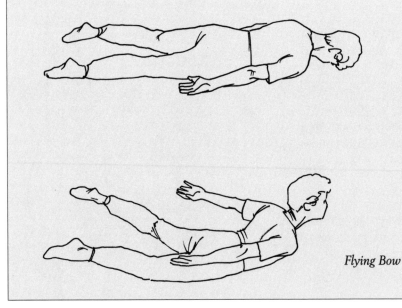

Flying Bow

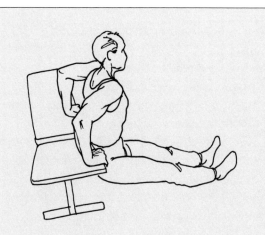

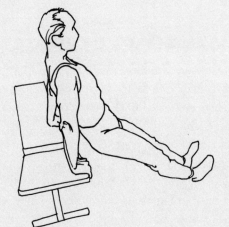

Dips

5. Pull-ups (Strengthens the Back, Shoulders, and Arms)

Install an inexpensive pull-up bar in a doorway, or use a pull-up bar at a playground or gym. The proper height will be low enough to reach but high enough so your legs don't quite touch the ground when you're holding on to the bar. Grab the bar with your arms spaced a little wider than your shoulders, palms facing away from you and thumb and fingers on the same side of the bar. Slightly

arch your back, look up, and pull yourself up until your chin is over the bar, then *slowly* lower yourself. Repeat as many times as you can. (If this is too hard, find a bar that is hip height. Grasp the bar so your hands are just

Pull-ups

outside your hips, palms toward you, and walk forward under the bar until it's even with your chest. With your knees bent, bend your elbows to pull your chest toward the bar, then lower.)

Variation 1: Reverse grip (a.k.a. chin-up) Perform exercise with palms facing toward you.

Variation 2: Close grip. Do pull-ups with your hands a fist's distance apart.

Variation 3: Wide grip. Do pull-ups with your arms out as wide as you can get them without discomfort.

6. Yoga Warrior Stance (Strengthens Legs)

Stand up straight and spread your legs wide. Turn your right foot out about ninety degrees and your left foot in about fifteen degrees. Your right heel should be in line with your left instep. Inhale, then exhale and bend your right knee until your right thigh is parallel to the floor, keeping your right shin perpendicular to the floor. Your right thigh and lower leg should form a right angle at the knee. Do not extend your knee beyond your ankle. Stretch your arms out as if two people were pulling you in opposite directions, palms down. (Your right arm should be over your right leg and left arm over your left leg.) Gaze at your right hand, and keep your torso vertical and your left leg straight. Hold this position for 20 to 30 seconds, breathing deeply. Then repeat on the other side. Work up to holding this position for at least one minute.

PART THREE: FLEXIBILITY

Stretching should be as relaxed and natural as a deep, satisfying yawn. Unfortunately, many men approach stretching with the same competitive mind-set they bring to sports. The idea isn't to get to some predetermined position—like touching your hands to your toes or your head to the floor. The idea is to focus on a muscle group and move your body to stretch that muscle to the point where you feel mild tension. Hold the stretch there for 5 to 10 seconds, breathing naturally and inviting your muscles to relax, then release. If it's painful, you're overstretching and need to back off.

Stretching will relieve muscle tension, boost circulation, and help prevent injury. When you stretch after exercise, it helps lengthen muscles that can get tight during activities such as running. When you stretch before exercise (after a gentle warm-up, like walking for a few minutes) it helps prepare your body for activity. When you stretch spontaneously throughout the day, it helps prevent stiffness.

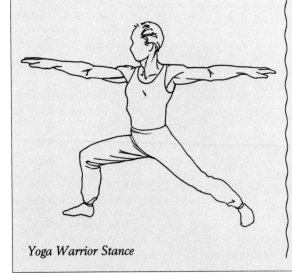

Yoga Warrior Stance

1. Wall Lean (Stretches Back of Legs)

Place both palms against a wall at about shoulder height and step away from the wall until your arms are fully extended with your palms flat against the wall. Bend your elbows and slowly bring your forehead toward the wall, being sure to keep both feet flat on the floor. Stop at the point where you feel mild tension and hold for 20 to 30 seconds, breathing naturally.

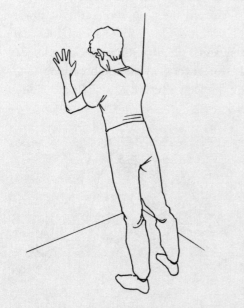

Wall Lean

2. Overhead Stretch (Stretches Triceps and Shoulders)

Stand tall, feet shoulder width apart. Raise your arms up over your head, then reach back so you hold your left elbow with your right hand. Gently pull your elbow behind your head until you feel mild tension in your shoulder or the back of your upper arm. Hold for 20 to 30 seconds, breathing naturally, then switch arms. (For an illustration, see page 45.)

3. Modified Hurdler (Stretches Hamstrings and Lower Back)

Sit on the floor with your legs out straight in front of you. Bend your right leg and place the sole of your right foot against the inside of your left thigh. Lean forward over your left leg and grab your toes, ankle, or shin as your flexibility permits. Keeping your spine straight, inhale, then exhale and bend your elbows as you gently pull yourself forward, focusing on bringing your lower rib cage to your left thigh. Hold for 20 to 30 seconds, breathing naturally, then repeat with the other leg.

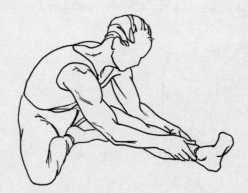

Modified Hurdler

4. Butterfly (Stretches Lower Back, Hip, and Groin)

Sit on the floor with your back straight and your legs in a "butterfly" position—knees bent and the soles of the feet touching. Grasp your feet and "flap your wings" by gently moving your knees up and down for a few seconds. Inhale, then exhale and bend forward from the waist, keeping your spine straight. Hold for 20 to 30 seconds, breathing naturally. (For an illustration, see page 47.)

5. Standing Spinal Twist (Stretches Back and Sides)

Stand with your hands on your hips, knees slightly bent. Inhale, then exhale and gently turn your body at the waist to the right, gazing over your right shoulder until you feel mild tension. Hold for 10 to 20 seconds, breathing naturally, then repeat on the other side.

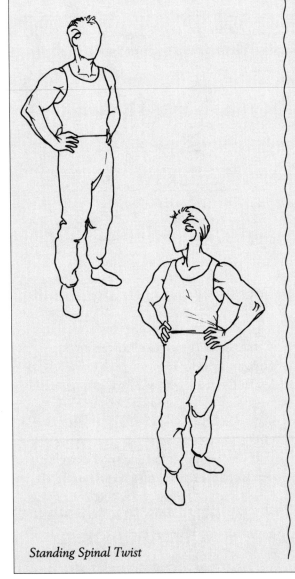

Standing Spinal Twist

6. Topsy Turvy (Stretches Shoulders, Legs, Arms, and Back)

Stand tall and step your feet out as wide as you can without discomfort, toes pointing forward, hands on hips. Inhale, then exhale and bend forward from the hips and touch the floor. (If you're flexible enough, let the top of your head touch the floor.) If this is easy, clasp your hands behind your back, straighten your arms, and let gravity pull your head down to the earth and your hands down toward the ground. Breathe naturally and let the muscles in the back of your legs soften and release without locking knees. Hold for several cycles of breathing, and enjoy the view. Return to standing, bending your knees.

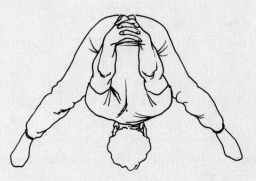

Topsy Turvy

PART FOUR:
RELAXATION/MOVING MEDITATION

This section is not about *doing*, but about *undoing* all the tension, pressures, and stress that build up in our lives. Those who think they can't take a few minutes to do some simple relaxation exercises are the ones who need them most. These practices can be integrated into your day—do them anytime and anyplace where you can take a few minutes to focus on your breathing.

1. Conscious Breathing

The essence of all relaxation and meditation techniques, a deep focused breath is one of the best things you can do to relieve tension and increase energy. The first step in learning the technique is to understand how to take a deep abdominal breath, as opposed to the common habit of taking a shallow, chest breath. To do this, lie on your back and place a book on your belly. Relax your stomach muscles and inhale deeply into your abdomen so that the book rises. When you exhale, the book should fall. You'll still be bringing air into your upper chest, but now you're are also bringing air down into the lower portion of your lungs and expanding your entire chest cavity.

Now sit up and place your right hand on your abdomen and your left hand on your chest. Breathe deeply so that your right, "abdominal" hand rises and falls with your breath, while your left, "chest" hand stays relatively still. Breathe in through your nose and out through your nose or mouth and spend a few minutes enjoying the sensation of abdominal breathing.

Place a timer or clock with a second hand in clear view. Breathe in slowly, filling your abdomen, as the timer counts off five seconds. Then breathe out slowly to the same count of five. Breathing in for five seconds and out for five seconds is an ideal pace that you can strive for whenever you want to relieve tension and increase energy. For example, take a conscious breath when:

✶ The phone rings. Before you pick it up, breathe deeply and smile.

✶ An angry or unkind remark is about to burst from your lips.

✶ You get stuck in traffic.

✶ You are about to make an important presentation.

✶ The boss calls you into his or her office.

✶ Your kids start fighting with each other.

You get the idea . . . (For more breathing exercises, see page 49.)

2. Qi Gong Internal Body Massage

Stand comfortably with your feet shoulder width apart and your shoulders relaxed. Place the backs of your hands on your lower back. Bend your knees so that you bounce gently up and down—but keep both feet flat on the floor. Let your shoulders and elbows relax completely so that your hands gently massage your back as you bounce. Exhale through your nose in little bursts as you bounce, until your lungs are empty, then inhale smoothly as you bounce. Repeat for five cycles of breathing.

3. Simply Standing

One of the best things you can do for your body is stand with good posture. Despite popular misconception, good posture isn't the "suck-in-the-gut-throw-out-the-chest" military stance. Proper body alignment should reflect a natural state of being centered and relaxed. To practice good posture be sure that you:

✶ Stand firmly on both feet, with shoulders and arms relaxed.

✶ Center your body, with your weight distributed evenly on both legs.

✶ Slightly tuck your pelvis, extend your

spine, and let your head float gently upward on your neck.

Whenever you find yourself standing—waiting in line, at a cocktail party—think about how you are standing. Is all your weight on one leg, back swayed, arms crossed? Take a conscious breath, plant both feet on the ground, and stand with good posture. Your body will thank you.

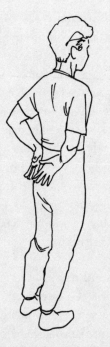

Qi Gong Internal Body Massage

4. Mind Games

Performance anxiety isn't limited to the bedroom. If you have a tendency to "choke" during a big presentation or important competition, try these mental relaxation techniques:

✳ Recognize that you're going to get nervous. Don't be worried about being worried.

✳ Focus on the task, not the outcome. Don't think about the trophy or the promotion; concentrate instead on the job at hand.

✳ "Rotten potato" unwanted thoughts. Treat negative notions like smelly potatoes and mentally throw them as far away as possible.

✳ Stick with self-affirming messages like "I've done all my homework, I can make it happen."

✳ Think about what you should do, not what you shouldn't do. For example, instead of thinking "Don't let my arms fly out" think "Keep elbows tucked in."

✳ Visualize success. Run a tape on the back of your eyelids where you see yourself accomplishing your goals.

✳ During competition, remain inwardly focused. Treat background noise like running tap water, and if it bothers you, turn off the tap.

✳ Remember that being nervous is not only natural, it helps release the adrenaline that can allow you to perform at a world-class level—if you channel it in a positive direction.

PART FIVE:
KEGELS FOR GUYS (OPTIONAL)

Many older men suffer from urinary incontinence, often related to an enlargement of the prostate gland from benign prostatic hypertrophy (BPH) or cancer. In many cases, behavioral techniques can help reduce or eliminate leakage. One of the most effective techniques is this easy exercise to strengthen the muscles of the pelvic floor:

1. Locate the pelvic floor muscles by standing naked in front of a mirror. Watch

your penis and try to make it move up and down without moving the rest of your body. If you can, you are using the right muscles. (If you have trouble isolating these muscles, ask your doctor for referral to a continence clinic, physical therapist, or biofeedback practitioner.)

2. Squeeze the pelvic floor muscles without tightening your abdominal muscles or buttocks. (Avoid the common mistake of straining or "bearing down," which does not isolate the right muscles. A properly done Kegel should feel like you're inwardly lifting and squeezing.) Squeeze the pelvic floor muscles as you count slowly to three, then relax them as you again count to three. Be sure to keep breathing! For the first two weeks, try to do 15 repetitions of "squeeze and relax," three times a day. Do one set of 15 while lying down, one set sitting, and one set standing.

3. Over the next ten weeks, work up to squeezing for 10 seconds, then relaxing for 10 seconds. Do 15 exercises at a time, three times a day, for a total of 45 exercises per day. Set a timer for 5 minutes (15 exercises × 20 seconds per exercise) or use an exercise diary if it's helpful.

4. Don't give up too soon. It takes about eight to ten weeks of exercising before you'll start to notice a difference.

5. Once your muscles become strong enough, you can do a maintenance program by fitting these exercises into your daily routine. Make it a habit to do Kegels while you're brushing your teeth, standing in line, sitting at a red light, or talking on the phone.

8

Women's Health

PREGNANCY

The Hebrew women are not as the Egyptian women; for they are lively, and are delivered ere the midwives come in unto them.
—*Exodus 1:19*

The idea that exercise benefits pregnant women and their babies is ancient. Back in biblical times, physically active Hebrew slave women gave birth more easily than did their less active Egyptian mistresses. In the third century B.C., Aristotle attributed difficulties in childbirth to a sedentary lifestyle.

Today, an emerging body of scientific data supports this long-standing notion that physical activity is good for the health of both mother and child. "Our studies show that women who exercise during pregnancy have shorter labors, gain less fat, require less medical intervention during delivery, and recover more quickly than pregnant women who were sedentary," says obstetrician-gynecologist James F. Clapp III of Case Western Reserve School of Medicine in Cleveland. After more than fifteen years of studying hundreds of exercising pregnant women and their children, he has found that "for most pregnant women, exercise has numerous physical and psychological benefits."

Yet during much of the last century, active pregnant women have been warned to cut back or stop their exercise entirely. Some of these cautions arose from societal mores regarding what was "seemly" during an expectant mother's "confinement." For example, a popular book of the Victorian era, the *Married Lady's Companion and Poor Man's Friend*, by Samuel Jennings, told readers: "It is common opinion that breeding women ought to live indolently and feast luxuriously as they are able, lest by exercise they should injure or by abstinence debilitate the unborn child."

In the 1930s, the respected guide *Modern Motherhood* offered this advice: "The expectant mother must, of necessity, curtail her usual physical activities because of her extra burden. She cannot exercise more than she is accustomed to; she should exercise less. She should not be persuaded to walk a lot [although] walking is supposed to make birth easier—this superstition is hundreds of years old and still prevalent."

These recommendations were unsubstantiated by any scientific data. In the 1970s and 1980s, however, some restrictions arose based on research done on pregnant animals. Concerned that exercise might divert blood flow toward the working muscles and away from the baby, scientists studied pregnant ewes and pygmy goats and found a link between intense exercise and fetal malformations. One study, reported in the 1980 *American Journal of Obstetrics and Gynecology*, found a 28 percent decrease in uterine blood flow in pregnant ewes during exhaustive exercise on a treadmill.

Although no such studies had been done on women and no cases of human fetal malformation from exercise had been documented, many physicians still feared that reduced blood flow could deprive the baby of oxygen and nutrients. As a result, they tended to be overly cautious and advised active women to limit their exercise to mild or moderate activity such as swimming and walking. Until 1994, the American College of Obstetrics and Gynecology (ACOG) was so concerned about the potential ill effects of intense exercise during pregnancy that it advised pregnant women to limit strenuous activities to no more than fifteen minutes in duration and to keep their heart rate to no more than 140 beats per minute.

But at a time when the fitness revolution had changed the lives of countless women, these limitations were anything but popular. Many women who relied on running, aerobics, and other intense activities for their physical and mental well-being felt these restrictions were unnecessary. Some simply ignored the advice and continued their workouts.

Olympic gold medalist Joan Benoit Samuelson, who won the first women's marathon in the 1984 Olympic Games in Los Angeles, continued to run enthusiastically throughout both her pregnancies, and bore healthy children three and five years after her Olympic victory. Under the guidance of fellow runner and sports medicine expert Joan Ullyot, M.D., Samuelson ran up until the day she gave birth. One of her best runs, a five-miler on snow-packed roads, occurred when she was "as pregnant as possible—for that evening I gave birth," she recalls in her book *Running for Women*.

Samuelson, however, was careful to follow two main, commonsense cautions: "not running to the point of breathlessness or getting overheated." Samuelson's experience highlights the general principle central to all of our exercise prescriptions: *Health is equilibrium. A person is healthy when his or her body is in balance and harmony. **Finding a comfortable balance between movement and rest** is crucial to using exercise to enhance health.*

An athletic woman accustomed to running twenty miles a week is likely to feel *unbalanced* and frustrated if forced to stop exercising vigorously when she becomes pregnant. Likewise, a totally sedentary woman would probably become upset and injured if she were instructed to begin intense activity during pregnancy. For this and other reasons, *exercise prescriptions during pregnancy must be individualized to take into account each woman's level of fitness as well as the specific conditions of her pregnancy.*

Especially during pregnancy, the extremes of exercise are to be avoided. Being completely sedentary (unless a complication necessitates bed rest) or pushing to exhaustion could both be unhealthy for mother and child.

This individualized approach to exercise during pregnancy received a boost in 1994, when ACOG lifted its heart-rate and intensity limits for women in low-risk pregnancies. In a "technical bulletin," ACOG acknowledged that "there are no data in humans to indicate that pregnant women should limit exercise intensity and lower target heart rates because of potential adverse effects." This new advice gave the green light to pregnant women without obstetric or medical complications to continue to exercise.

As a result, "active women sighed with relief," says Judy Mahle Lutter, president of the Melpomene Institute, a Minneapolis-based organization specializing in health issues affecting physically active women. For years, female athletes had been calling Melpomene for advice about exercise and pregnancy that they felt they weren't getting from their doctors.

"Many pregnant women had stopped dis-cussing their exercise with their obstetricians," Lutter says, "because they felt their doctors were being unnecessarily restrictive." As examples, she points to a bored and frustrated ultramarathoner who was told by her doctor to stop running because "running pounds the baby" and the unhappy aerobics instructor who was "tired of hearing about a maximum heart rate of 140 when you're pregnant."

ACOG's new recommendations allowed women to have honest discussions with their doctors about exercise. But even though most physicians today recognize the health benefits of exercise for women with uncomplicated pregnancies, Lutter says, "there are still mixed messages being given." Many physicians remain "overly cautious," she says, from concerns that strenuous exercise will harm the fetus.

One of the first studies to examine the effects of vigorous maternal exercise on humans found "no deficits" in the children. Case Western physician Clapp tested offspring of twenty women who ran, cross-country skied, or did aerobics at least three times a week for at least 30 minutes and compared them with the offspring of twenty women who only walked during pregnancy. After testing the children as newborns and retesting them five years later, Clapp found that children of the mothers who exercised vigorously were as healthy as or healthier than the controls.

The study, published in the December 1996 *Journal of Pediatrics*, noted that "the exercise offspring performed significantly better" on tests of intelligence and oral language skills. They were also leaner, although their heights and weights were well within the normal range. "It is not that the offspring of the exercising women are unduly lean at age 5 years," Clapp concluded, "rather that the offspring of the control subjects are a bit on the fat side."

The reasons for these differences are unclear, says Clapp, who suggests one factor may be that exercise stimulates growth of the placenta, making more nutrients available to the baby. Also, it's difficult to draw conclusions from research on such a small population, which is why Clapp is continuing to follow these children and is currently expanding on this research by studying 250 pregnant woman exercising at a variety of different intensities and comparing them with 250 controls. Clapp has also received a grant from the National Institutes of Health to examine how exercise may help prevent premature labor and low birth weight in populations at risk.

But while he is a firm believer in the benefits of exercise for most pregnant women, Clapp shies away from offering general guidelines for exercise during pregnancy. "This is a highly individualized matter that must take into account a variety of issues, such as the woman's past conditioning and the status of her pregnancy," he says. "One set of recommendations cannot be used for all women."

In general, advice about physical activity has become "more liberal, and physicians are more pro-exercise during most pregnancies," notes Philadelphia obstetrician-gynecologist Mona Shangold, who is preparing a patient-education pamphlet on exercise and pregnancy for the American College of Sports Medicine. Many physicians now encourage their pregnant patients to be active, since a good program of regular exercise can help relieve some of the common problems associated with pregnancy, such as excessive weight gain, swelling of the hands and feet, leg cramps, varicose veins, insomnia, fatigue, backache, and constipation. Plus, exercise helps improve mood, energy level, and self-image, and may reduce the risk of pregnancy complications such as gestational diabetes and pregnancy-induced hypertension.

"I tell my patients that it's better to become fit before they become pregnant," Shangold says. "But if they haven't already begun to exercise regularly, it's not too late to start."

EXERCISE R_x

An exercise program for pregnancy must recognize that virtually every bodily system will change over the course of nine months. Hormonal changes affect respiration, circulation, digestion, and even the musculoskeletal system. The heart adapts to its increased demands by increasing cardiac output, blood volume, and resting heart rate, which makes the conventional concept of exercising at a "target heart rate" unreliable during pregnancy. Ligaments become lax, which helps the pelvis widen for delivery, but also makes a pregnant woman's joints unstable and increases her risk of injury.

In addition to accommodating these physical changes, an exercise prescription for pregnancy should take into account two main factors:

1. *Prepregnancy fitness level.* Athletic women who have been training in an activ-

ity can generally continue in most sports, with some commonsense cautions. However, sedentary women who want to become active when pregnant are advised to stick with mild to moderate activities such as walking, swimming, and beginners' aerobics classes designed for pregnant women.

2. *The status of her pregnancy.* Certain medical or obstetric conditions can make exercise inadvisable. These include:

✳ Incompetent cervix

✳ Persistent second- or third-trimester bleeding

✳ Intrauterine growth retardation

✳ Preterm rupture of membranes

✳ Preterm labor during prior or current pregnancy or both

✳ Pregnancy-induced hypertension

Remember: If complications arise during pregnancy, an exercise program may need to be modified.

For these reasons, it's essential that each pregnant woman discuss her exercise plans with her doctor and get advice that is as individualized and specific as possible. An excellent screening tool to help physicians determine an appropriate exercise prescription is the *PARmed-X for Pregnancy*, developed by the Canadian Society for Exercise Physiology. (See Additional Resources at the end of this section.) The Canadian Academy of Sports Medicine (CASM) released a new position statement on exercise and pregnancy in 1998 because "previous advice has been too restrictive for most women," says obstetrician-gynecologist Julia Alleyne, medical director of the sports medicine clinic at Women's College Hospital in Toronto.

For *previously inactive women in low-risk pregnancies*, the CASM guidelines recommend:

✳ Wait to start a program of mild to moderate exercise until after the thirteenth week of pregnancy.

✳ Use perceived exertion as a guide to how hard to work out—stick with mild to moderate intensities and be sure you can talk while exercising.

For *already active women in low-risk pregnancies*, the guidelines advise:

✳ Continue to exercise at your accustomed level during the first trimester. If desired, it's okay to increase exercise slightly during the second trimester, but decrease the level slightly during the third trimester.

✳ Rely on perceived exertion to determine intensity. Trained women can push to a level they consider moderate to somewhat hard but should avoid working out so intensely that they become breathless.

✳ Women who have been training in most noncontact jumping or running sports may continue their activity as long as they proceed with caution.

All exercising pregnant women should:

✳ *Avoid high-risk sports* that could result in falls (downhill skiing, water skiing, and karate) and *activities that involve pressure changes* (scuba diving, mountain climbing).

✳ *Avoid lying on the back after the fourth month of pregnancy*, since the enlarged uterus may decrease the flow of blood returning from the lower half of the body as it presses on a major vein. Exercises normally done in the supine position, such as sit-ups, should be altered.

✳ *Avoid holding the breath while working against resistance* (the Valsalva maneuver), which can cause a decrease in blood pressure. Breathe continuously throughout exercise, being sure to exhale on exertion and inhale on release.

✳ *Be aware that postural changes and joint laxity may lead to injury.* Pay special attention to balance and avoid overstretching.

✳ *Avoid participating in highly competitive sporting events.*

✳ *Eat properly.* Pregnancy requires an additional 300 calories a day, so women who exercise (and burn even more calories) should be particularly careful to eat an adequate diet.

ELEMENTS OF GOOD PRENATAL EXERCISE PROGRAMS

Check with fitness centers, YMCAs and YWCAs, and community hospitals for exercise programs for pregnant women. Be sure the instructor is certified by a reputable organization such as the American College of Sports Medicine or the American Council on Exercise and has specialized training in prenatal exercise.

A good prenatal exercise program will have these components:

1. **A warm-up,** to slowly increase breathing and heart rates and to protect joints and muscles from injury.
2. **Cardiovascular conditioning exercises,** to build and maintain heart and lung capacity and endurance. Good choices for previously inactive women include walking, swimming, water aerobics, riding a stationary bicycle, and prenatal aerobics. Previously athletic women can continue in most activities they're accustomed to, such as jogging, golf, and tennis (be careful of balance and sudden stops). Avoid activities that have serious risks of falling, abdominal blows, or pressure changes.

   Water exercise, such as swimming and aqua-aerobics, is particularly well suited to pregnancy, since the buoyancy of the water places the muscles in a relaxed, non-weight-bearing position. This can make pregnant women feel more comfortable by reducing feelings of clumsiness and eliminating fear of falling.
3. **Muscle-strengthening exercises** to build and maintain strength. Easy exercises that use a women's body weight or use light resistance such as elastic tubing or dumbbells are the best choices for previously inactive women. Women who have been lifting weights regularly prior to pregnancy may continue as long as they **switch to lighter weights and avoid maximal lifting,** since relaxed ligaments make the joints more susceptible to injury. In general, weight machines are safer than free weights, since altered balance and posture can lead to injury.
4. **A cooldown** to ease the cardiovascular system back into its normal level.
5. **Relaxation techniques** to release muscular tension and stress.

Prenatal exercise classes may also include discussion periods to provide women with a supportive environment in which to air questions and concerns about their pregnancies.

MATERNAL MOVES

Certain body parts need special attention during pregnancy. In particular, the stresses caused by the expanding uterus make it important to strengthen the muscles of your back and pelvic floor. The special pregnancy exercises in Healing Moves for Women, page 279, can help.

CAUTIONS

Pregnant women who exercise should always be aware of the **Three Don'ts:**

1. **Don't get exhausted.** Listen to your body and exercise within a zone that feels good to you. "No pain, no gain" does *not* apply during pregnancy.
2. **Don't overheat.** Avoid exercising outdoors in hot, humid weather; wear comfortable, appropriate clothing; and stay out of saunas and hot tubs.
3. **Don't dehydrate.** As a rule of thumb, drink eight ounces of fluid both before and after exercise. You may also want to drink every 15 to 20 minutes during exercise. Water is fine, or you may choose a sports drink to maximize absorption and supply you and the baby with fluids, carbohydrates, and electrolytes.

If you experience any of the following symptoms, stop exercising and call your doctor:

* Vaginal bleeding
* Increased uterine contractions
* Gush or leakage of fluid from the vagina
* Feeling dizzy or faint
* Shortness of breath
* Heart palpitations
* Persistent nausea or vomiting
* Back or hip pain
* Difficulty walking
* Swelling of the hands, feet, legs, ankles, or face
* Numbness anywhere in your body
* Excessive fatigue
* Unexplained abdominal pain
* Persistent, severe headaches and/or visual disturbances

If any of your risk factors change during pregnancy—for instance, if you develop elevated blood pressure or gestational diabetes—be sure to ask your physician's advice about modifying your exercise program.

PRESCRIPTION PAD

* Consult your physician for individualized guidelines based on your fitness level and pregnancy status. In general, it's advisable to do regular, moderate aerobic activity —such as walking or swimming.
* Perform easy muscle-strengthening exercises two or three times a week.
* Do relaxation exercises daily.
* Do Kegel exercises for the PC (pubococcygeus) muscles of the pelvic floor daily. (See page 279 for detailed instructions.)
* Stay hydrated.
* Avoid overheating.
* Don't work to exhaustion.

ADDITIONAL RESOURCES

✳ *The Melpomene Institute* for Women's Health Research offers an information packet on exercise and pregnancy for $14 plus $4.50 shipping and handling. Write to the institute at 1010 University Ave., St. Paul, Minn. 55104, or visit the Web site at www.melpomene.org.

✳ *PARmed-X for Pregnancy*, contact the Canadian Society for Exercise Physiology, 185 Somerset St. West, Suite 202, Ottawa, Ontario, Canada K2P OJ2; 877-651-3755.

✳ *The Bodywise Woman*, by Judy Mahle Lutter and Lynn Jaffe (Human Kinetics, 1996).

✳ *Essential Exercises for the Childbearing Year*, by Elizabeth Noble (Houghton Mifflin Company, 1988).

✳ *Exercising Through Your Pregnancy*, by James F. Clapp, III, M.D. (Human Kinetics, 1998).

PREMENSTRUAL SYNDROME

"She has two different sorts of mood," the Greek poet Semonides wrote of his wife in the sixth century B.C. "One day she is all smiles and happiness. . . . Then, another day, there'll be no living with her . . . she flies into a rage."

Some twenty-six hundred years later, both men and women are still struggling to cope with these Jekyll-and-Hyde female mood swings that are a classic symptom of premenstrual syndrome, or PMS. In recent years, PMS has become recognized as one the most common health problems affecting women. Yet it remains one of the most poorly understood.

An estimated 40 to 60 percent of reproductive-age females—some ten to fourteen million women—experience a cyclic reoccurrence of troublesome symptoms such as irritability, bloating, breast tenderness, and food cravings. Theories abound as to what causes these distressing physical, psychological, and behavioral changes, and hundreds of scientific papers have been published on the topic. But there is still no comprehensive explanation.

Yet while scientists don't know precisely what causes PMS, they do know what doesn't: PMS is not a result of "raging hormones" and it is not an imaginary ailment that is "all in a woman's head." Rather, the complex constellation of symptoms associated with PMS stem from a temporary physiologic imbalance that some women experience during the two-week period between ovulation and menstruation. Some experts classify PMS as a "reproductive endocrine disorder" in which a woman's hormones interact with brain chemicals and other body systems differently during the luteal phase (days 15 to 28) of her cycle. Others call it a "metabolic imbalance" or "biochemical disorder."

A small proportion of women—3 to 5 percent of reproductive-age females—experience PMS that is so severe its symptoms become temporarily disabling. In 1987, the American Psychiatric Association classified severe PMS as a depressive condition called premenstrual dysphoric disorder, or PMDD. Yet not all experts agree that severe PMS should be considered a psychiatric disorder. For example, a 1998 study reported in the *New England Journal of Medicine* challenged this classification by suggesting that women with PMDD have altered estrogen and progesterone receptors in their brains. This highlights both the scientific and the political controversies that have surrounded PMS for decades.

PMS BASICS

The menstrual cycle is regulated by a complex and delicate series of interactions among the female hormones, which include estrogen, progesterone, FSH (follicle-stimulating hormone), and LH (luteinizing hormone). Menstruation represents the first phase in the cycle and typically lasts about five days. Next comes the follicular phase, from about days 6 to 12, when estrogen levels begin to rise. Days 12 to 13 are the proliferative phase, when estrogen production surges, and around day 14 comes ovulation, when a ripe egg is released from the ovary. During the second half of the cycle, called the luteal phase, progesterone levels rise, peaking on about day 22, then dropping off. By day 27 or so, estrogen, progesterone, and other hormones are at their lowest levels, triggering menstruation. *PMS symptoms occur during this second half of the menstrual cycle, in the luteal phase.*

Virtually all reproductive-age women experience minor physical and/or psychological symptoms that forewarn them about impending menstruation. These normal changes, called *premenstrual molimina*, are typically milder versions of the more intense, troublesome symptoms we call PMS. For example, slight breast soreness that doesn't bother you is considered molimina. But if your breasts are so sore that you cry out in pain if someone hugs you, that's PMS.

Over 150 clinical symptoms have been linked to PMS, from well-known ones like moodiness, headaches, and acne to less-recognized changes such as shakiness, nightmares, forgetfulness, insomnia, clumsiness, constipation, and breathing difficulties. Generally, PMS symptoms are grouped into one of four categories:

1. Breast tenderness and/or enlargement
2. Fluid and abdominal bloating
3. Appetite change and/or carbohydrate craving
4. Mood changes: increased anger, anxiety, frustration, or depression.

Not every woman has trouble with all four types of symptoms, and usually symptoms vary in intensity from month to month. In fact, some experts say that a woman who doesn't feel at least one of these normal premenstrual symptoms the week before her period probably isn't ovulating. Many women don't realize that it's possible to still bleed monthly, yet not release an egg. Slight breast tenderness close to the armpit is considered a sign of ovulation, as is a brief, sharp abdominal pain—known as *mittelschmerz*—that occurs midcycle. But not all ovulating women experience either of these symptoms.

Psychologically, PMS is often characterized by a sense of "things always falling apart," and some women are vulnerable to extremes in behavior during this time. Medically, PMS is linked with "flares" of numerous ailments, such as asthma, allergies, and rheumatoid arthritis. Other chronic medical conditions known to recur or intensify during particular phases of the menstrual cycle include epilepsy, migraine headaches, sinusitis, genital herpes, and vaginal yeast infections. Diabetes and glaucoma also may worsen in association with female hormonal fluctuations.

PMS can affect everything about a woman's life, from how she looks to how she thinks, acts, and feels. Still shrouded in mystery, the syndrome also is associated with numerous surprising changes, including:

✳ *Heightened sensitivity to some drugs.* Premenstrual changes may make a woman more sensitive to caffeine, alcohol, and other drugs, including psychotropic medications such as lithium.

✳ *An increased caloric need.* As a woman's temperature rises with ovulation, she needs about 300 extra calories per day, which may explain why some women experience premenstrual food cravings.

✳ *Heightened sensory perceptions.* Some women report a premenstrual sensitivity to noises, odors, light, and touch, which can result in symptoms such as shakiness, handwriting changes, and eye difficulties. In some women, this heightened sensitivity prompts positive changes such as increased creativity, energy, and sexual interest.

✳ *Euphoria after menstruation.* As soon as monthly bleeding stops, some women experience a heightened sense of well-being at least as great in magnitude as the lows of PMS.

Despite new understanding about premenstrual changes, there is no test per se to determine whether or not a woman has PMS. Even the clinical diagnosis is a judg-

ment call, influenced largely by the individual's perception of her problem. The key to identifying PMS is not the symptom itself but *the cyclic regularity of its occurrence.* If symptoms occur solely or primarily during the two weeks prior to menstruation (the luteal phase of the menstrual cycle) the problem could be PMS. *Moreover, women with PMS should be symptom-free during the week after menstrual flow.*

The best way to determine whether or not you have PMS is to keep a monthly chart documenting your symptoms. Only about half of women who think they have PMS actually show a pattern when they chart, say experts, who note that some women may prefer to blame their problems on PMS rather than face marital conflicts, alcohol abuse, or other difficulties. But for those women whose bizarre, "personality-transforming" symptoms lead them to fear that they're crazy, charting can be a great relief because they can finally see the cyclic nature of their problem.

It's important to chart for at least two months, beginning at the first day of menstruation. Keep track of specific symptoms and whether they occur mildly, moderately, severely, or not at all. *It's also important to get a thorough physical exam to rule out thyroid disease, endometriosis, or other possible causes of troublesome symptoms.*

Another reason why PMS is so difficult to diagnose is that, typically, it doesn't strike suddenly but develops gradually and progressively over time. Often, a young woman will experience some mild symptoms occasionally during some cycles; then over the years, these symptoms will worsen, new ones will arise, and they will all become increasingly troublesome during most cycles. While even teenage girls can have PMS, it is much more common in women over thirty and it can be especially disturbing during the perimenopausal years, as a woman's hormones shift toward menopause. By the time women finally seek treatment, many feel like they're being affected nearly half their lives—two weeks out of every month.

RISK FACTORS

One of the most puzzling questions about PMS is why some women have nonexistent or mild symptoms while others battle monthly with disabling symptoms. While the answer is not entirely clear, many experts think PMS relates to hypothalamic maturity, exercise, and body fat. PMS is known to occur more frequently in the third and fourth decades of life, among sedentary women, and in populations whose food intake tends to be generous.

Several factors can exacerbate PMS, including stress, birth of a child, stopping oral contraceptives, and having surgery. Some researchers suggest that PMS is worse in Western cultures, where dieting, sedentariness, and dual-career lifestyles exacerbate symptoms. But studies document typical premenstrual symptoms in a variety of races, cultures, and socioeconomic groups. PMS-like behavior has even been observed in other primates, including baboons and chimpanzees, who, like the human female, have a twenty-eight-day menstrual cycle. Still, in cultures where women experience few menstrual cycles because of repeated episodes of pregnancy and breast-feeding, PMS is uncommon.

Many women don't experience PMS until a "trigger" event occurs in their life and affects their hormonal balance. These precipitating factors for PMS include:

* Pregnancies—including those that end in miscarriage or abortion
  * Tubal ligation
  * Hysterectomy
  * Use of oral contraceptives
  * Being over thirty

Other risk factors for PMS include:

* Sedentary lifestyle
* Overweight
* Stress

HOW EXERCISE HELPS

Although scientists have yet to find the specific cause of PMS or any magic-bullet cure, numerous studies indicate that most women can control their symptoms with several important lifestyle strategies. They are: regular exercise, a healthy diet, stress management, and eliminating alcohol, caffeine, and nicotine.

Regular exercise is one of the most powerful of these strategies because it exerts positive effects on both mind and body, which helps bring all the organ systems—including the reproductive system—into balance. Some researchers theorize that regular exercise helps relieve PMS by altering hypothalamic activity in the brain, possibly through changes in core body temperature. This activity in turn may signal the pituitary gland and ovaries to bring a woman's system into a more comfortable balance. While all this is speculative, scientists clearly know that regular exercise eases PMS by:

* Improving the flow of blood and fluids throughout the body, which can decrease fluid-related symptoms such as abdominal bloating and constipation.
* Increasing the flow of oxygen to all the body's organs.
* Helping women lose fat and maintain a healthy weight.
* Increasing the effectiveness of insulin, which helps stabilize blood sugar levels and decrease food cravings.
* Strengthening back and abdominal muscles, which can reduce back pain and cramping.
* Exerting a strong stress-reducing effect, reducing anxiety, relieving depression, and boosting mood.

This stress-reduction factor may be one of the most important, since stress is frequently a major component of PMS. One reason PMS is so prevalent in our culture may be the high levels of stress experienced by American "supermoms" who work full-time while raising children and running a home.

Stress often triggers PMS because the hormonal shifts that occur after ovulation can make women less resilient at that time than during the rest of the month. Minor irritants can send normally tenacious women into tailspins: crying when the post office turns out to be closed, shouting at children for misbehaving, or feeling overwhelmed by financial worries that are manageable the rest of the month.

Exercise can help relieve this stress and boost mood, exerting an anti-depressant and anti-anxiety effect that can counter the negative, "catastrophizing" mind-set characteristic of PMS. As an effective way to process energy of many types, exercise can help women avoid the "buildup" of negative energy that leads to the "stressed-out" mentality that frequently characterizes PMS.

EXERCISE ℞

Two kinds of exercise appear to be particularly effective in reducing troublesome symptoms: aerobic activities and mind-body exercises.

Numerous studies indicate that aerobic exercise decreases both physical and mental symptoms of PMS. Most experts recommend that women exercising to prevent or treat PMS follow the same guidelines offered for cardiovascular fitness: *Do some form of aerobic activity (such as walking, stair climbing, cycling, or swimming) three to six days a week, at about 55 to 90 percent of your maximum heart rate, for 20 to 60 minutes.*

But in addition, to help counter PMS, be sure the exercise is:

* ***Pleasurable.*** Do something you like. If you hate running but force yourself to run because you think you should, that's an added stress than may exacerbate your PMS. Doing an enjoyable aerobic activity will directly help relieve your symptoms, and taking time out for yourself to do something fun will indirectly help, too.
* ***Done daily, or almost daily, throughout your cycle.*** Don't wait until PMS strikes to start exercising. For many women, a chicken-or-the-egg phenomenon may occur, where being "stressed out" may interfere

with a routine of regular exercise, which leads to becoming more stressed out and even less able to exercise. Breaking this pattern by making exercise a regular habit throughout your cycle may result in dramatic improvement in mood.

✳ *Uninterrupted.* While accumulating short, 10-minute bouts of exercise can boost cardiovascular fitness, when it comes to PMS, activity should last for at least 20 to 30 uninterrupted minutes to achieve maximum physical and mental benefits.

✳ *A priority.* In addition to boosting physical and mental health, the daily practice of taking time out for yourself and your health is an important skill that can help you protect yourself during stressed-out PMS days. Women suffering from PMS must learn to make their own health a priority if they want to effectively fulfill all their other roles as mothers, wives, and workers. Remember what the flight attendants always warn: *In an emergency, place the mask over your own nose and mouth before trying to help children, older people, or others around you who may need assistance.*

You may also want to consider exercising outdoors whenever possible. Fresh air and sunlight can help exert additional positive effects, as can experiencing the varied cycles of nature as you go through your own natural cycle. But more important than where or when or how you exercise is simply the quality of the experience. Strive for a daily "play break," where you move your body continuously for at least 20 minutes, doing something you enjoy.

Mind-body exercises such as tai chi and yoga can also be extremely helpful for women with PMS. Not only do these activities help unite mind and body, restoring emotional and physiologic balance, but specific yoga poses can improve circulation in the groin area and strengthen muscles in the abdomen and back, which can help alleviate cramping and pain. While a regular practice of yoga or tai chi can be helpful throughout the cycle, specific yoga poses—such as the Lying Down Cobbler's Pose (see page 284)—can be helpful during times of PMS to relieve specific symptoms.

CAUTIONS

While enjoyable, daily activity can be beneficial to overall health and relieve PMS discomfort, an extremely intensive program of vigorous exercise may cause menstrual irregularity. Women who train vigorously and excessively for competitive sports, such as gymnastics and running, sometimes menstruate less often or stop entirely—a condition known as athletic amenorrhea. Typically, women who experience these menstrual irregularities have extremely low body fat, and sometimes the condition is also associated with eating disorders.

As with all conditions, PMS requires using good common sense and listening to your body to maintain a balance between not doing enough and doing too much. If you begin suffering from repeated injuries, are chronically tired, and/or stop menstruating you are probably exercising too much.

Be aware, too, that competitive exercise may not be the best choice for some women experiencing PMS. If you find competition exhilarating, great. But if you find competition particularly stressful, consider doing noncompetitive activities during your vulnerable weeks.

Start your exercise program when you are *not* premenstrual, since the "nothing is right" mind-set characteristic of PMS can doom a new exercise program to failure. Try many different kinds of exercise—dancing, gardening, skating, martial arts—to find ones you enjoy. Don't worry about exercising for a particular goal, such as losing weight. Instead, exercise daily solely for the pleasure it brings.

PRESCRIPTION PAD

✳ Do an aerobic activity that you enjoy three to six days a week, for at least 20 to 60 uninterrupted minutes.

✳ Exercise outdoors, in fresh air and sunlight, when possible.

✳ Practice several yoga poses a few times each week, then perform specific poses as needed during PMS days to relieve certain symptoms.

ADDITIONAL RESOURCES

✳ Melpomene Institute for women's health research offers information on PMS; write to the institute at 1010 University Ave., St. Paul, Minn. 55104, or visit the Web site: www.melpomene.org.

✳ Susan M. Lark, M.D., *PMS: Premenstrual Syndrome Self Help Book*, (Celestial Arts, 1993).

✳ Stephanie DeGraff Bender and Kathleen Kelleher, *PMS: A Positive Program to Gain Control* (Perigee/The Body Press, 1991).

✳ Michelle Harrison, M.D., *Self-Help for Premenstrual Syndrome* (Random House, 1985).

MENOPAUSE AND PERIMENOPAUSE

Menopause is a natural life event that represents a woman's passage from her reproductive to her nonreproductive years. Historically misunderstood as a disease of "estrogen-deficiency" or "ovarian failure," it is neither a sickness nor a taboo topic, as it was in years past. In fact, there has been a surge of interest in the mental and physical changes surrounding menopause as the first wave of female baby boomers reach the end of their childbearing years. Best-selling books, TV talk shows, and support groups have all emerged to help America's 38 million female boomers grapple with the complex changes surrounding this biological landmark.

Technically, the word *menopause* means the end of all menstrual bleeding, and *refers to a single day in a woman's life after she has not had a menstrual period for 12 consecutive months* when no other biological or physiological cause can be identified. In general usage, however, the term *menopause* describes the broader transitional period surrounding this one-day event. During this time, decreasing production of the female sex hormones estrogen and progesterone frequently prompts a variety of physical and psychological effects, including hot flashes, weight gain, mood swings, and unpredictable menstrual bleeding.

In recent years, the term *perimenopause*—which literally means "around menopause"—

has come into vogue to describe the years leading up to menopause. Perimenopause is loosely defined. Some say it begins as soon as a woman's menstrual periods start changing, which can occur more than a decade before menopause. Others confine it to the immediate three to six years prior to the last menstrual period.

For some women, this transition is smooth and uneventful. For others, it's an emotionally charged time akin to riding a hormonal roller coaster, an experience some women describe as "puberty in reverse." In our culture, perimenopause and menopause can be a complex time with physical, psychological, social, and political overtones that include:

* The physical complexity of adjusting to a new hormonal equilibrium.
* The psychological aspects of dealing with aging and the end of fertility
* The societal pressures of growing older in a youth-oriented culture
* The political issues of the "invisibility" of older women in contemporary society.

MENOPAUSE BASICS

At birth, a woman's ovaries contain all the eggs she will have throughout her lifetime. At puberty, the ovaries begin to release eggs periodically, and menstruation begins. During the initial years of menstruation, as this intricate hormonal symphony "tunes up," periods are often irregular and are accompanied by psychological and physical changes, such as mood swings and acne. These troublesome symptoms generally diminish as a young woman's body adjusts to the delicate hormonal balance that orchestrates her monthly cycles.

Just as adolescence can be a volatile time of hormonal fluctuation, so too can perimenopause. When the hormones that regulate fertility begin to "wind down" prior to menopause, periods often become irregular, and other unsettling effects can occur. Psychologically, many women are surprised at how early these changes can occur, and also at how far ranging their effects can be. Physically, endocrinological and biological changes can affect a woman's entire body, from thinning hair to joint and muscle pain, vaginal dryness, hot flashes, itchy skin, and fatigue.

The most obvious changes are those in the menstrual cycle itself, with shorter or longer periods, lighter or heavier flow, and frequently skipped cycles. While most of these changes are natural, women should contact a health-care provider if they notice abnormal uterine bleeding, such as periods more often than every three weeks, heavy periods with "gushing" and clots, or bleeding after intercourse.

At menopause, the ovaries no longer produce enough estrogen and progesterone to build up the lining of the uterus each month, so monthly flow stops. Menopause can only be identified retrospectively, since it marks the date on which a woman has not menstruated for a full year. In industrialized societies, most women experience menopause between the ages of forty-five and fifty-five, with the average age around fifty-one. Some women stop menstruating as early as their late thirties, while in rare cases women have periods into their sixties.

Despite popular myths, the timing of

menopause is unrelated to race, pregnancy, breast-feeding, fertility patterns, use of birth-control pills, height, weight, or age of menarche (first period). One factor known to influence the timing of menopause is cigarette smoking. Smokers and even former smokers may reach menopause two years earlier than nonsmokers, according to the North American Menopause Society. There is also some evidence that women who have had a hysterectomy—surgical removal of the uterus but not the ovaries—may experience earlier onset of menopause. Genetics play a key role in determining the timing of menopause, so family history is often a good clue as to when a woman will reach the end of her reproductive years.

Although most women experience "natural" menopause, some women go through an "induced" menopause as a result of medical interventions such as the surgical removal of both ovaries or cancer treatments, including chemotherapy and radiation, that can damage the ovaries. The sudden loss of ovarian hormones frequently causes these women to experience menopausal changes. Also, some drugs used to treat endometriosis or severe PMS suppress menstruation. This creates a kind of "reversible menopause," since periods resume when a woman stops taking the medication.

Since modern women may expect to live into their eighties, and increasing numbers are reaching one hundred, many will live nearly half their lives "postmenopause." During this postmenopausal period, with diminished levels of the protective hormone estrogen, women are at increased risk for numerous life-threatening diseases, including heart disease and osteoporosis.

As a commanding landmark of physical and psychological transition, perimenopause and menopause represent an ideal time to reassess health habits and lifestyle strategies, especially those that might affect troublesome symptoms and reduce the risk of serious ailments common in postmenopausal life. With the possible exception of quitting smoking, no single habit or health strategy addresses the range of mind-body-spirit issues more than adopting a regular program of physical activity.

HOW EXERCISE HELPS

Women experience a broad range of changes during perimenopause and menopause that can affect much more than just their reproductive system. Hormonal fluctuations can also influence the functioning of organs and tissues throughout their entire bodies, from their bones to their skin, heart, blood, and brain. Some are temporary, such as hot flashes and night sweats. Some are annoyances, such as vaginal dryness and frequent urination. Others can be permanent, disabling, or fatal conditions, such as coronary artery disease and osteoporosis.

Hormone replacement therapy (HRT) is a standard treatment for many of these conditions, yet these drugs remain controversial and many women are reluctant to take them. Hormone therapy is inadvisable for some women with an increased risk of cancer, and the potential side effects of these drugs are frequently a concern. Many women raised in the generation that pioneered natural childbirth worry that pharmaceutical companies are pushing drugs to "medicalize" a natural life stage. "Only 30 percent of women who are given prescriptions for HRT ever fill them," writes surgeon Susan Love in *Dr. Susan Love's Hormone Book*. Important studies, such as the Women's Health Initiative, which will conclude in 2008, are examining the safety and effectiveness of HRT. Until more is known, women need to make individualized decisions based on their risk factors for osteoporosis, heart disease, and cancer.

Whether or not a woman chooses to take HRT or other "designer estrogens" at menopause, *regular exercise is itself a powerful medicine that helps mitigate virtually all the negative changes women experience at midlife and beyond*. These include:

✳ **Increased cholesterol levels.** As estrogen levels go down, total cholesterol levels go up, increasing the risk of heart disease. Regular aerobic exercise elevates the level of HDL, "good" cholesterol, lowers the triglyceride level, improves the total cholesterol-to-HDL ratio, and lowers the level of LDL, "bad" cholesterol.

✳ **Weight gain.** Most women's waistlines expand during menopause, although it's unclear whether this results from aging, decreased activity, increased intake, or hormonal changes themselves. The average woman gains about ten to twelve pounds during the menopausal years, according to some experts. Regular exercise can help eliminate or minimize this midlife weight gain. Strength training can boost muscle mass, which increases the metabolic rate so that a woman will burn more calories, even at rest. Aerobic exercise is an unsurpassed calorie burner.

✳ **Hot flashes.** An estimated 85 percent of perimenopausal and menopausal women have hot flashes, some just two or three times a day and some as often as once an hour. These three- to ten-minute flashes of heavy sweating and increased heart rate can be annoying and embarrassing by day, and frustrating at night, since night sweats can disturb sleep, contributing to the irritability and depression common at this life stage. Relaxed, slow abdominal (yoga) breathing has been shown to cut in half the number of hot flashes a woman experiences. In addition, research suggests that regular aerobic exercise also may reduce the frequency and severity of hot flashes.

✳ **Insomnia.** Regular exercise helps people go to sleep more easily and also deepens sleep. Fit people typically take less time to go to sleep, have fewer awakenings, and experience more delta sleep, which is the nondreaming sleep that promotes the greatest amount of body recovery. Also, exercise that reduces night sweats can aid sleep, since these middle-of-the-night awakenings are often associated with insomnia.

✳ **Anxiety and depression.** Regular physical activity can help relieve mild to moderate anxiety and depression and is associated with a variety of positive psychological outcomes, including improved self-esteem, reduced stress, enhanced feelings of energy, and elevated mood.

✳ **Bone loss.** The dramatic drop in estrogen at menopause prompts women to lose bone at an accelerated rate, with some women losing up to 20 percent of their bone mass in the eight years after menopause. Weight-bearing activities and resistance exercise can help build and maintain bone, with some research suggesting that it may be as effective a bone builder as HRT. "Physical activity, through its load-bearing effect on the skeleton, is likely the single most important influence on bone density and architecture," concludes the *U.S. Surgeon General's Report on Physical Activity and Health.*

Regular exercise can exert such a powerful effect on virtually all aspects of women's midlife health that many experts say that, next to eliminating cigarettes if she's a smoker, *getting adequate physical activity is the single most important thing a menopausal woman can do to feel and look better now and for the rest of her life.* Women who can't or won't take synthetic estrogens may find that exercise can provide many similar benefits, while those who are on HRT can use exercise as an adjunct therapy to enhance the medication's effects on bone and the cardiovascular system while potentially minimizing some of the drug's side effects.

EXERCISE ℞

Three kinds of exercise are particularly helpful in reducing troublesome symptoms of perimenopause and menopause:

1. *Aerobic activity.* Helps with weight loss and maintenance, relieves negative psychological symptoms such as anxiety and depression, improves cardiovascular fitness, and has been shown in a study of Swedish women to reduce the number and severity of hot flashes. In addition, weight-bearing aerobic activity, such as running and walking, can reduce the risk of osteoporosis.
2. *Strength-training exercises.* Helps with weight loss and maintenance by boosting muscle mass and metabolic rate and can reduce the risk of osteoporosis by strengthening bones.
3. *Deep abdominal breathing.* Can reduce the frequency of hot flashes by 50 to 60 percent, according to extensive studies by psychologist Robert Freedman, professor of psychiatry and behavioral neurosciences at Wayne State University School of Medicine.

Here are menopause-specific guidelines for each of these three types of exercises. (For details of individual exercises, see Healing Moves for Women, page 272.)

Aerobic Exercise

Do some form of rhythmic activity that uses the large muscles of the body—such as walking, dancing, or running—three to six days a week, for 20 to 60 minutes. Be sure to pick an activity you enjoy—especially if you're interested in the stress-reducing, mood-elevating effects. If osteoporosis is a concern, choose a weight-bearing exercise such as running or walking rather than a non-weight-bearing activity such as swimming or cycling. (See the section on osteoporosis, page 127.) If hot flashes are a concern, try an hour of aerobic exercise, three times a week. Brisk walking can meet all these criteria, which may be why many women say they "walk" through menopause. (For instruction on starting a walking program, see Healing Moves for Heart Health, page 214.)

Strength Training

Lift weights or use strength-training machines two to three days a week. Do one set each of eight to ten exercises that strengthen the major muscle groups—arms, shoulders, chest, back, abdominals, hips, and legs. Younger women can work up to a weight they can lift at least eight but no more than twelve times. Older and more frail women (ages fifty and above) may find it more appropriate to choose a lighter weight they can lift as least ten but no more than fifteen times. While one set of each exercise is sufficient to boost strength and prevent loss of muscle mass in most adults, a three-set regimen may provide slightly greater benefits for those who have time.

Deep Abdominal Breathing

Also known as paced respiration or yoga belly breathing, deep abdominal breathing is an effective technique to relieve stress. Researchers at Wayne State University have shown in numerous published studies that focused breathing can cut in half the number of menopausal hot flashes a woman experiences. First, women are taught the technique, which involves learning to cut the breathing rate in half. For example, the average rate of respiration is fifteen to sixteen breaths per minute, but by paying attention to the breath and deliberately trying to slow the breathing rate (with deep, slow inhalations that fill up the belly and long, smooth exhalations), women can learn to breathe just seven to eight times per minute. Researchers found that when a woman begins this kind of breathing as soon as she feels a hot flash is coming on, she can interrupt the flash, eliminating it entirely or reducing its severity. (For more detailed instructions, see Healing Moves for Women, page 282.)

Consider enrolling in a yoga or tai chi class to learn and become skilled at focused breathing. In the ancient tradition, people often did not begin the practice of these meditative disciplines until their fifties, when the children were grown, the business was handed over to "new blood," and they could turn their attention to self-awareness and the meaning of life. It is a simple fact that most women experience the physical, emotional, and spiritual transitions of perimenopause and menopause at about this age. A woman who directs her attention to fitness and good health, proper nutrition, deep breathing, and relaxation is far more likely to embrace the changes of menopause as a natural part of life.

CAUTIONS

Precautions about exercise during this life stage are not related to menopause itself but to the increased risk of certain medical conditions that occurs when estrogen levels diminish. The most common of these are heart disease and osteoporosis.

Women in midlife need to be aware *that heart disease is not just a "guy thing." It is also the leading cause of death in women.* Strenuous physical exertion by women with uncontrolled heart conditions can cause serious cardiovascular events. *If you are planning to start a program of vigorous exercise, it is essential that you consult a physician immediately if:*

* You have two or more risk factors for heart disease. These include high blood pressure, high blood cholesterol, diabetes, smoking, family history of the ailment, and obesity.

* You are a sedentary woman over age fifty (or a man over age forty).

* You have a known heart condition.

Osteoporosis also is of special concern to women at midlife, especially since it's a "silent disease," which means that a significant number of people with low bone density are unaware they have a problem until a minor fall results in a major fracture. Women approaching menopause—especially those with family history of osteoporosis—should consider having a bone-density test to determine their risk. If you already have low bone density of the spine or osteoporosis—particularly if you've suffered a fracture—consult a physician or physical therapist for an individualized exercise program. (See the section on osteoporosis, page 127).

Remember: Some exercise is better than no exercise.

If you've been inactive, be sure to start any new exercise program slowly and progress gradually. Begin with as little as a 5-minute walk and each week add another 5 minutes until you're walking continuously for 30 to 60 minutes. Always warm up before activity, stretch gently, and cool down at the end of exercise.

PRESCRIPTION PAD

* Do some form of enjoyable aerobic activity (preferably a weight-bearing one) for 20 to 60 minutes, three to six days a week.

* Lift weights or use a strength-training machine two or three days a week.

* Practice deep, abdominal breathing whenever you feel under stress or can sense a hot flash coming on.

* Consider taking a yoga or tai chi class to learn and become skilled in relaxation breathing techniques.

ADDITIONAL RESOURCES

* The North American Menopause Society (NAMS) has a multidisciplinary membership of menopause experts from diverse health-care fields and provides free and low-cost menopause-related information to consumers and professionals. Visit the Web site at www.menopause.org or write to NAMS, P.O. Box 94527, Cleveland, Ohio 44101.

* The Melpomene Institute for women's health research offers information on menopause on its Web site: www.melpomene.org and by mail: 1010 University Ave., St. Paul, Minn. 55104.

* The American College of Obstetricians and Gynecologists (ACOG) Resource Center can provide information about a variety of women's health concerns, including menopause. Visit the Web site: www.acog.org or call 800-762-2264 or send a self-addressed, stamped envelope with your request to ACOG Resource Center, P.O. Box 96920, Washington, D.C. 20090.

* Healthfinder, an Internet site for health-related government agencies, such as the National Institutes of Health and the Department of Health and Human Services,

can provide a wealth of information about menopause and associated conditions. Access the Web site at www.healthfinder.gov, then follow the "search" cues to find information about specific disorders.

✳ *Menopause Naturally*, by Sadja Greenwood, M.D. (Volcano Press, 1996).

✳ *Strong Women Stay Young* and *Strong Women Stay Slim*, both by Miriam Nelson, Ph.D., with Sarah Wernick, Ph.D. (Bantam Books, 1997 and 1999).

✳ *Outsmarting the Midlife Fat Cell*, by Debra Waterhouse, M.P.H., R.D. (Hyperion, 1998).

✳ *Dr. Susan Love's Hormone Book*, by Susan Love, M.D., with Karen Lindsey (Times Books, 1997).

✳ *The Menopause Self Help Book*, by Susan M. Lark, M.D. (Celestial Arts, 1990).

✳ *The Bodywise Woman*, by Judy Mahle Lutter and Lynn Jaffee (Human Kinetics, 1996).

✳ *The Change: Women, Aging and the Menopause*, by Germaine Greer (Fawcett Columbine, 1991).

✳ ✳ ✳

HEALING MOVES FOR WOMEN

✳

Many of us grew up in a world where women were considered "too delicate" for vigorous exercise. Yet in just a generation, women have trampled these notions of being the "weaker sex," with success as professional basketball players, Olympic marathoners, champion rock climbers, and karate black belts. Not only are these athletic accomplishments vital to women's self-esteem, but they are central to optimum health. When we look back at outdated medical texts that prescribed confinement during pregnancy and bed rest for menstrual discomfort, it's clear that women have come a long way.

Regular physical activity is essential throughout the female life cycle, from puberty and pregnancy through menopause and beyond. In fact, women's lives contain many gender-specific phases—such as menstruation, childbirth, and perimenopause—that may be positively affected by exercise. The specific exercises a woman performs may need to vary according the unique demands of her cycles and stage of life. For example, during menstruation, certain inverted yoga poses are inadvisable and can be substituted with other postures. During pregnancy, a woman may find that her daily run has become uncomfortable, so she may benefit more by switching to swimming. If troublesome symptoms of PMS or menopause flare, breathing exercises may provide the best relief.

That's why our Healing Moves for Women contain a varied menu of options to help each woman individualize a program that suits her preferences, abilities, needs, and place in the life cycle. The three main components of this workout are:

Part One: Aerobic Activity

Aerobic activity strengthens the cardiovascular system, helps maintain a healthy weight and positive self-image, and helps regulate the endocrine system, balance the emotions, and boost mood. Regular aerobic activity is particularly important for pregnant women and those dealing with troublesome symptoms of PMS and menopause. For best results, aerobic exercise should be performed three to six days a week.

Part Two: Strengthening Exercises

Strengthening exercises preserve bone density, build muscle mass and strength, boost metabolism, improve balance, and enhance the quality of daily life. Strengthening exercises are vital to women in midlife and beyond, since declining levels of estrogen put postmenopausal women at increased risk of osteoporosis. Pregnant women also can benefit from the special set of strengthening "maternal moves" included here. Do these activities two or three days a week.

Part Three: Mind-Body Practice

Mind-body practice helps relieve stress and counters troublesome symptoms related to the menstrual cycle and menopause. Women under stress may especially benefit from these exercises. Do the basic breathing exercises daily, or even several times daily, and the other practices as needed.

Women are said to be the more adaptable sex, possibly because females' lives—and their bodies—are constantly changing. This flexibility also is important when it comes to exercise, since at different points in her monthly cycle and in her life cycle a woman may want to adapt her physical-activity program.

The main point to remember is this: *Do something active most days of the week.* You can do just one part of this workout each day or do two or all three. In general, it's best to plan your workouts over the course of a week, so that in a seven-day period you do at least three aerobic workouts and two strengthening ones, plus daily relaxation breathing. As an example, here's the weekly schedule of a perimenopausal woman who enjoys walking:

Monday: 30-minute walk, 5 minutes relaxation breathing
Tuesday: 20-minute strength-training workout, 10 minutes mind-body practice
Wednesday: 45-minute line-dancing class, 5 minutes mind-body practice, 5 minutes relaxation breathing
Thursday: 20-minute walk, 20-minute strength-training workout, 5 minutes relaxation breathing
Friday: 30-minute walk, 5 minutes relaxation breathing
Saturday: 15 minutes mind-body practice
Sunday: 60-minute walk in the country with friend, 5 minutes relaxation breathing

Women dealing with PMS may want to chart their exercise program on the calendar, making sure to schedule in ample aerobic activities and mind-body practices during their symptomatic weeks. If PMS is your main health concern, you may substitute aerobic activities and/or mind-body practices for the strengthening routines, since these forms of exercise are especially important in combating PMS.

PART ONE: AEROBIC ACTIVITY

Any physical activity that uses the large-muscle groups of the legs, back, and arms in a continuous and rhythmic manner is considered an aerobic exercise—which means that you have lots of choices. The two most important criteria in picking the one—or ones—that you'll do regularly are:

✳ *Enjoyment.* Pick an activity you like, so you'll do it regularly and it can become a stress-reducing "play break" in your day. This may also mean picking an exercise, like walking or in-line skating, that you can pair with something else you enjoy, such as listening to music on a personal stereo.

✳ *Safety.* Pick an activity that you can perform without undue risk to yourself or your baby (if you're pregnant). Pregnant women should be sure to read the guidelines in the pregnancy section (page 252) and consult their physician before embarking on any workout. If you have other health problems, such as hypertension or arthritis, see those chapters in this volume, and discuss an optimal exercise program with your doctor. (See Pre-Participation Checklist, page 29.)

In selecting an aerobic activity, it's important to consider the amount of impact involved. High-impact exercises like running or racquet sports can be good choices for women who want strong bones, since the greater the impact, the greater the strengthening effect on the bones. But high-impact activities may be a poor choice for pregnant women or women who have advanced osteoporosis, with increased risk of fracture.

Here is a menu of aerobic options, categorized by degree of impact:

High-impact: Running, jogging, volleyball, basketball, soccer, karate, rope skipping, step aerobics, high-impact aerobics, racquet sports

Low- to Moderate-Impact: Line dancing, walking, in-line skating, cross-country skiing, low-impact aerobics, stair-stepping machine

No-Impact: Swimming, cycling, water walking, aqua-aerobics, rowing

Older women who enjoy high-impact activity, such as running, but find it stressful on their joints may want to alternate running with a low- or no-impact activity like line dancing or swimming. In general, alternating activities—such as going to an aerobics class one day and cycling the next—is a good way to get an all-around workout while minimizing your risk of injury and avoiding boredom. Known as cross-training, this practice relies on doing different activities that use different muscle groups on different days. It's fine to vary your specific aerobic exercise to suit the weather, your preferences, your fitness level, or other needs. For example, if you like hiking in good weather but want to take an aerobics class in bad weather, that's fine. Just be sure to *do some form of aerobic exercise from three to six days per week.*

If you're devoted to just one form of aerobic exercise, such as walking, and want to walk every day, that's fine, too. (For instructions on starting a daily walking program, see Healing Moves for Heart Health, page 214.)

Women with PMS may want to consider picking an outdoor activity, whenever possible, since fresh air and sunlight can exert additional positive effects on cyclic symptoms. But more important than where or when you exercise is ensuring that your activity is an enjoyable experience. If you're having trouble picking something "fun," think back to your childhood and consider activities you used to enjoy, such as dancing, table tennis, or hiking. Try them again. Think about whether you prefer solo or social activity, whether you prefer mellow motion or competitive sports, and design your program accordingly.

If you need an extra boost to jump-start your program, consider getting instruction at a YMCA or YWCA or with a personal trainer. (For referral to a certified trainer in your area, contact the American Council on Exercise's consumer hotline, 800-529-8227.)

Once you've picked your aerobic activity or activities, start slowly and progress gradually. Warm up first by doing your activity at a slow pace for 5 to 10 minutes, then stretch gently. (Stretch routines are outlined in Healing Moves for Health and Fitness, page 44, and Healing Moves to Strengthen Muscles and Bones, page 146.) Then do as little as 5 minutes more of your selected activity at a quicker pace before slowing back down for a 5-minute cooldown and 5-minute stretch. Each week, add on 5 more minutes of quicker-pace activity until you're performing your aerobic activity for 30 to 60 minutes at an intensity you consider moderate to somewhat hard. Be sure to stretch out the muscles you've worked at the end of your workout.

If you're pregnant, you may want to exercise at a comfortable to moderate pace. Good aerobic activity choices during pregnancy include: walking, riding a stationary bicycle, prenatal aerobics classes, water aerobics, or swimming.

This section is divided into "basic strength," for women who are *not* pregnant, and "maternal moves" for pregnant women.

BASIC STRENGTH

These exercises will help you strengthen your body's major muscle groups. Some use a modest amount of equipment. If you don't have a padded weight bench, improvise by placing blankets or towels on a piano bench, picnic bench, or coffee table, or lie on a bed or on the floor. If you don't have dumbbells, improvise with soup cans, shampoo bottles, or socks filled with pennies or sand. Your goal will be to work your way up to using a weight heavy enough for you to do at least 10, but no more than 15, repetitions of each exercise. If you've been sedentary, it's advisable to start out by using an obviously light weight—or no weight at all—to perform each exercise. When you can perform 15 repetitions easily, you can increase the amount of weight you're using gradually, by no more than 10 percent per week. Younger, stronger women may use a weight they can lift at least 8 times but no more than 12 times. (When these exercises have become easy and you're ready for more variety, try the strengthening exercises in Healing Moves for Health and Fitness on page 38 or Healing Moves to Strengthen Muscles and Bones on page 140.)

1. Dumbbell Bench Press (Works Upper and Midchest Muscles)

Lie on a padded weight bench with your feet flat on the floor about shoulder width apart. Hold a dumbbell in each hand. Keep the dumbbells at chest level, holding them with an inward grip (palms facing toward each other). Inhale, then exhale and raise the dumbbells until your arms are fully extended. Pause slightly at the top, then inhale as you lower the weights back to your chest. Do one set of 10 to 15 repetitions to start, then work up gradually to doing three sets of 10 to 15 reps.

2. Single-Dumbbell Pullover (Works Lower-Chest Muscles)

Lie on a bench with your feet flat on the floor, shoulder width apart. Grasp one end of a dumbbell with both hands and raise it directly overhead with your arms extended and your elbows slightly bent. Inhale deeply into your rib cage as you lower your arms backward until the dumbbell is just about level with—or slightly lower than—your back. Pause slightly, then exhale as you return the dumbbell to its original overhead position. Do one set of 10 to 15 repetitions to start, then work up gradually to doing three sets of 10 to 15 repetitions.

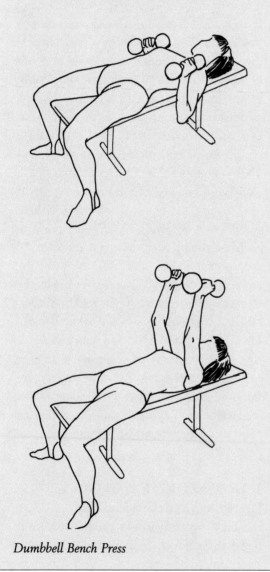

Dumbbell Bench Press

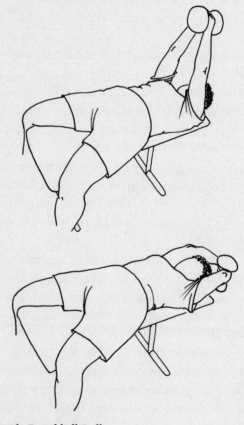

Single-Dumbbell Pullover

3. Biceps Curl (Works the Front of the Upper Arm)

Stand erect with your feet shoulder width apart. Grasp a dumbbell in each hand, palms facing inward and arms fully extended so the dumbbells rest lightly against your thighs. Inhale, then exhale and raise the dumbbell in your right hand, turning your wrist so your palm faces up. Keep your elbows and upper arms in to your sides as you lift the dumbbell to about shoulder height. Inhale as you slowly lower the dumbbell back to the starting position. Repeat with the left arm, making sure to lift and lower in a slow,

controlled manner. Do one set of 10 to 15 repetitions with each arm to start, then work up gradually to doing three sets of 10 to 15 with each arm.

4. Triceps Curl (Works the Back of the Upper Arm)

Stand with your feet about shoulder width apart. Hold a dumbbell with both hands and raise it over your head with arms extended, elbows slightly bent. Inhale as you slowly lower the dumbbell behind your head as far as possible, being sure to keep your arms close to your head with elbows pointed upward. Exhale as you raise the dumbbell back to the starting position. Pause slightly, then repeat. Do one set of 10 to 15 repetitions to start, then work up gradually to doing three sets of 10 to 15 repetitions.

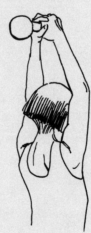 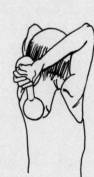

Triceps Curl

5. Front Lunge (Works the Thighs, Buttocks, and Hips)

Stand erect with your feet shoulder width apart and your hands on your hips. Keeping

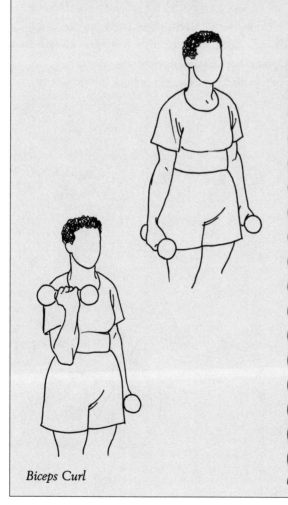

Biceps Curl

your back straight and your head up, inhale as you step forward with your right foot as far as possible, continuing until your upper right thigh is almost parallel to the floor. Exhale as you step back to the starting position. Repeat on the other side, stepping forward with the left leg. (You may hold lightly on to a countertop for balance if you like.) Do just two lunges on each side to start, then add a few more lunges each week until you're doing 10 to 15 lunges with each leg. When this is easy, do the exercise holding a light dumbbell in each hand.

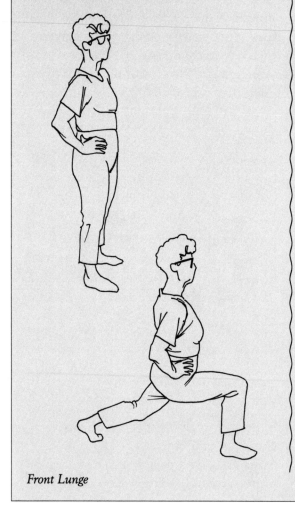

Front Lunge

6. Core Crunch (Works the Abdominal Muscles)

Lie on your back with your knees bent and your feet in the air, resting on a chair or a bench if you prefer. Leave your arms at your sides, if you're a beginner. (The farther away your arms are from your belly, the harder the exercise will be. As you get stronger, you may want to cross your arms over your chest or place your fingertips behind your ears.) Contract your abdominal muscles, squeeze your buttocks together, and tilt your pelvis up so that your lower back presses into the floor. Slowly curl your head up, just until your shoulder blades lift off the floor. Do not swing your elbows forward and yank on your head, since this can place harmful stress on your neck. Concentrate on working your abdominal muscles. Ease back down. Do just

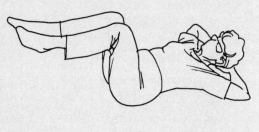

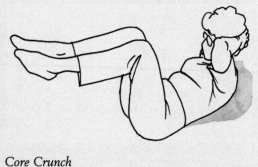

Core Crunch

three to start, being sure to exhale as you curl up and inhale as you release. Then add a few more crunches each week until you're doing 25 repetitions. (When this gets easy, try the crunch variations in Healing Moves to Strengthen Muscles and Bones, page 145.)

7. Pelvic-Floor Power Squeeze (Kegels; Works the Muscles of the Pelvic Floor)

Many women know these exercises as Kegels because they're named after Arnold Kegel, the Los Angeles gynecologist who developed them in the 1940s to help relieve one of the most common health problems for women of all ages—incontinence. Since the once taboo topic of leaking urine has come out of the closet in recent years, many people know that more than 40 percent of women over sixty (and 20 percent of men over sixty) have this problem. But many women don't realize that about one-third of college-age female athletes also report leaking urine during high-impact sports. These exercises are also essential for pregnant women, since childbirth puts women at greater risk of incontinence.

Locate the pelvic floor muscles by sitting on the toilet, spreading your legs apart, and trying to stop the flow of urine without moving your legs. If you can slow or stop the flow, you're using the right muscles. (Be sure not to strain or "bear down," which does not isolate the right muscles. A properly done Kegel should feel like you're inwardly lifting and squeezing.)

Squeeze the pelvic floor muscles as you count slowly to three, then relax them as you again count to three. Be sure to keep breathing! For the first two weeks, try to do 15 repetitions of this squeeze and relax, three times a day. Do one set of 15 while lying down, one set sitting, and one set standing.

Over the next 10 weeks, work up to squeezing for 10 seconds, then relaxing for 10 seconds. Do 15 exercises at a time, three times a day, for a total of 45 exercises per day. Set a timer for five minutes (15 exercises × 20 seconds per exercise) or use an exercise diary if it's helpful.

Don't give up too soon. It takes about eight to ten weeks of exercising before you'll start to notice a difference.

Once your muscles become strong enough, you can do a maintenance program by fitting these exercises into your daily routine. Make it a habit to do Kegels while you're brushing your teeth, standing in line, sitting at a red light, or talking on the phone.

MATERNAL MOVES

During pregnancy, certain body parts need special attention. In particular, the stresses caused by the weight of your expanding uterus make it important to strengthen the muscles of your back and pelvic floor. (Kegel exercises are presented on this page, so since you probably skipped that section, go back and do the *pelvic-floor power squeeze*.) The following exercises are designed to help your body meet the challenges of pregnancy:

Standing Pelvic Tilt

Stand comfortably with your feet shoulder width apart and your knees slightly bent. Squeeze your buttocks and tighten your abdominal muscles. Rock the pelvis gently forward while rotating the pubic bone upward. Hold for 10 seconds, then release. Repeat 10 times.

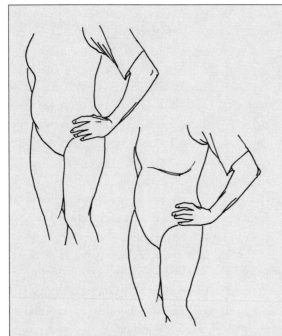

Standing Pelvic Tilt

Cat Stretch

Kneel with your weight equally distributed between your hands and knees. Be sure your arms and legs form right angles at the shoulder, hip joints, and floor. Exhale while curling your head and buttocks down and arching your back up. Inhale while reversing this curve so that your head and buttocks curl back up and your back relaxes back down. Be sure to relax just back to a neutral position—don't let the spine sag. Repeat 10 times.

Cat Twist

Kneel with your weight distributed evenly on your hands and knees. Exhale and look back toward your right hip, so that you feel a stretch at the left side of your waist. Inhale and return to the center. Exhale and look backward toward your left hip, so that you feel a stretch at the right side of your waist. Inhale and return to the center. Repeat, alternating sides, 10 times.

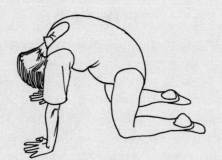

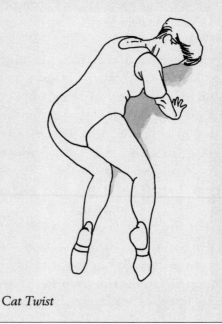

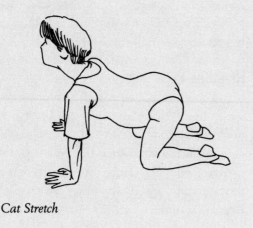

Cat Stretch

Cat Twist

Supported Squat

Stand next to an immovable object, such as a railing or a doorjamb, with your feet flat and wide apart. Grasp the immovable object firmly, then bend your knees as you descend slowly and gradually into a squat. Be sure you keep your heels on the floor. Shift your weight to the outsides of your feet, keeping your arms straight and your head up. Hold for 15 to 20 seconds, working up to holding for up to 3 minutes. Get out of the squat by lowering yourself to a sitting position, slowly and carefully.

Half Wall Hang

Place your palms against a wall at shoulder height, shoulder width apart. Slide your hands down the wall while slowly walking backward until your arms are straight and your spine is parallel to the floor. (If you

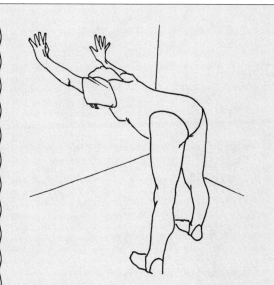

Half Wall Hang

can't get your spine straight and your back wants to round, place your hands higher on the wall.) Move your feet a little farther apart, until you're comfortable. The distance will widen as your belly grows. Keep your feet parallel and legs straight, but don't hyperextend your knees. Be sure they're slightly bent, then lift your kneecaps and keep your thigh muscles active, while pressing against the wall with your hands. Imagine space opening up between each of the vertebrae in your spinal column. Feel your shoulders open, let your abdomen drop, and breathe slow, long, easy breaths. Breathe comfortably in this position for one or two minutes, then inhale deeply as you step toward the wall to stand up. Be sure to inhale as you stand to avoid getting dizzy.

PART THREE:
MIND/BODY PRACTICES

Hot flashes, mood swings, and other troublesome symptoms linked to women's hor-

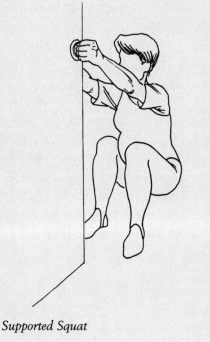

Supported Squat

monal fluctuations can both cause and be greatly affected by stress. In fact, one theory about why certain women get PMS relates to a hypersensitivity of the autonomic nervous system, which regulates the body's fight-or-flight reactions, putting these women in a near constant state of tension. Mind-body practices don't eliminate stress, but they help process it by connecting physical and mental energies. That's why these exercises are so important for women who are "hormonally challenged."

Paced Respiration (Yoga Belly Breathing)

One of the single most important healing exercises in this book, paced respiration can be effective for anyone, anywhere, who is slammed with a sudden onslaught of stress. In any tense situation—from a traffic jam to a work deadline to childbirth—taking a controlled, calming breath can be wonderfully therapeutic, bringing healing oxygen and connecting energy flow throughout the body, while expelling fatigue and tension. Paced respiration is particularly effective in combating menopausal hot flashes. Studies at Wayne State University in Detroit showed that controlled breathing cut the frequency of hot flashes in half. By teaching women to slow down their breathing rate from its average of fifteen to sixteen cycles (inhaling and exhaling) per minute to seven or eight cycles per minute, psychologist Robert Freedman has demonstrated that women can abort a flash or at least reduce its severity.

Known in yoga as "belly breathing," paced respiration involves sitting quietly, focusing on the breath, and allowing air to completely fill the lungs right down to the abdomen. Many women discover that only their chest expands when they breathe, often because our culture continually urges women to hold in their stomachs. That's why the first step in learning the technique is teaching women to stop being "chest breathers" and start being "abdominal breathers." To do this:

1. Lie on your back and place a book on your belly. Relax your stomach muscles and inhale deeply into your abdomen so that the book rises. When you exhale, the book should fall. You'll still be bringing air into your upper chest, but now you're are also bringing air down into the lower portion of your lungs and expanding your entire chest cavity.

2. Sit up and place your right hand on your abdomen and your left hand on your chest. Breathe deeply so that your right, "abdominal" hand rises and falls with your breath, while your left, "chest" hand stays relatively still. Breathe in through your nose and out through your nose or mouth, and spend a few minutes enjoying the sensation of abdominal breathing.

3. Place a timer or clock with a second hand in clear view. Breathe in slowly, filling your abdomen, as the timer counts off five seconds. Then breathe out slowly to the same count of five. Breathing in for five seconds and out for five seconds is an ideal pace that you can strive for whenever you feel a hot flash—or other stressful event—coming on.

(Once you've mastered this technique, try the enhanced variations featured in Healing Moves for Health and Fitness, page 49.)

Child's Pose

This yoga posture, which brings the body into a comfortable fetal position, gently stretches the lower back and improves circulation to the brain and pelvic region. It is excellent for calming anxiety and irritability and can help relieve menstrual cramps.

Sit on your feet with your knees together and slowly bend forward, stretching your spine long, until your torso rests on your thighs and your forehead rests on the floor. (Pregnant women can do this pose by opening the knees to make room for the belly.) Relax your arms so they rest at your sides, elbows slightly bent, palms up. Breathe deeply and make any small adjustments necessary for your comfort. If your head is uncomfortable, try folding your arms in front of your forehead and resting your hands on your arms. Close your eyes and hold the position through several cycles of breathing.

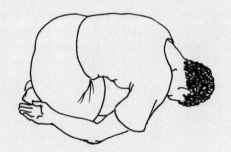

Child's Pose

Wide-Angle Legs-Up-the-Wall Pose

This exercise opens up the pelvic region, boosts circulation to the female reproductive system, helps varicose veins, and relieves fluid retention in the legs and feet.

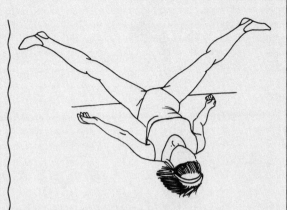

Wide-Angle Legs-Up-the-Wall Pose

Lie on your back with your legs up against the wall and your arms out comfortably at your sides, palms facing up. (Pregnant women shouldn't do this or any exercise lying on the back after their fourth month.) Be sure your hips are as close as possible to the wall, with your buttocks resting on the floor. Extend your legs out gently as far as possible, so that they form a V. Allow the inner thighs to relax, and stay in this position through 5 to 10 cycles of breathing. Then gently bring your legs together and hold for a few cycles of breathing.

Cobbler's Pose

This pose can be helpful in relieving menstrual discomfort, since it opens up the pelvic region and improves circulation to the reproductive tract.

Sit on one or two folded blankets with your legs stretched out straight in front of you. Extend your spine so that you're "sitting tall" and keep your head straight, gazing forward. Bend your knees and place the soles of your feet together, holding on to your toes or ankles and bringing your heels as close as possible to your body. Focus on pressing

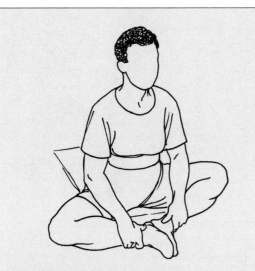

Cobbler's Pose

your knees down toward the ground, while stretching your torso up and opening your chest. Hold this position through several cycles of breathing, then release.

Lying-Down Cobbler's Pose

This is a restorative version of the cobbler's pose.

Sit facing a wall with the soles of your feet together and knees apart. Curl your toes back and press them against a wall. Place a bolster or several rolled blankets lengthwise behind your back and gently lie back over it with an extra blanket under your head if you want. Keep your arms out gently to your sides, or raise them over your head, palms facing up. Hold for several cycles of breathing. When you are ready to get up, turn gently onto your side and push against the floor with your hands.

Wall Hang

This pose reverses gravity's usual pull on the head and back, relaxing those muscles, improving circulation to the brain, and stimulating the pituitary gland, which may relieve some perimenopausal symptoms.

Stand about twelve inches from the wall, with your feet about hip width apart, then lean back and rest your buttocks against the wall. Inhale, then exhale and bend forward. Fold your elbows and let the weight of your arms and torso gently pull your upper body down. Relax your head so it hangs without effort. Lift your toes and spread them out

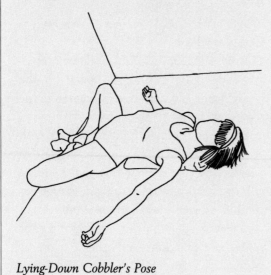

Lying-Down Cobbler's Pose

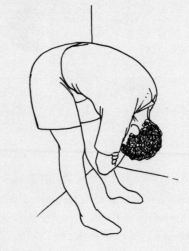

Wall Hang

against the floor to fully support your weight. Be sure to keep your legs straight and activate the quadriceps muscles in the front of your thighs to support your knees. Breathe deeply as you feel the muscles in the back of your legs release. Allow your spine to lengthen and gently shake your head to release tension in your neck. Relax in this position for a minute or two, and when you are ready to rise, inhale as you walk your hands up your legs until you're in a standing position.

9

Respiratory Disorders

ASTHMA AND CHRONIC OBSTRUCTIVE PULMONARY DISEASE

For most of us it's automatic—something we do without thinking, awake or asleep, every minute of every day: *Breathe in, breathe out.*

But for the more than 30 million Americans who suffer from a chronic respiratory disease, this most basic of bodily functions can become a terrifying struggle for air. Many breathing disorders—such as asthma, emphysema, and chronic bronchitis—result in obstruction to normal airflow, producing oxygen starvation. A sense of suffocation may produce panic, making the breath quicken and the airways constrict. With normal lungs, these changes promote a more efficient fight-or-flight physiology. But with abnormal lungs, these changes make

breathing less efficient, compounding the oxygen deficiency. Furthermore, in a progressive struggle to breathe, the mechanics of the chest cavity and the sheer work of moving air inefficiently through abnormal airways may compromise heart function. This can make the fight for air even harder and the sense of terror greater.

Restoring and promoting more normal breathing patterns is one of the dramatic benefits that certain forms of exercise can offer people with these conditions. Frequently, mind-body activities, such as yoga or relaxation exercises, are the first steps by which physical movement can play a therapeutic role for individuals suffering from respiratory disorders.

In addition to helping combat psychological distress, physical activity also may help remedy many of the physiologic abnormalities of breathing disorders. Regular aerobic activity can help boost heart and lung efficiency and build endurance. Fear of exercise, however, is a common problem for people with respiratory disorders. Many asthmatics are afraid to exert themselves because physical activity can trigger an attack. People with chronic bronchitis or emphysema may be so short of breath just getting through the activities of daily living that they assume they don't have enough "wind" to benefit from additional movement or even gentle exercise.

Inactivity promotes a vicious cycle. People who are sedentary get progressively more out of condition. Muscles weaken, the heart and lungs lose tone and efficiency, and self-esteem deflates to the point where exercise may seem impossible. Additionally, myths still abound about breathing disorders, including the false notion that people with respiratory ailments shouldn't exercise. Years ago, standard medical advice cautioned people with respiratory conditions to avoid exertion, which could trigger symptoms such as coughing, breathlessness, and wheezing. Over the past several decades, however, the benefits of movement in improving abnormal breathing have been widely recognized. Currently, supervised and self-administered exercise programs have become an integral part of treatment programs. With the development of self-care strategies and medications to help control symptoms, most people with breathing disorders can participate in exercise programs to improve their general health and help manage their disease. Regular exercise can boost airflow and blood flow, increase strength and stamina, improve the efficiency of the cardiorespiratory system, relieve

stress, enhance energy, improve sleep, and brighten mood. And for some breathing disorders, including asthma, becoming fit may even decrease the need for medication and reduce the frequency of symptoms.

In this chapter we'll explore how to apply healing moves to two main forms of respiratory disease:

✳ *Asthma.* An inflammatory condition of the lungs, asthma is characterized by overly sensitive airways that react to a wide range of triggers, including allergens, temperature change, stress, exertion, and hormonal fluctuations. One of the most vexing modern health problems, the incidence of asthma is increasing at an alarming rate throughout the developed world.

✳ *Chronic obstructive pulmonary disease (COPD).* This umbrella term includes two main conditions, chronic bronchitis and emphysema, which manifest as obstruction of airflow and restriction of air movement, respectively. Many people with this diagnosis have both disorders. Unlike asthma, the abnormalities underlying COPD syndromes are largely irreversible. A progressive lung disease, COPD is frequently caused or worsened by smoking, infection, or exposure to pollutants.

THE ASTHMA-ACTIVITY CONNECTION

Some say it's like trying to suck peanut butter through a straw. Others describe it as feeling like their lungs are on fire or that a demon is crushing their chest or choking their neck. Sufferers cough, wheeze, and gasp in an often-panicked attempt to simply take a breath.

Asthma attacks can be frightening and, at their worst, fatal. More than five thousand Americans die annually from this chronic lung inflammation, which has become one of the fastest-growing, most pervasive public health problems in the nation. Since 1980, asthma cases have more than doubled, affecting an estimated 5.3 percent of adults and 6.3 percent of children, making it the most common chronic illness of childhood and the leading cause of hospitalization for youngsters. Current estimates are that 15 million Americans suffer from asthma, compared with just 6.8 million in 1980. Asthma mortality increased by 45 percent between 1985 and 1995, with the death rate for black Americans almost three times that of whites.

Why this dramatic rise? Health officials are scrambling to find out. While many theories exist, increasingly experts are calling asthma a disease of civilization, because it's virtually unheard of in preindustrial societies. With increasing urbanization comes increasing incidence of asthma, typically more common in cities than in rural areas. While some blame urban air pollution, experts note that outdoor air pollution levels have actually *improved* in many areas over the last few decades. *Indoor* air pollution, however, may be a prime culprit since our modern, tightly sealed, energy-efficient homes are often packed with allergens— such as dust mites, molds, pet dander, and cockroach droppings—which can trigger asthma attacks.

Not only are our homes and offices full of allergens but we're spending more and more time indoors sitting and less and less time outdoors moving. One of the newest theo-

ries to explain the explosive growth in asthma incidence points to our increasingly sedentary lifestyle, with its resulting epidemic of obesity. Harvard Medical School assistant professor Carlos Camargo studied the connection and found that during the same time period that asthma rates skyrocketed, so did obesity. "Both diseases follow an intriguing pattern," Camargo notes. "The richer the country, the more obesity and asthma. But within the richer countries, it's the poorer people who have more asthma and obesity."

When Camargo explored this link, he found that obesity increases the risk of asthma in adult women and in children. His study of 16,862 children, ages nine to fourteen, concluded that the most overweight kids were two to three times as likely to have asthma as the least overweight kids. His research on 116,678 adult women found similar results.

Exactly how obesity increases asthma risk is unclear, Camargo says, "but it may be related to a sedentary lifestyle. In the lab we've shown that if you take really shallow breaths your airways can close down. When kids sit and watch TV for hours on end, their breathing tends to become shallow, which may increase bronchial reactivity and airway irritation."

This notion represents a startling reversal of past assumptions about obesity and asthma. Physicians have long recognized that people with asthma tend to be overweight. But the conventional wisdom has been that weight gain occurs because many asthmatics avoid exercise, since physical activity can trigger symptoms. Today, however, new evidence suggests that sedentary lifestyles and excess weight may not simply be the *result* of asthma, but a *cause* of this increasingly common disease.

BREATHING BASICS

The primary function of breathing is an exhange of gases, bringing nourishing oxygen into the body and eliminating carbon dioxide waste. In normal respiration the action of muscles in the chest, diaphragm, and abdomen makes the lungs expand, drawing in fresh air. Oxygen molecules in the air pass through delicate membranes that line both the airways and tiny blood vessels called capillaries. These oxygen molecules are retained by hemoglobin proteins in blood cells, which are then pumped by the heart to all the organs and cells of the body as oxygenated ("red") blood. In the presence of needy tissues, hemoglobin releases the oxygen molecules. The deoxygenated blood cells are then pumped by the heart back to the lungs to be reoxygenated, in the continuous blood movement called circulation. During this process, other by-products of cell metabolism, such as carbon dioxide, are passed from the cells out to the airways as gaseous waste for elimination. This breathing in of oxygenated air, percolation of air and blood cells, and breathing out of carbon dioxide waste is the central activity of the normal process of respiration.

In people with respiratory disorders, as lung tissue and airways become progressively abnormal, very high pressures in the chest may develop. This can reduce the flow of blood through the lungs and decrease the amount of fresh air pulled through the airways. Changes in pressure and airflow can result in the fresh air going to one section of the lungs, while the needy, "blue" blood percolates through a different section, an abnormality called ventilation-perfusion mismatch. With compromised airflow, gas by-products like carbon dioxide may not be exhaled efficiently, and may therefore take up space in the airways, preventing inhaled fresh air from reaching the blood vessel capillaries altogether. Combined, these abnormalities of respiration can result in symptomatic or dangerous drops in blood oxygen levels, compromising muscle activity, energy levels, and organ function and, at extremes, causing death.

ASTHMA BASICS

Asthma is an inflammatory condition of the lungs in which there is at least a partially reversible obstruction of airflow. People with asthma have hyperreactive, easily irritated airways, so that certain individualized "triggers"—such as an allergen or cold, dry air—can set off an immune response that narrows these breathing passages and can shut them down. During an asthma "attack," three changes take place that make breathing difficult:

1. Muscles surrounding the bronchial tubes constrict and become "twitchy" with spasms, which may make it hard to exhale through the narrowed air passages.
2. The tissues that line the bronchial tubes become irritated and swollen, just as your skin does when you get scratch or scrape, further narrowing the air passages.
3. Mucus that normally lubricates and cleans the airways is produced in excess.

This thick, sticky substance tends to clog up and even close off the breathing passages.

Asthma attacks can range from severe, persistent, and life threatening to mild, intermittent, and merely annoying—with the entire spectrum in between. Someone having a severe attack may have trouble talking and their lips and fingernails might turn a grayish or bluish color from lack of oxygen in the blood. With severe asthma, if they don't take medication immediately or if they wait too long to get to an emergency room for treatment, the condition can progress and even be life threatening.

Much more common are moderate and mild attacks, which produce symptoms such as chest tightness, breathlessness, coughing, and wheezing (the air makes a whistling sound when you breathe). Asthma episodes sometimes clear up on their own, but often medication is necessary to open, or "dilate," the airways. Attacks can last from a few minutes to several hours or even days. Sometimes people experience a "second wave" attack after the first appears to ease up.

No one knows why people get asthma, although heredity appears to plays a strong role and asthma tends to run in families. While about half of those with the condition get their first symptoms before age ten, asthma can develop at any age. The condition is very different from one person to another, and from one attack to another. Each person's symptoms and triggers are so unique that some experts refer to an individual's asthma "fingerprint"—their personal profile of stimuli that can set off an asthma attack. The number one asthma trigger is allergy, and the most common allergens include dust mites, animal (especially cat) dander, cockroach droppings, molds, pollen, smoke, aspirin, environmental irritants (such as paints, perfumes, and detergents), sulfites, and other food additives. Other asthma triggers include colds and other respiratory infections, temperature change, exertion, stress, and strong emotional responses such as laughing, crying, and yelling.

Asthma is often difficult to diagnose and is sometimes called the "great pretender" because its symptoms are similar to a wide range of ailments, from bronchitis and heart conditions to panic attacks. As a result, asthma often goes undetected and untreated. In a physician's office, a device called a spirometer, which tests free air movement, is used to detect airway obstruction. At home, or on an athletic field, a handheld gadget called a peak-flow meter can measure airflow and help make the diagnosis. While there is no cure, asthma is very controllable today, largely through modern medications, self-care strategies, elimination of asthma triggers from the environment, and structured exercise programs.

EXERCISE-INDUCED ASTHMA

Most people with asthma will experience symptoms when they exercise very vigorously. Some people *only* experience asthma symptoms during or after vigorous exercise. When strenuous activity triggers asthma, the condition is called **exercise-induced asthma (EIA)**. EIA affects an estimated 70 to 90 percent of asthmatics and roughly 12 to 15 percent of the general population—many of whom aren't aware they have the disorder. Since many people assume that breathlessness during exercise means that they're out of shape, EIA frequently goes undetected, even among Olympic athletes. For example, when champion swimmer Nancy Hogshead would pass out after a hard workout or when her face would turn purple from exertion, she attributed the problem to not trying hard enough or being out of condition—even though she swam up to eight hundred laps a day. It wasn't until after she won three gold medals and a silver at the 1984 Olympics that a doctor recognized that her breathing difficulties came from the increasingly recognized condition EIA.

"I was stunned and thought the man was crazy," Hogshead recalls in her book *Exercise and Asthma* (Henry Holt, 1990). But when she tried medication before exercise, she was "amazed that people could breathe this easily, so effortlessly." Like many people with EIA (including an estimated 11 percent of all Olympic-level athletes), Hogshead controls her condition by taking two puffs from a prescription drug inhaler twenty minutes before swimming, playing tennis, or beginning any other vigorous activity.

EIA can be tricky to diagnose because some people experience symptoms only seasonally. Allergic individuals may have problems just during the summer, when pollen counts rise. Others may experience EIA only in winter, since aerobic activity in cold, dry air is one of the strongest triggers for the disorder. Some people's symptoms emerge only when they're tired, under stress, or fighting a cold. Frequently active people don't—or won't—acknowledge that their symptoms may indicate asthma. It's not uncommon for athletes to resist seeking help, in part because numerous myths still surround asthma, including the notion that it's a debilitating, limiting condition. Some competitors think EIA is a weakness on their part that they'd rather not acknowledge. Yet many world-class athletes use medication to control their asthma. With proper medical management, there is virtually no sport or exercise that a person with asthma can't do. And there's no limit to their success, as evidenced by the forty-one medals won by athletes with EIA on the 1984 U.S. Olympic team.

HOW EXERCISE HELPS

It seems like a paradox: Exercise can trigger asthma, yet it also can help prevent attacks. For many years, concern about provoking symptoms led physicians to advise asthmatics to avoid exertion. Yet today experts acknowledge that—*unlike other asthma triggers—physical activity should not be avoided.* Even though vigorous exercise may trigger asthma, the condition can be controlled through medications and other strategies. And the benefits are so important that asthmatics are now typically encouraged to exercise at least moderately for overall good health and to help relieve their symptoms. Numerous studies have shown that regular physical activity can decrease the frequency and severity of asthma attacks, reduce the use of medications, cut down on absences from school and work, and improve the quality of life. "Exercise is not only safe if done properly, it's an integral part of [asthma] treatment," notes the *Physician and Sportsmedicine Journal* in a special guide to exercising with asthma. "Regular work-outs will make you stronger and more ener-getic . . . [and] your asthma is likely to improve."

Exercise is medicine for people with asthma for a variety of reasons. Predominant among them is the recognition that much of the abnormality causing symptoms with asthma stems from *reversible physiological reactions*. Exercise can be a powerful way of influencing the reversible components of this physiological response. For example, regular exercise promotes conditioned responses that dilate the airways. In addi-tion, other elements of exercise, such as structured warm-ups, positive feelings of relaxation and enjoyment, and the general health and positive self-image associated with fitness, may reduce or prevent the abnormal airway response called asthma.

Regular exercise also conditions and strengthens the heart and lungs, which boosts endurance, breathing efficiency, and stamina. The normal response to exercise is that your airways will open or dilate. Being fit enhances this bronchodilating effect, while being out of condition can weaken it. A sedentary lifestyle can also lead to shallow breathing, which may play a role in devel-oping the condition. And less fit people are more likely to be overweight, which may put them at increased risk for asthma. Excessive weight can make it harder to expand the lungs, restricting the contribu-tion of the abdominal muscles to breathing mechanics. Exercising to lose and maintain weight may also help people breathe easier.

Regular exercise can be a positive influ-ence on many other factors that can con-tribute to ill health for people with this complex condition. As a group, people with asthma tend to be physically unfit, often because they avoid exercise to keep from triggering symptoms. The vicious cycle of inactivity, mentioned earlier, leads not only to a weak cardiorespiratory system and weight gain but to psychological issues such as depression, anger, and low-self esteem—all of which can trigger asthma symptoms and attacks.

Regular physical activity can enhance mental health and help boost mood (see chapter 3, Mental Health Conditions, page 89). In particular, physical activity helps relieve stress, which *itself* can be a trigger for asthma. "Letting off steam" and balancing emotions through exercise also may provide relief, since strong emotions—such as rage and hysteria—can provoke symptoms. Yoga can be particularly helpful for asthma suffer-ers, since it centers on deep, focused breath-ing and tension relief. Yoga breathing can help people deal with the "fear factor" in asthma, by providing calming strategies to relieve tension and enhance airflow. Other physical activities that center around mind-body balance and breath control—including karate, qi gong, and tai chi—may also bene-fit people with asthma. Learning relaxation techniques and breathing skills can help counter the panic that can trigger and accompany an asthma attack.

By boosting confidence and enhancing self-image, exercise can keep people with asthma in the mainstream of society. This can be especially critical for youngsters with the condition, who—in years past—frequently were restricted from participat-ing in active games at recess or in physical education classes. And by improving overall fitness and reducing the risk of other chronic diseases, regular physical activity can play a uniquely therapeutic role in the lifestyle of all children and adults with asthma.

EXERCISE ℞ FOR ASTHMA

The exercise goal for people with asthma is similar to the recommendation for anyone who desires basic good health: Work your way up to doing at least 30 minutes of an aerobic activity—such as walking or swimming—most days of the week. *It's particularly important for people with asthma to discuss their exercise program with their health-care provider, especially if vigorous exercise tends to bring on symptoms.* Many people with chronic asthma benefit from taking preventive medications, and those with EIA are often advised to take a few puffs from a prescription inhaler before strenuous activity. (Also, if you've been sedentary and plan to start a program of *vigorous* exercise, it's essential that you check with your doctor.)

In addition to medications, there are many self-care strategies that can help people with asthma avoid symptoms during physical activity. A central strategy is picking a form of exercise that is less likely to induce symptoms. Swimming and aqua-aerobics are often recommended as ideal for people with asthma because the water tends to moisten the air that is inhaled, making it less likely to trigger symptoms. It's important to recognize that, for many people with EIA, symptoms occur most often about five to ten minutes after they begin doing a continuous, vigorous activity. This is the point at which many people begin to breathe through the mouth instead of the nose. The nose serves as a sort of "air conditioner," humidifying and filtering inhaled air. The mouth can't perform these functions, which means that air inhaled through the mouth tends to be dryer and cooler. Cool, dry air tends to irritate the airways of sensitive individuals, prompting an asthma attack. The moist, humid environment of the swimming pool or open water minimizes these problems.

Sports that involve brief intervals of activity, with rests in between, also may be less likely to provoke symptoms. Examples of these "stop and go" activities include racquet sports, football, volleyball, half-court basketball, softball, gymnastics, golf, and wrestling. Many people with EIA find vigorous activity, such as running, more problematic than moderate activity, such as walking. Allergic individuals may need to consider indoor options during pollen time, such as racquetball instead of outdoor tennis.

But the most important factor in choosing an activity is to *pick something you enjoy.* If you enjoy and have fun doing your activity, you're more likely to do it regularly and receive both the physical and mental benefits of exercise. So while it's important to take your condition into consideration, remember that many athletes with asthma have succeeded in sports that can provoke attacks (such as outdoor running) by working with their physician and being conscientious about taking medication and following other strategies to keep their symptoms under control.

Other important self-care strategies for exercising with asthma include:

* **Start slowly and progress gradually.** If you've been sedentary, don't try to exercise for 30 minutes all at once. Do as much as you comfortably can, even if it's just 2 minutes. Then gradually add a few more minutes each week until, eventually, you're exercising for 30 minutes. (See Healing Moves to Breathe Easy, page 298.)

* **Don't skip the warm-up or the cooldown.** Important for everyone, these "exercise-adjustment periods" are especially critical for people with asthma because they gradually prepare the body for exertion. Workouts should always start with a warm-up of at least 5 to 10 minutes, consisting of light and easy activity—such as walking or slow laps—and gentle stretching. Many people with EIA report fewer symptoms if they've had a good warm-up. An adequate cooldown also is essential to avoid rapid changes in blood pressure, which can strain the heart. It may also help prevent asthma symptoms that can occur immediately following an exercise session.

* **Check the climate.** The temperature, humidity, and quality of air may all affect your symptoms. If you know that cold air triggers coughing, consider wearing a mask or scarf over your nose and mouth to humidify the air you breathe before exercising outdoors in cold weather. If pollution "sets you off," walk in a park or on a trail instead of along a road or highway, or try walking early in the morning before traffic and heat raise pollutants to their highest levels.

* **Plan for "bad-air" days.** Having a "backup workout" can help you keep your exercise habit, even on bad-air days. For example, if the pollen count is too high for you to go for your daily walk or if there's a smog alert, don't just skip exercise entirely. Do an exercise video inside in the air-conditioning, or consider buying a summer membership to your local gym.

* **The nose knows.** Whenever possible, try to breathe through your nose, to keep air moist and filtered.

* **Pace yourself.** Get to know your asthma "fingerprint" and try to regulate the intensity and duration of your activity to avoid symptoms, especially during times of stress or fatigue. For example, if you're under work pressure or exhausted, you may want to skip your regular aerobics class and go for an easy walk instead. When symptoms are particularly bothersome (if you're wheezing or coughing) or if you're fighting a cold, it may be advisable to skip exercise.

* **Consider self-monitoring.** People with moderate to severe asthma, and competitive athletes who want to train intensively, can consult their physician about using a peak-flow meter to monitor their condition themselves.

* **Stay well hydrated.** Don't wait until you're thirsty to drink. Good hydration keeps airway secretions thinner so they can lubricate the airways. Thick, dry secretions, on the other hand, may plug up airways. Guidelines from the American College of Sports Medicine recommend drinking seventeen ounces of fluid two hours before exercise and drinking five to twelve ounces every fifteen to twenty minutes during activity. Also, rehydrate after exercise to replenish fluids lost during activity.

✳ *Practice breathing and relaxation exercises daily.* Pick a convenient time (such as first thing in the morning or upon getting home from work) and get in the habit of taking a few minutes for deep-breathing and relaxation practices. Use these strategies anytime you need to quiet your mind and reduce stress.

COPD BASICS

Chronic obstructive pulmonary disease, or COPD, is a general term used to describe progressive lung diseases such as emphysema and chronic bronchitis. Characterized by predominantly irreversible obstruction to airflow, COPD affects an estimated 15 million Americans and is responsible for 200,000 deaths annually. Cigarette smoking is by far the most common cause, although some disease results from infection and exposure to environmental irritants. Ideally, the irreparable injury to the lungs that produces COPD would be prevented by avoiding cigarette smoking or other toxic exposures. In men over forty, COPD is second only to coronary heart disease as a cause of disability.

Most people with COPD have both chronic bronchitis and emphysema, although some people have more of one than the other. Here are some basic facts about each of these lung diseases:

✳ *Chronic bronchitis.* About five percent of Americans, or 14 million people, have this condition, which is characterized by a recurrent inflammation of the lining of the large airways, called the bronchial tubes. The main cause is irritation from cig-

arette smoke, although it can also result from exposure to industrial dusts and fumes, air pollution, or infection. (Coal miners, grain handlers, and other workers who constantly breathe in dust are at high risk for the disease.) When this lung irritation continues over a long period of time, the bronchial wall linings thicken and secrete excess mucus and an irritating cough develops as people try to bring up phlegm. Airflow is obstructed and the bronchial tubes become a festering breeding ground for infection.

Many people develop a brief attack of bronchitis when they have a cold. The disease is classified as chronic bronchitis when someone has a mucus-producing cough most days of the month, three months a year, for two successive years without other underlying disease to explain the cough.

✳ *Emphysema.* Characterized by an enlargement of the lungs and progressively worsening breathlessness, emphysema results from destruction of the walls of the smallest airways, the alveoli, or air sacs, in the lungs. As air sacs are destroyed, the lungs lose their elasticity and are able to transfer less and less oxygen into the bloodstream, causing shortness of breath and difficulty in exhaling. Coughing is a common symptom, but there is little sputum. As people work harder to get the same amount of air into their lungs, they burn substantially more calories and often lose weight. In severe cases, people become emaciated, with enlarged chests.

Typically, the disease is caused by smoking, but a small percentage of cases are linked to a genetic deficiency of a protein known as alpha₁-antitrypsin (AAT), which can lead to an inherited form of emphysema. The condition comes on gradually, usually after years of exposure to cigarette smoke. The first sign is often breathlessness during exercise, but over time even the activities of daily living can cause shortness of breath. An estimated two million Americans have emphysema, which historically has mostly afflicted men. It is becoming more common among women, however, as the rate of female smokers increases.

HOW EXERCISE HELPS

Quitting smoking and eliminating exposure to environmental irritants are obviously the two most important factors in relieving COPD. But getting regular physical activity can also play an important role. While exercise cannot reverse the damage done by the disease, it can reduce disability by improving endurance and breathing efficiency, especially in severely impaired patients. Aerobic activity, such as walking or dancing, strengthens the heart and lungs, as well as other muscles. Breathing exercises can also help tone and condition the muscles involved in respiration, while teaching people with COPD how to move air in and out of their lungs with less effort.

With regular aerobic exercise, even people with severe impairments have been able to increase their exercise tolerance. For example, in one study, people with COPD who participated in an exercise program for eight weeks nearly doubled the amount of time they were able to walk on a treadmill—from 12.5 minutes to 23 minutes. Plus, regular exercise can also help by enhancing appetite. This can be particularly important for COPD patients, who often have problems with poor nutrition because the disease frequently interferes with their ability to eat properly.

The benefits that result from regular exercise reflect both physiological and psychological factors, since the decline in function associated with COPD can be emotionally devastating. As COPD progresses and people find activity increasingly difficult, many stop moving. This exacerbates the problem because they get out of condition, which makes exercise even harder. This vicious cycle of inactivity (similar to that mentioned earlier involving people with asthma) results in further weakening and fatigue, often accompanied by depression and low self-esteem. As regular exercise boosts people's ability to do more physical activity, it also typically enhances mood and self-confidence. Some research indicates that COPD patients who exercise regularly can work out at harder levels before experiencing shortness of breath. Since breathlessness can be related to emotions—such as fear and anxiety—this increased tolerance for dyspnea (the medical term for shortness of breath) may reflect the patients' enhanced confidence in their ability to exercise and carry out the activities of daily life.

Exercise also can play an important role in helping people with COPD break their dependence on cigarettes. Amazingly, many people with advanced lung disease continue to smoke, unable to quit even though they know the habit makes their condition worse. Growing evidence shows that engaging in a regular exercise program can help people kick cigarettes, most likely as a result of varied physiologic and psychological changes that accompany getting fit. A rehabilitation program with exercise is one of the most helpful steps people with COPD can take to break their smoking habit and enhance their health.

EXERCISE ℞ FOR COPD

People with COPD should discuss their exercise programs with their health-care provider, who may recommend using prescription medications, monitors, or supplemental oxygen during exercise. Since most people with COPD tend to be older, they frequently have other chronic conditions that may affect their ability to exercise, which makes it even more crucial that they design an exercise program in partnership with a physician. People with severe impairment may be directed to a supervised rehabilitation program, where a doctor, nurse, respiratory therapist, or physical therapist will help them become physically active. Often these patients can "graduate" to independent exercise after as little as six weeks of guidance.

Walking is one of the easiest, best physical activities for people with COPD, although other forms of aerobic activity, such as stationary cycling, swimming, or water aerobics, may also be effective. Discuss your exercise plan with your physician and ask him or her how much exercise is right for you. For many patients with COPD, an appropriate goal is to work your way up to doing an aerobic exercise for 20 to 30 minutes, three days a week.

Be sure you:

✳ *Wear supportive, appropriate athletic shoes and loose, comfortable clothing.*

✳ *Choose a well-ventilated environment*—outdoors on a nice day or in your home, a wellness facility, or shopping mall.

✳ *Start slowly and progress gradually.* For example, begin by taking a short walk as far as you can go without getting breathless. If you can walk for only 2 minutes at first, that's fine. Add a few more minutes each week, and as long as you're consistent, improvements will come. (If you can only go less than 5 minutes without getting short of breath, you may want to consider doing two short sessions on your exercise days.)

✳ *Always warm up and cool down.* Prepare your body for exercise with some easy movements. Then stretch gently before you do your aerobic activity. Don't stop moving abruptly. Cool down at the end of your session with some gentle movements.

✳ *Practice breathing and relaxation exercises daily.* Pick a convenient time each day to do some simple breathing and relaxation techniques. (See Healing Moves to Breathe Easy, page 298.) Use these practices anytime during the day when you feel agitated and short of breath.

✳ *Quit smoking.* Instead of lighting up, try getting moving.

CAUTIONS

If you have a chronic respiratory disease, it is essential that you discuss your exercise with your health-care provider. He or she can help you establish an appropriate exercise program and prescribe necessary medications and devices that can allow you to be active enough to reach your fitness goals. People with severe impairment and/or other chronic diseases may benefit from starting a physical-activity program in a supervised setting.

PRESCRIPTION PAD

✳ **Exercise ℞ for asthma:** Work your way up to doing at least 30 minutes of an aerobic activity—such as walking or swimming—most days of the week. (Be sure to use prescribed medications, if necessary, before activity.) Practice breathing and relaxation exercises daily.

✳ *Exercise ℞ for COPD:* Work your way up to doing aerobic exercise for 20 to 30 minutes three days a week. Practice breathing and relaxation exercises daily.

ADDITIONAL RESOURCES

✳ The Asthma and Allergy Foundation of America Helpline, 800-7-ASTHMA; Web site: www.aafa.org.

✳ National Heart, Lung, and Blood Institute Information Center, 301-592-8573; Web site: www.nhlbi.nih.gov.

✳ National Jewish Medical and Research Center, 800-222-LUNG; Web site: www.njc.org.

✳ The American Lung Association, 800-LUNG-USA; Web site: www.lungusa.org.

✳ American Yoga Association, P.O. Box 19986, Sarasota, Fla. 34276. For information about yoga for asthma, send a self-addressed, business-sized envelope, stamped with 55 cents postage.

✳ ✳ ✳

HEALING MOVES TO BREATHE EASY

✳

Many years ago you were an expert. In fact, most babies are masters of the gentle art of breathing. To study a pro in action, watch a sleeping infant: the inhalation and exhalation are deep and even, slow and easy, with the abdomen ballooning out and in, the rhythmic flow as steady and constant as waves on sand.

Yet many of us lose these breathing skills with age as stress, poor posture, tight clothing, cultural influences, and health problems take hold. By the time we're adults, most of us have developed unhealthy habits, such as unconsciously holding and restricting our breath or breathing shallowly from the chest, instead of deeply from the abdomen. Stressful and tiring for the average person, these disordered breathing patterns can be especially problematic for people with respiratory diseases who are, all too often, locked in a desperate struggle for air. That's why a foundation of treatment for people with breathing-related ailments is breaking bad breathing habits and relearning this most basic of bodily functions.

Our Healing Moves to Breathe Easy are designed to relieve symptoms of respiratory disease, boost lung capacity, and increase the efficiency of your cardiorespiratory system through three practices:

Part One: Breathing Lessons

Most people know that the way they breathe affects two of their body's systems: respiratory and cardiovascular. But many are unaware that their *breathing patterns also affect virtually every system in the body*, including the neurological, gastrointestinal, muscular, and metabolic. Enhancing breathing can benefit the entire body and provide the optimum setting for physical and mental well-being. This section explores some of the most common breathing problems and provides a step-by-step approach to healthy breathing technique.

Part Two: Aerobic Activity

Aerobic literally means "with oxygen," and *aerobic activity* refers to any form of exercise (such as walking or swimming) that demands large quantities of air for prolonged periods. When you do aerobic exercise regularly, it stimulates your body to strengthen the systems responsible for transporting oxygen. The result is a stronger, more efficient heart and lungs, increased endurance, and more stamina—helpful for anyone, but particular beneficial for people with respiratory disease. Since exercise can trigger symptoms for people with breathing disorders, we offer a "pros and cons" list of aerobic options to help you pick the best form of exercise for your particular condition.

Part Three: Mind-Body Moves

An important contributor to breathing problems is the psychological impact of stress, which can both trigger and result from the symptoms of respiratory disease. We present several mind-body moves designed to help you calm and center yourself, relax tight muscles, open airways, and restore your entire being to a harmonious balance.

PART ONE: BREATHING LESSONS

Breathing isn't something most people think about, partly because it's so easy you can do it in your sleep. But yogis have known for centuries—and modern studies confirm—that breathing provides a powerful link between body and mind. In times of stress, be it childbirth or work deadlines, proper breathing is an unsurpassed tension buster. Concentrating on the flow of air in and out of the body can help you focus attention, improve performance, and even relieve pain.

As yoga master B. K. S. Iyengar explains in his classic guide *Light on Yoga: "Regulate the breathing, and thereby control the mind."*

Yogis teach that the way people breathe influences every part of their physical and mental health. Proper breathing is the foundation of health, while disordered breathing can contribute to a wide variety of ailments, including depression, insomnia, headache, and asthma. Some breathing experts estimate that up to half of all adults in industrialized, Western cultures are dysfunctional breathers, which may help explain the prevalence of these health problems in urbanized society.

The most common breathing problem is the tendency to be a *chest breather* rather than an *abdominal breather*. To test yourself, take a deep breath and notice what happens. If you're like many Americans, you'll suck in your gut and throw out your chest. That's because our culture teaches people to hold their stomachs tight, which impairs breathing. *Proper breathing expands the abdomen, allowing the deepest part of the lungs to fill.* The ribs and chest also swell out as the lungs inflate fully, much like twin balloons.

Another common breathing problem is shallow, rapid breathing. This can be a result of chest breathing, which doesn't allow the lungs to fill completely, or it may occur as a reaction to stress or other forms of emotional distress. Rapid breathing is just one of the many physiological changes that are triggered when tension strikes and the body's sympathetic nervous system prepares you to "fight or flee": your heart rate speeds up, blood pressure rises, muscles tense, blood vessels constrict, and respiration accelerates.

Deep breathing can break this stress pattern and help restore a peaceful equilibrium to body and mind. Because of all the varied responses to stress, *respiration alone is both involuntary and voluntary.* Your body will breathe by itself, without conscious effort. But you also can control your breathing, which can help you control these other reactions as well. Taking a deep, slow breath will help lower your blood pressure and heart rate, relax your muscles, and ease your mind. And for people with respiratory disorders, such as asthma, taking several slow, calming breaths can help relieve—and sometimes prevent—an attack.

Inhaling through the nose (avoiding "mouth breathing") also can be helpful for people with respiratory disorders. The nose functions as an "air conditioner" that humidifies and filters inhaled air. When air comes into the body from the mouth, it doesn't gain the benefit of this filtration process and may be drier or contain more pollutants, which can trigger symptoms in susceptible people. (People with COPD may find that

exhaling through the mouth with pursed lips when they feel short of breath helps reduce anxiety and sensations of breathlessness.)

A related problem that affects breathing is our tendency to have bad posture and sedentary habits, which keeps us from being able to fill our lungs deeply and fully. Sitting slumped over a computer keyboard all day compresses the lungs and impairs respiration. Plus, when people are inactive for long periods of time, their breathing often becomes shallow, which may increase bronchial reactivity and airway irritation. Proper posture—plus stretching and breathing breaks—can help "air out" our bodies and minds. Similarly, standing with good posture and even sleeping properly (on the back or side) is important to allow the lungs to expand fully and completely. (For a detailed explanation of proper posture and posture exercises, see Healing Moves to Strengthen Muscles and Bones, page 149.) Breathing fully and deeply also keeps the chest mobile and can help prevent the decrease in flexibility of the rib cage that can occur with age.

Today, medical science confirms what the ancients have known for thousands of years: Breathing properly enhances the body's capacity for total well-being. Follow these steps to learn the essentials of proper breathing:

1. Pay attention to posture. If you're sitting, place both feet on the floor and sit tall on your "sit bones"—don't slouch. If you're standing, keep your weight evenly distributed on both feet, slightly tuck your pelvis, extend your spine, and let your head float gently upward on your neck.

2. Place both hands on your belly, with your index fingers touching each other near your navel. Inhale and expand your belly, so it pushes against your hands. Exhale and tighten your abdominal muscles. Inhale again and allow your stomach muscles to relax as the air flows into your abdomen. Exhale deeply and visualize the air being pushed out from the bottom of your lungs.

3. Place both hands on the lower part of your rib cage, with your fingertips barely touching. Inhale and feel the air fill your abdomen, then expand into your rib cage as your fingertips move slightly apart. Exhale and feel the air flow out of your rib cage and abdomen, so that your fingertips touch again.

4. Place both hands on your chest. Inhale and feel the air expand your abdomen, then your rib cage, then your chest. Your shoulders may lift slightly as the air fills your chest. Exhale and relax the shoulders, letting the air flow out of the chest, then the rib cage, then the belly, which will tighten.

5. Relax your arms, let your hands fall gently to your sides or rest on your knees, close your eyes, and practice drawing a complete breath, being sure to inhale through your nose. Inhale from the bottom up, so that air first fills your abdomen, then rib cage, then chest. Exhale from the top down, so that air flows out of your chest, then rib cage, then belly, which will tighten at the end of the exhalation. Don't hold your breath at either the in or the out extremes, and try to make the transition as smooth and even as possible. See if you can breathe for about the same length of time both ways—in and out—but don't strain or force your breath. Concentrate on the sound and feel of the air flowing into and out of your body. If your attention wanders, gently bring it back to your breath.

6. Once you've got the hang of taking a complete breath, repeat step 5, but this time *concentrate only on breathing out*. Sometimes, too strong a focus on breathing in can make you tense. When you concentrate on breathing out and exhaling all the air from your body, you will naturally breathe in fully and completely. Your goal is to take complete breaths in a relaxed and natural state.

At first, practice this good breathing technique for 5 minutes a day. Then, when it becomes more natural, incorporate this "breathing lesson" into your daily life. Breathe consciously at regular intervals throughout the day—for example, when you're driving to work, standing in the shower, or waiting in line. Try using a regular occurrence—such as a ringing telephone or a beeper going off—to remind you to take a slow, complete breath.

(For more breathing lessons, see "relaxation breathing" in Healing Moves for Health and Fitness, page 48, and "paced respiration" in Healing Moves for Women, page 282.)

PART TWO: AEROBIC ACTIVITY

Aerobic exercise often frightens people with respiratory disorders because exertion can trigger symptoms. That's why it's essential that you develop an exercise program in partnership with your health-care provider, who may prescribe medication or devices to help you engage in activity safely. A helpful option, especially for people with severe disease, is to begin an exercise program in a supervised setting and work with an instructor who is skilled and sensitive to the concerns of people with respiratory disorders. An added benefit is the camaraderie of exercising with others who share your health concerns. For a referral to an appropriate group, ask your physician, contact a hospital-based wellness center near you, or call the resource groups listed at the end of the respiratory disorders section (page 298).

Most people with respiratory ailments can also do an appropriate aerobic activity on their own. Again, your health-care provider can help you determine how much activity is right for you and which form of aerobic exercise to choose. *Remember: The most important quality in the activity you choose is that it be fun.* If you enjoy your exercise, you're more likely to do it regularly and gain both the physical and mental benefits it can provide. Here's a list of some of the most popular aerobic exercises, with pros and cons for people with respiratory disease.

1. **Swimming.** *Pro:* This is a top choice for people with asthma, because it is the aerobic activity least likely to trigger symptoms in most people. The air near a pool or open water is moist and humid, which makes it less likely to irritate airways. A program of regular swimming can greatly increase the lung capacity. *Con:* Lap swimming may be too strenuous for people with COPD and doesn't allow the use

of supplemental oxygen that may be required. Some people may find heavy chlorination irritating.

2. **Aqua-aerobics or water walking.** *Pro:* Water exercise is another excellent choice for people with respiratory disorders because the moist, humid air is less likely to cause symptoms. For frail, older people and those with other conditions—such as obesity or joint problems—exercising in water is an excellent way to gain cardiovascular benefits with a minimum of orthopedic risk. *Con:* Water workouts don't allow use of supplemental oxygen that may be required for people with COPD.

3. **Walking.** *Pro:* This moderate form of activity is easy, convenient, and inexpensive and may be less likely to trigger symptoms than a more strenuous activity. *Con:* Outdoor walking may be problematic during bad-air days, when a switch to indoor walking on a treadmill or in a shopping mall may be preferred. (For instructions on starting a walking program, see Healing Moves for Heart Health, page 214.)

4. **Running.** *Pro:* An excellent cardiovascular workout. *Con:* Running may be too intense for people with severe disease, and outdoor running, especially longer distances—or runs during pollen season or on cold, dry days—can be the aerobic activity most likely to trigger symptoms. If you experience problems, try switching to shorter sprints, moving indoors to a treadmill, or wearing a scarf or mask to help filter and moisten inhaled air.

5. **Cycling.** *Pro:* An excellent, impact-free cardiovascular workout, cycling can be

done at varied intensities to suit an individual's conditioning and preferences. Indoor stationary bikes are particularly suited to frail people, those who need supplementary oxygen, and those with other health problems, such as obesity or osteoporosis. *Con:* Outdoor cycling during bad-air days may trigger symptoms in allergic people, who may need to use a mask to filter air or may prefer to move indoors to a stationary bike.

6. **Racquet sports:** *Pro:* The stop-and-go nature of these sports may make them less likely to provoke symptoms in susceptible people. *Con:* During pollen season or cold weather, people with respiratory conditions may find it necessary to use indoor courts to avoid triggering symptoms.

7. **Group fitness classes:** *Pro:* Usually set to music, led by a motivational instructor, and done with others, these classes typically offer an enjoyable, all-around workout that includes aerobic, strengthening, and stretching components. Because they're done indoors, in well-ventilated clubs, the air quality is good, and the presence of an instructor can help allay fears in apprehensive individuals. *Con:* Some classes may be too strenuous, so it's important to pick an appropriate level. Avoid "mob scene" workouts and those led by unqualified instructors.

8. **In-line skating.** *Pro:* An excellent, nonimpact cardiovascular workout. *Con:* May be too difficult for older, frail people and usually must be done outdoors, which may be problematic on bad-air days.

9. **Dancing.** *Pro:* A dance class that keeps you moving continuously provides a good cardiovascular workout that can also help improve balance. Typically done indoors, in well-ventilated rooms, it also provides the added motivation of music and social interaction. Line dancing is a good option for people who don't have a partner. If there is no class available or convenient, you can also just play some music at home and dance. *Con:* May be too difficult for frail people or the "choreographically challenged."

Once you've chosen your activity—or activities—here are some guidelines to starting and staying active:

1. *Discuss your exercise program and goals with your health-care provider.* Let him or her know the activity you plan to do and ask for help in setting realistic goals. Appropriate short-term goals may include: being able to walk for 10 or 15 minutes without stopping or being able to carry your groceries into your house or climb the stairs without becoming winded. Long-term goals may include: Losing 10 or 15 pounds, participating in a 5K or 10K walk or run, pedaling the equivalent of a coast-to-coast trip on your bicycle in one year.

2. *Start slowly and progress gradually.* Begin by doing a short, comfortable chunk of your activity, then add a little bit more each week so that you gradually work up to doing 20 or 30 minutes of continuous activity. Don't worry if when you start you can walk for only a few minutes, and you can add only a few feet to your exercise session each week. As long as you exercise regularly, you *will* make progress.

A reasonable amount of activity for most people with asthma is to work your way up to doing 30 minutes of aerobic activity on most days of the week. For many people with COPD, a reasonable goal to aim for is doing 20 to 30 minutes of aerobic activity three days a week

3. *Don't skip warm-ups and cooldowns.* All exercisers should warm up before activity to prepare their body for exercise and cool down afterward to help their system return to normal. This practice is particularly important for people with respiratory disorders, since many find that a good warm-up helps lessen symptoms. To warm up, do easy, gentle movements similar to what you'll be doing in your activity. For example, pedal your bike slowly, do some easy splashing around in the water, or stroll gently. This is a good time to do breathing exercises, too, being sure to take full, complete breaths. Add movement to your breathing, such as raising your arms when you inhale and lowering them when you exhale. Do some light stretching, then begin your "formal" activity session. And don't forget to cool down at the end of your workout to slow your cardiovascular system back to its resting rate. The same motions you use to warm up can help you cool back down. The end of your exercise session is also a great time to stretch, since muscles are warm and pliable.

4. *Have a backup plan so you can stick with exercise regularly.* It's all too easy to let too hot or too cold weather, lack of daylight, or other factors deter you from exercise. But regular exercise is essential to your health, so it's important to determine a fallback plan for times when you can't do your preferred activity. Here are some stumbling blocks and solutions:

Problem: There's too much pollen in the air to go outside for a walk.

Backup: Do an exercise video indoors, or walk laps around the shopping mall.

Problem: The community swimming pool is closed for repairs.

Backup: Find an alternative pool at a health club or Y, or do another activity, such as walking or dancing.

Problem: It's too cold and dark outside to bicycle.

Backup: Ride a stationary bike at home or in a wellness facility, or do another activity such as water aerobics or working out on a home exercise machine like a treadmill or cross-country ski machine.

5. *Stay well hydrated.* Drink water before and after your activity and every fifteen to twenty minutes during exercise.

6. *Protect the joy.* The physical and mental exhilaration of moving your body through space can be one of life's great joys, enhancing body, mind, and spirit. Yet all too often people wind up forcing themselves to exercise, an experience that can be an unhealthy stress. To ensure that your activity stays enjoyable, remember to:

   a. Do a form of exercise that you like
   b. Seek help from a health professional or qualified personal trainer if you need assistance in starting or sticking with your program
   c. Find an exercise buddy (human or canine)

d. Vary your activities if you start to get bored

e. Consider adding music for added motivation

f. Don't overdo it. A good rule of thumb is to increase the weekly intensity or duration of your activity by no more than 10 percent over your previous level.

g. Give yourself a weekly rest day, especially if you do a strenuous activity. Pushing yourself hard all the time is a setup for physical injury and mental burnout.

h. Listen to your body. Symptoms may flare up if you're tired or stressed, so on days when you're not "up to par," it may be advisable for you to modify and "downshift" your workout. For example, take a leisurely stroll instead of an intense bike ride. If you're wheezing or coughing or fighting a cold, consider skipping exercise entirely.

PART THREE: MIND-BODY MOVES

In many cultures, breath is understood to be much more than merely the air that goes in and out of our bodies—it is the essence of our spirit, the measure of our vitality, and a tangible manifestation of our very soul. The first action we take at birth and the final one at death, breathing is considered a sacred act that connects us with the divine.

In Chinese, the character for *breath* is comprised of three characters that mean "of the conscious self or heart." In Japan, the breath is the key to unlocking the powers of a universal energy and individual life force known as *ki*. Learning to develop and extend *ki* is central to martial arts practices—including karate and tae kwan do—and is crucial to performing "superhuman" feats, such as breaking concrete blocks or stacks of boards. Developing *ki* is also central to the healing aspects of the softer martial arts—such as qi gong and tai chi—which are designed, in part, to help strengthen the flow of *ki* (or *chi* in Chinese) throughout the body and activate our innate curative powers.

In India, an essential component of the healing art of Ayurveda is *prana*—a Sanskrit concept that is translated variously as air, life force, soul, and breath of life. Ayurveda regards breathing as especially important because it brings *prana*, or life energy, into our body from the environment. The physical postures of hatha yoga are an integral part of this healing art and are designed, in part, to use the breath to unite all the energy currents running through the body. Yoga postures, called asanas, are just one of the eight limbs (or stages) of yoga, which is designed ultimately to link the individual with the divine. The fourth limb of yoga is a practice called *pranayama*, which teaches control over all the functions of breathing—inhalation, exhalation, and retention or holding of breath. Breath is, says yoga master B. K. S. Iyengar, "the hub around which the wheel of life revolves."

Breathing is the central focus of these mind-body moves, which are inspired by these Eastern practices. They all involve *moving in harmony with the breath* and are designed to strengthen the body, soothe the nervous system, enhance respiration, and help quiet the constant "chatter" of the mind. The result is a buoyant feeling of well-being, which can help lift the depression and anxiety that is all too common in people with respiratory disease.

Seated Calming Fold

This is an easy, tranquilizing exercise for people who feel agitated and breathless.

Sit in a chair with your feet flat on the floor. Exhale completely as you bring your head down toward your knees. Count to three. Sit back up and air will rush into your lungs naturally, since your "unfolding" body acts as a kind of pump.

Child to Cat

Kneel on a comfortable mat or blanket with your weight distributed equally between your hands and knees. Be sure your arms and legs form right angles at the shoulders, hip joints, and floor. Inhale, then exhale as you move your buttocks back to your heels and fold your body so that your forehead touches the floor. Inhale as you come back to all fours, then arch your back so that your head and buttocks lift up and eyes gaze toward the ceiling. Exhale as you reverse the curve and

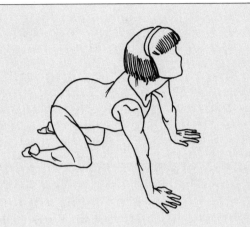

bring your buttocks back to your heels and forehead to the floor.

Repeat this sequence several times, slowly and evenly, being sure to move your body in time with your breath.

Drawing a Bow

This qi gong exercise emphasizes the chest and improves the circulation of blood and oxygen through the heart and lungs.

Stand with your feet shoulder width apart, knees slightly bent, shoulders relaxed, and arms in a circle in front of your chest with palms facing in, as if you were holding a giant ball. Inhale, then exhale as you turn your head to the left and move your left arm to the left with your fingers pointed upward and palm flat as if pressing against a wall. At the same time, make a fist with your right hand and bring it in toward your chest, while bending your right arm and extending your right elbow out toward the right, as if you were pulling a giant bow string. Inhale and return your hands to the starting "holding the giant ball position." Exhale and repeat the movement to the opposite side.

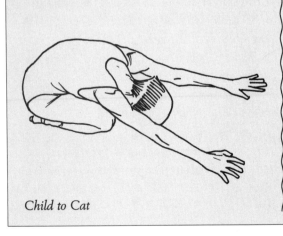

Child to Cat

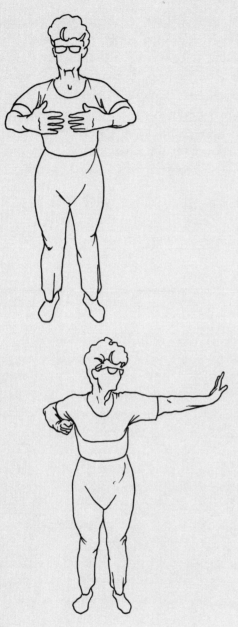

Drawing a Bow

Repeat this sequence several times, being sure to alternate sides and to move your body with your breath. (This exercise can also be done seated.)

Greet the Sun

This movement eases neck and shoulder tension while aiding respiration.

Sit on the edge of a chair with both feet flat on the floor, spine "tall" (don't slouch), and arms resting comfortably at your sides. Gaze forward. Exhale, then inhale as you extend your arms out and up in a wide circle over your head until your palms touch. Gaze up at the space between your thumbs. Exhale as you return to the beginning position.

Repeat the sequence several times, slowly and evenly, moving your body in time with your breath. (This exercise can also be done standing.)

Basic Relaxation Pose with Chest Opening

This meditation exercise is a variation of the basic relaxation practice (see Healing Moves for Health and Fitness, page 48) but uses a folded or rolled blanket to help open the chest. To set up, you'll need three blankets. Fold one and place it under your head, fold or roll another and place it under your back along your shoulder blades, and roll the third and place it under your knees. Take a minute to adjust the blankets' height and

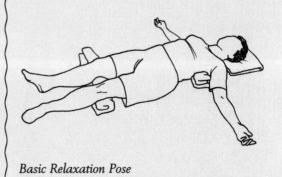

Basic Relaxation Pose

placement, so that when you lie down you can relax completely, with your body supported in total comfort. If you want, place a blanket over you for warmth and use an eyebag to shut out light and still the movements of your eyes.

Once you're comfortable, imagine yourself as innocent and uncomplicated as a sleeping child. Then bring your attention to your breath. Focus on the easy, natural flow of air in and out of your body, abdomen relaxed and rising gently on inhalations and falling softly on exhalations. Stay in this position for 5 to 10 minutes. When you're ready to come out of it, bend one knee and slowly roll to one side. Rest in this position for several breaths, and when you're ready, push against the floor with your hands to slowly bring yourself to a seated position.

Movement Is Medicine

10 STEPS TO HELP HARNESS THE HEALING POWER OF PHYSICAL ACTIVITY

When most people think of medicine, they visualize something material like a pill to be popped, a liquid to be swallowed, or an injection to be endured. Some might also consider surgery, tests, or procedures to be medicine, since these high-tech maneuvers can help diagnose and treat disease.

But by now you're well aware that one of the most potent forms of medicine isn't something you buy at a pharmacy or get at the doctor's office. No one else can give you this medicine or perform its magic for you. It's movement, simple physical activity that can have profound healing effects. And *it's something only you can do for yourself*.

In many ways, movement is the ideal medicine. It's extremely effective, free (or at least inexpensive), low risk, abundantly available, socially acceptable, simple to do, and flexible enough to suit your personal preferences and needs. When compared to traditional treatments, such as drugs and surgery, the risk-benefit profile frequently is far superior. In our remote-control culture, movement is the perfect prescription both for prevention and treatment of America's epidemic of inactivity-related diseases.

Unfortunately, most adults approach movement with the same aversion they express toward a hypodermic needle or the stinky, awful-tasting medicine we sometimes have to swallow to "feel better." As children we didn't feel this way about moving our bodies. Kids typically view physical activities like skipping, jumping, and running as exciting play to be enjoyed. That's why, throughout *Healing Moves*, we've emphasized the importance of *making movement fun*. In fact, joy in movement may be even more healing than the physical elements of movement per se. Thus our primary principle for integrating the medicine of movement into your life: *Approach exercise as enjoyable play.*

But even with this attitude adjustment, becoming active in our sedentary society isn't easy. In our hyperbusy, car-oriented culture, barriers to exercise abound. It's not uncommon for cities and towns to have no sidewalks or bike paths, for buildings to prohibit the use of stairs, for parks and playgrounds to be unsafe, and for electronic devices to automatically do everything for us—from opening doors to compacting trash. Long workdays, difficult commutes, and balancing family and job obligations leave many Americans chronically exhausted, with little energy for anything more demanding than channel surfing.

No one said becoming fit and healthy would be easy. But with the right attitude and the proper information, it can be fun. In fact, the time you spend moving is generally repaid in full by the energy, relaxation, and pleasure that physical activity brings. Better health and fitness is well within virtually anyone's grasp. All it takes is awareness and dedication to put the curative power of exercise to work for you.

To help you become—and stay—physically active, we've outlined 10 steps to make the joyful medicine of movement a regular part of your life:

1. *Recognize that your body needs movement to be healthy.* We know that when we're hungry we should eat, and when we're tired we should sleep. But when we get stiff, achy, and sluggish, we generally don't recognize these signals as cues that our body craves movement. Instead, we misinterpret these symptoms as the body's need for rest, which makes us stiffer, achier, and even more sluggish. In our sedentary society, many adults have smothered their body's natural "Move me!" impulses and have forgotten that exercise is essential to good health. Instead of always living "in your head," learn to take your awareness out of your mind and into your body, so you can recognize the signals it sends you.

2. *Make the active choice.* In general, when you're faced with the choice of moving more or moving less, *move more*. For example, if you approach an escalator alongside a staircase, choose the stairs. If you have a choice between a leaf blower or a rake, choose the rake. Get rid of the negative mind-set of trying to expend as little energy as possible and adopt a "proactive attitude" that eagerly looks for opportunities to move: Park in the farthest spot, dig in the garden, wash your car, turn off the TV, and go for a walk.

3. *Make a commitment to healing moves.* Design your own personal healing moves program from the options presented in this book, and schedule your plan into your week. The possibilities are endless, depending on your needs and goals—and we've outlined many strategies in each of our nine healing moves programs. But the important point is to make a commitment to practice your healing moves and set aside time to make it happen. You may find it

helpful to keep a healing moves journal. Once a week, plan ahead the activities you'll do for that week. Each day, jot down what you've done and how you feel. Consider adding music to your session, to boost your motivation and enjoyment.

4. *Understand the importance of attitude.* If you say "I can't," you won't. Belief in your ability to achieve your goals is one of the most important predictors of success.

5. *Avoid sitting for prolonged periods.* Whenever you must sit for an extended length of time, be sure to take regular stretch breaks and quick "walk-abouts," and stand or shift positions when possible. If you're confined to a cramped sitting position, as in an airplane, do some stretching exercises in your seat and walk the aisles when permitted.

6. *Never answer the phone on the first ring,* and use the "captured" time for a brief breathing meditation. Telephone calls frequently disrupt our already harried lives. So instead of racing for the receiver, take a six-second tranquilizer (about two rings) before picking up the phone. Use that time for this simple "telephone meditation": Breathe deeply into your abdomen. Exhale completely as you smile. Then answer the phone.

7. *Consider an exercise buddy—human or canine.* Fitness experts regularly advise people to work out with a buddy, because studies show that those who exercise with a partner are more likely to stick with their program. While friends and family members make great exercise partners, scheduling a workout

with another human can be difficult. Dogs, however, are *always* ready to go for a walk or a run, providing wonderful camaraderie and motivation to be active while adding an extra measure of safety and a huge serving of fun. And unlike a human workout buddy, your dog won't cancel on you at the last minute. If circumstances make a canine companion impossible, borrow a neighbor's pet or just walk your "inner dog."

8. *Strive for balance.* Remember that health is equilibrium. A person is healthy when his or her body is in balance or harmony. So while it's important to keep moving, it's also crucial to strike a healthy balance between exercise and rest. As with any medicine, it's possible to overdose on movement by doing too much. How much is "too much" varies widely, depending on your health status and fitness level. In general, it's better to do a modest amount of movement every day rather than knock yourself out with a big bout of exercise once a week.

9. *Remember that doing something is better than doing nothing.* All too often, people think that if they don't have at least 30 minutes to exercise it's not worth moving. Not true! Five minutes of calisthenics, 3 minutes of stretching, a 2-minute walk, even a 30-second deep breath all can contribute to better health.

10. *Find the joy.* Let go of thinking how you're going to look from the exercise you're doing today, and just go outside—or inside—and play. Be present in the moment and relish the sensations of moving your body through space, as opposed to watching the clock and

thinking, "I'll get through this." Fitness is an attitude toward the exciting journey of life, not an elusive quest for physical perfection or immortality.

We've called these 10 strategies "steps," not "commandments," for a reason: They are *not* carved in stone. They are simply tools to help you fully embrace the curative power of exercise. Use those that work for you; ignore the rest. Just remember: *The most important aspect of healing moves is that you do them regularly.* And whatever else you do, remember to breathe. A deep, purposeful inhalation and a slow, complete exhalation—*with a smile*—are perhaps the most healing moves of all.

Index

Hamstring exercises. *See* leg exercises/stretches
hatha yoga. *See* yoga
HDL. *See* cholesterol level
health clubs, 16, 100
heart disease, 190–223
   aerobic exercise as prevention, 26
   cholesterol and, 61, 62, 63, 65
   diabetes and, 51
   as postmenopausal risk, 267, 270–71
   risk factors, 26, 29, 62, 107
   upper body fat and, 231
heart rate
   resting, 18, 195
   target, 216, 217
   training zone, 16, 20, 36
heat sensitivity, 76
high blood pressure, 11, 191, 194, 202–14, 231
   risk factors, 206–7
high-density lipoprotein. *See* cholesterol level
hip exercises/stretches, 47–48, 148, 247, 277–78
hip fractures, 128
Hispanics, 54
HIV/AIDS, 164, 165, 175–78
home exercise, 16
hormone replacement therapy (HRT), 131,
   267–68
hormones. *See* estrogen; testosterone
hot flashes, 268
human immunodeficiency virus. *See* HIV/AIDS
hyperglycemia, 53
hyperlipidemia, 11, 60–67
hypertension. *See* high blood pressure

Immune system, 19, 163–64, 166, 167
immunological conditions, 163–89
immunosurveillance theory, 170, 171
impotence, 226, 227
inactivity. *See* sedentary lifestyle
indigenous peoples, 52–53
injury prevention, 19, 21, 26, 75–76
   excessive exercise, 25
   high-intensity/high-impact exercise, 24, 80
   stretching, 22
in-line skating, 101, 240, 303
insulin, 51, 53, 54, 56
insulin resistance, 54
ischemic heart disease, 193–94

Job stress, 91
jogging, 117, 133, 139
ju ching, 104
jumping rope, 241
junk-food diets, 11, 51, 52

Karate, 100, 305
Kegel exercises
   for men, 237, 250–51
   for women, 279
ki, 186, 305
Klinefelter's syndrome, 132
knee-strengthening exercises, 161–62
kyphosis (spine curvature), 127

LDL. *See* cholesterol level
lean tissue mass, 22, 65, 77, 138
leg exercises/stretches
   Dumbbell Lunge, 141–42
   Knee Extension, 87, 142
   stretches, 45, 147–48, 149, 247, 248
   Yoga Upper-Body Strengthener, 43
   Yoga Warrior Stance, 246
libido loss, 225–26
life expectancy, 6, 224–25
lifting, back pain avoidance and, 115
love handles, 232, 233
low-density lipoprotein. *See* cholesterol level
lung cancer, 169

Magnesium, 212
manic depression, 92
mantra breathing, 49
martial arts, 5, 100, 305
medications
   immune suppression, 164
   interactions with activity, 25
   osteoporosis risk, 132
   premenstrual cycle and, 261
   sexual dysfunction and, 226
meditation, walking, 101–4
meditative exercises, 180, 186–88, 307–8
melancholic depression, 94
men, 224–51
   abdominal fat, 225, 231–33
   bone loss, 137
   cholesterol levels, 63, 64
   high blood pressure, 206
   Kegel exercises for, 237, 250–51
   life expectancy, 224–25
   muscle building, 233–35
   posture, 149
   prostate cancer, 169, 170–71, 173, 225, 229–31
   sexual dysfunction, 225–29
menopause, 265–72
   and bones, 127, 129, 130, 131, 137
   and cholesterol levels, 63
menstruation
   amenorrhea, 25, 132, 137, 229

running (*cont.*)
  immune system and, 164
  sex drive increase and, 228

Salt intake, high blood pressure and, 207,
    212
San Shin Kai (breathing), 180, 188
seasonal affective disorder, 93
sedentary lifestyle
  asthma and, 288–89, 292
  back pain and, 114
  breathing effects of, 300
  cancer risk from, 170, 173
  demographics, 14
  diabetes and, 51, 52–53
  health problems from, 3, 11, 51, 107, 131
  heart disease and, 191, 192
  high blood pressure and, 206
  immune system decline from, 164
  muscle loss from, 138
  obesity and, 69
  results of, 11–12, 51, 116, 149, 191, 194
  technology factor, 3, 69
self-efficacy, 8
self-esteem, enhancing, 7, 70
sexual dysfunction, male, 225–29
shoulder exercises/stretches
  Chin In, 151
  Dumbbell Shoulder Shrug, 41
  Flying Bow, 244
  Pull-ups, 245–46
  Seated Side Lateral Raise, 40–41
  Shoulder Strengthener, 85, 86
  stretches, 44–45, 147, 247, 248
  Wall Reach, 151
  See also push-ups
sitting precautions, 115, 123–24, 311
  posture and, 149
sit-ups, 42–43, 243–44
  fitness level test, 30–31, 33
skating. *See* in-line skating
sleep, 8, 19, 93, 115
smoking
  back pain and, 117
  body-fat distribution and, 231
  cancer and, 170
  cholesterol and, 64
  chronic obstructive pulmonary disease and, 287,
    295, 296–97
  emphysema and, 295
  heart disease and, 26, 191, 194
  high blood pressure and, 207, 212
  menopause and, 131, 267

sexual dysfunction and, 226
  weight gain and, 7–8
spare tire. *See* abdominal fat
spinal fracture, 127–28
spine curvature, 127
split sets, 140–41
spot reducing, 233
stationary bicycling, 111
stomach exercises. *See* abdominal exercises
strength training exercises, 38–44, 100–101
  for muscle and bone building, 16, 19, 20–21, 26,
    38–44, 74, 79, 85, 129, 133, 140–46
  for osteoporosis, 135
  for repetitive stress injury, 125–26
  split sets, 140–41
  See also specific body regions
stress, 89–98
  back pain and, 117, 118, 154
  hardiness, 8, 94
  heart disease and, 191, 195
  high blood pressure and, 207
  immune system and, 166
  posture and, 149
  relief measures, 7, 48, 56, 70, 196
  repetitive stress injury and, 124
  sexual dysfunction and, 227
stress response, 102
stretching
  exercises, 44–48, 247–48
  flexibility and, 21–22, 26
  for muscle and bone strengthening, 146–49
  for repetitive stress injuries, 124–25, 156–58
stroke, 51, 61, 208–9
suicide, 91
Sun Salutation (Surya Namaskar), 179, 181–86
swimming, 99–100, 117, 133, 175, 240–41, 302

Tae kwon do, 100, 305
tai chi, 96, 99, 100, 111–12, 199, 211, 264, 305
target heart rate, 216, 217
technology, health effects of, 3, 13, 69, 82
tendinitis, 120
tennis players, 129
testosterone, 170–71, 225, 226, 228
thermogenic hypothesis, 93
thigh exercises/stretches
  Chair Squat, 39
  Front Lunge, 277–78
  Step-ups, 43–44
  stretch, 46
training effect, 20, 216
  chart of heart rates, 217
training zone, 16, 20, 36, 216

triceps exercises. *See* arm exercises/stretches
trigger finger, 120
triglycerides, 65, 196
Turner's syndrome, 132
type I and II diabetes. *See under* diabetes

Underweight, 233–35
urinary incontinence, 237, 250–51

Vitamin D, bone health and, 129, 131

Waist-to-hip ratio, 231
walking, 99, 111
    as aerobic exercise, 16, 74, 81, 117, 175, 302
    calories burnt during, 24, 80
    as cancer risk reduction, 173
    as diabetes therapy, 55
    improved cholesterol profile from, 65
    meditation, 101–4
walking breaks, as repetitive stress injury prevention, 125
warm-ups, pre-exercise, 20, 21, 26, 38
water exercise, 111, 118, 302. *See also* swimming
weight
    cancer relationship, 170
    management, 7–8, 24–25, 56, 72
    menopause-related gain, 268
    mid-life gains, 232
    See also body fat; obesity; underweight; weight loss
weight-bearing activities, 129, 133, 134–35, 137, 139–40
weight loss, 24, 70, 71–72, 232–33
    amount of aerobic exercise needed for, 66
    calorie deficit needed for, 24, 26, 74, 82
    cholesterol levels and, 65
    exercise as best means of, 67
    regaining after, 71
    underweight problems, 233–35
weight training. *See* strength training exercises
white-coat syndrome, 205
women, 252–85
    cancer and, 169, 170, 173
    carpal tunnel syndrome and, 121

cholesterol level and, 63–64
heart attack risks, 190
high blood pressure and, 206
life expectancy, 224–25
obesity and, 68–69
posture and, 149
premenstrual dysphoric disorder, 91–92, 259
sexuality and exercise, 228
See also menopause; menstruation; osteoporosis; pregnancy
workplace
    back pain avoidance, 116
    job stress, 91
    repetitive stress injury, 120–27, 156–58
wrist exercises, 43

YMCAs, 100
yoga, 5
    Belly Breathing, 48–50, 270, 282
    Bird Play, 222–23
    Chaturanga Dandasana Pose, 43
    Child's Pose, 283
    Cobbler's Pose, 283–84
    Essential Breath, 220
    Frog Pose, 220–21
    health and fitness benefits, 124, 133, 199, 211, 264, 292
    Legs up the Wall, 223
    limbs or stages of, 305
    Lying-Down Cobbler's Pose, 284
    as mind-body unification, 96, 99, 100
    Plank Pose, 43, 184
    pranayama, 305
    Restorative Pose, 189
    Savasana Pose, 105–6
    Spinal Twist, 221–22
    Sun Salutation, 179, 181–86
    Upper Body Strengthener, 43
    Wall Hang, 284–85
    Warrior Stance, 246
    Wide-Angle Legs-Up-the-Wall Pose, 283

About the Authors

CAROL KRUCOFF, a karate black belt and yoga devotee, is an award-winning health columnist for the *Washington Post*, the founding editor of the *Post*'s health section, and a frequent contributor to a variety of national magazines, including *Reader's Digest*, *Self*, and the *Saturday Evening Post*. Her *Bodyworks* column appears in newspapers around the country. She is certified as a personal trainer by the American Council on Exercise.

MITCHELL KRUCOFF, M.D., F.A.C.C., an internationally renowned clinical researcher and pioneer in electrocardiographic monitoring, is a senior staff cardiologist and the director of the Ischemia Monitoring Laboratory at Duke University Medical Center.

The Krucoffs have been married since 1974 and have two children, Max, fifteen, and Rae, twelve.